METHODS IN
TOXICOLOGY

EDITED BY

G. E. PAGET

M.D. B.S. D.C.H.

*Smith, Kline & French
Laboratories Ltd,
Welwyn Garden City
Herts, England*

BLACKWELL SCIENTIFIC PUBLICATIONS

OXFORD AND EDINBURGH

SBN 632 06830 2

FIRST PUBLISHED 1970

Printed and bound in Great Britain by
WILLIAM CLOWES AND SONS LTD
BECCLES, SUFFOLK

Contents

List of Contributors

G.E. PAGET
Smith Kline & French Laboratories Ltd, Welwyn Garden City, Hertfordshire

H. HURNI
Der Tierfarm A.G., Sisseln, Switzerland

T. BALAZS
Department of Toxicology, Smith Kline & French Laboratories, Philadelphia

K.-F. BENITZ
Toxicology Research Section, Lederle Laboratories Division, American Cyanamid Company, Pearl River, New York. Now Associate Professor of Toxicology, Institute for Experimental Pathology and Toxicology, Albany Medical College, Albany, New York

The late C.S. DELAHUNT
Department of Pharmacology, Chas Pfizer & Co. Inc, Groton, Connecticut

P.N. MAGEE
Courtauld Institute of Biochemistry, Middlesex Hospital Medical School, London

G.E. DAVIES
I.C.I. Ltd, Pharmaceuticals Division, Research Department, Alderley Park, Macclesfield, Cheshire

R.E. LISTER
Inveresk Research International, Inveresk, Scotland

J.C. GAGE
I.C.I. Ltd, Industrial Hygiene Research Laboratories, Alderley Park, Macclesfield, Cheshire

M.W. PARKES
Pharmacological Laboratory, Roche Products Ltd, Welwyn Garden City, Hertfordshire

F.T. PERKINS
Director, Immunological Products Control, National Institute for Medical Research, Hampstead Laboratories, Holly Hill, Hampstead, London

A.E. STREET
Huntingdon Research Centre, Huntingdon

S.R.M. BUSHBY
Head of Department of Chemotherapy, Wellcome Research Laboratories, Beckenham, Kent

Preface

The practice of toxicology is not a discipline in its own right but comprises many different disciplines, ranging from physiology to pathology and requiring very different technical skills. No one individual can be equally familiar with all the skills required nor can most organizations afford to employ individuals of the necessary diversity of skills. It is always desirable, of course, for an individual in charge of toxicity experiments to consult those having particular skills that may become relevant to the toxicological experiments. However, this is not always possible and in any event an expert in a particular discipline may not always have considered how his discipline might be applied to the study of toxicity.

This book is intended to provide an expert opinion in many areas that are particularly relevant to toxicology as to how a particular discipline may best be applied to that study. It is hoped that these expert views will serve to guide experts from other disciplines in their use of skills with which they are not familiar and to give them some insight into what can be achieved in particular fields and to indicate the various complexities that surround the subject. Each chapter is intended to be complete in itself and there is, therefore, necessarily some repetition of material covering common points as, for example, the types and numbers of animals used in various experiments. It is hoped that this repetition will enable a particular expert's views to be consulted without the necessity of frequent cross-reference to other parts of the book.

For the most part the chapters are in the form of practical advice on the actual conduct of experiments. In some cases the subjects covered are too complex for such detailed advice and there, guidance is given to literature sources of experimental details.

All the authors are experts and are in day-to-day practice of their subjects. The book is, therefore, addressed primarily to the scientific worker in toxicology rather than to the administrator or regulator with only a peripheral interest in the subject. It is hoped that the chapters will be interpreted as guidance rather than as strict rules that should not be transgressed. Guidance is surely frequently needed by anybody engaged in this subject whereas strict rules would strangle any possibility of further development in it.

G.E.P.

CHAPTER 1

The Design and Interpretation of Toxicity Tests

G.E. PAGET

The history of the invention of new drugs is one of increasing technological complexity. The reasons for this are, of course, many, but from every aspect a major cause of this complexity is the realization by those who are concerned with the discovery and use of drugs that the issues involved are far more complicated than was realized by the earliest workers in the field. In no area has this increasing complexity been more evident than in that which is the concern of this volume, namely the examination of the potential toxicity of new drugs intended for trial and use in man.

The earliest investigators were content with simple, brief, and superficial examinations of this question and everybody in the field will be aware of the limitations of the studies of such drugs as digitalis, salvarsan, and the earliest sulphonamides. The increasing clinical recognition of the potentiality of new drugs to cause undesirable reactions has led to the development of a more sophisticated attitude to such studies in the laboratories of firms discovering and developing new drugs. The growth of this attitude has been materially hastened by the occurrence of major and widely reported mishaps in the use of drugs, which, it was generally felt, might have been avoided if the study of drug toxicity had been more extensively developed or more widely employed.

Unfortunately a number of difficulties beset this laudable desire to determine the potential toxicity of a drug in advance of its use. The most fundamental difficulty is that the study of drug toxicity is not a technical discipline in its own right. The toxicity of potential drugs must be studied by a large number of different techniques, all or any one of which may be relevant to a particular situation.

1

Thus, the drug toxicologist is but a scientist of another discipline masquerading under a professional title because of the use to which he puts his primary discipline. Even in the largest organizations concerned with the study of the undesirable effects of drugs, it will prove impossible to assemble sufficient experts of sufficient diverse disciplines to design the necessary experiments from a basis of expertness in all those disciplines. One purpose of the present volume is to ensure that the individual who must design experiments in a particular field that would be relevant to the study of the toxicity of a drug and who does not have the advantage of expert advice in that field, may have a work to which he may refer and from which he will obtain advice equivalent to what a local expert might have given him. It is felt that although this process cannot substitute for the working collaboration of an expert in a particular field, it will certainly be an improvement over the solitary investigator developing methods for himself from scratch.

One hazard of collecting a compendium such as the present volume is that the mere assembly of methods that may in appropriate circumstances be applied to a particular problem, may give rise to the attitude that all those methods must be applied to every problem. This danger is particularly severe since the climate of thought about the application of toxicity tests seems to be moving in the direction of comprehensive testing rather than of selective experiment, although the latter is surely to be preferred.

The reasons for this disquieting development are easy to see. A number of people are concerned in determining whether a compound has been demonstrated as being safe enough to investigate in man or to exploit more widely. Unfortunately, but inevitably, only a minority of these people have any expertise in the techniques by which compounds are evaluated from this point of view, and indeed a majority of these individuals may well be laymen in this respect. All of them are, however, aware of the public scrutiny that must necessarily follow a failure in the evaluation of the safety of a drug. In these circumstances it is not surprising that the mere existence of a test will suggest to them that the test should be applied, not so much to determine whether the drug does or does not possess a particular property, but rather to provide a climate of assurance, either political or legal, should future events bring their actions into question. This is so much the case that a number of regulatory agencies are now known or thought to have checklists of tests that should, in their estimation, have been applied to a drug, and should the checklist be incomplete, the drug is rejected without enquiry being made as to why a particular group of tests was omitted. It is additionally difficult to sustain a contrary attitude, since many of the tests that are applied have been developed in response to a particular need. Instances of this are many and obvious, as for example, the extensive use of tests involving the pregnant female developed in response to the thalidomide episode or the considerable interest taken in ocular toxicity following experience with Mer-29. No doubt other specific tests will be developed following calamities we have not yet encountered.

Nevertheless, despite these facts, any thinking scientist must argue strongly against this attitude of mind, although the counter-arguments are more subtle than those in favour of completely comprehensive testing. Perhaps the most obvious counter-argument concerns the amount of effort which it is sensible to put into the safety evaluation of drugs. It is the case that 20 years ago a drug firm that employed one or two graduates and a handful of technicians on safety evaluation was considerably in advance of its time and was regarded as being highly advanced in this aspect of drug development. Nowadays, the largest firms may have enormous departments of drug toxicology and may devote to that subject as much as one third of their total development resources. This growth is obviously continuing and must in the present climate of opinion continue and even increase. This is because no test once described and found to be generally useful is ever dropped but is applied to an increasing range of substances, while new tests and techniques are developed at an increasing rate. To carry the process to absurdity, one could imagine the situation where all the resources available were devoted to safety testing and none to the discovery of new entities. This would plainly be a ridiculous and untenable situation. Somewhere considerably short of that situation a balance must be struck between the discovery of new drugs and the evaluation of their safety. It must be generally recognised that if new drugs are to be developed and if mankind is to have the benefit of those drugs, some hazard is inescapable and no proliferation of safety testing will ever remove it.

The second point arises from the fact that the scientific basis of safety testing is dubious, since all such tests are designed to demonstrate a negative, which, by definition, cannot be achieved. Nevertheless a point is readily reached where the size of the operation involved, the number of tests that have been performed, and their complexity give rise to a feeling of assurance in everyone concerned that safety has truly been demonstrated. The inertia of this process may be such that those whose responsibility is the evaluation of safety may be convinced that they have, in fact, achieved a demonstration of it. It is commonly remarked, in fact, that the toxicity tests that had been carefully carried out on thalidomide without exception had demonstrated it to be an almost uniquely safe compound. What was required in this instance, and I think it true to say in many other instances, was not a further proliferation of tests but rather an awareness in those concerned that situations might exist in which hazards might arise that were not covered by the extensive tests they had performed. Such awareness can only arise when the mind of the investigator is open to the possibility and when individual investigators have sufficient time to consider the whole of the problem rather than being overwhelmed by its numerous and substantial parts.

I have noted above that the scientific basis of the study of drug safety is dubious. Most of the tests that have been developed and that are described in this volume were originated as rule-of-thumb methods that were intuitively thought to possess some validity but which it would be difficult to substantiate from any basis of scientific principle. An essential point in the development of more satisfactory methods, and one which is demonstrated in all the contributions to this volume, is a research approach to the problems. On many occasions this will demand going outside accepted methods in order to develop new and more satisfactory ones. This can only be possible if time and facilities are available to the investigator and if the management of pharmaceutical firms, and even more the civil servants in regulatory agencies, are sufficiently flexible to see that new methods may be more relevant and more informative than the blind application of old ones. The mere existence of those new methods, however, should not suggest to the regulator that they must forthwith be applied across the board, since this would be to compound the fault which I have already criticized.

Similarly, regulatory agencies must recognize that often the application of a new method or experimental technique will give rise to information which may not be easily evaluated when it is obtained.

whatever its ultimate use may be. A real and powerful reason for the failure of many pharmaceutical firms to mount investigations of problems of toxicity employing techniques new to this field is that, should they obtain information of which the significance cannot be evaluated, they anticipate severe difficulties with the regulatory agency to which that information must be disclosed. They are often, therefore, placed in the anomalous and scientifically ridiculous situation of preferring not to obtain new information in case they are saddled with impossible requirements by a regulatory agency as a result. This attitude has certainly materially held up the development of techniques that undoubtedly in the long run will prove to be of use.

From all the foregoing, it will be clear that I believe that the evaluation of the potential toxicity of a drug is a scientific problem that is not to be resolved by the blind application of a set of standard tests, and it is not the intention of this volume to recommend the use of such standard tests. When it becomes relevant to determine whether a chemical compound may be tested in man after it has been demonstrated that it may possess useful properties, a number of questions should arise in the mind of the responsible investigator long before a single test is carried out. These concern the mode of action by which it is presumed to bring about its desired effects. Consideration of this mechanism of action, even when it is only partly understood, should enable many predictions about the safety of the drug in use in man to be made. In the case of novel mechanisms of action, some consideration of the total biological situation and how it is affected by the new drug may give rise to apprehensions about its safety in particular respects. Drugs that are analogous to known drugs are an easier problem, and here too specific circumstances of hazard may be defined.

A number of questions will remain and answers to these questions must be sought before it is sensible to commence designing elaborate, long-continued, large scale tests. In their very nature such tests are to be carried out in animals, and it is, therefore, important to decide what species of laboratory animal is to be used for the test. This question is perhaps the most fundamental of all those that must be answered before experiments are designed. The considerations that affect this choice are discussed in Dr Benitz' chapter. Often enough the question of the ideal species must be left unresolved because of inadequate information. There is, however, a growing tendency to believe that procedures permitting the choice of a species, which in some respect or other may be thought to resemble man more closely than others that might be used, are desirable. Perhaps this point is one on which major advances are to be expected.

Another point that must be determined before major experiments are designed is what aspects of the action of the drug warrant particular attention during the definitive and prolonged toxicity experiments. Often if it is known that a particular organ or system is liable to be damaged by a drug, particular observation of that organ during the course of other experiments will be desirable. There is much to recommend a short, preliminary experiment using small numbers of animals as a method of determining how the main experiment is to be monitored.

It is increasingly possible to measure in animals some parameter to which drug effects are likely to be more closely related than they are to such simple measures as the dose actually administered. The tendency is, of course, to believe that effects are more clearly related to blood level of the agent than to any other measurement. While this is often true, it is by no means exclusively true and the measurement of blood levels, although desirable, should not be allowed to obscure the fact that other measures are sometimes more relevant, such as the concentration of the material in a particular tissue or the concentration in blood or tissues of some material related to the action of the compound. It may be, for example, that the compound exerts its action by depleting or increasing some normal tissue constituent and a measure of this may well be more relevant than a measure of the actual compound. A particular case of this is, of course, compounds which inhibit particular enzyme systems where the toxic effects are often related to the degree of inhibition rather than to the actual level of the compound present.

These measurements and many others that will undoubtedly be developed offer the opportunity of increasing quantification and sophistication in the monitoring of all types of toxicity experiments while they are in progress. No measure, however quantifiable and 'scientific' will ever replace the supervision of the experiment by a skilled and experienced experimentalist. No schedule of necessary tests, no automation of numerical results of such tests, and no intervention of specialist technologists should obscure the need for intimate supervision of all toxicity experiments by an individual who is concerned with the totality of the experiment and with its purpose. Only in this way will the unexpected and significant observation ever be made. The same consideration is also true of procedures used to assess the experiment at its conclusion. The various contributors to this book have pointed out the various observations that are regarded as essential to the correct assessment of toxicity tests. The most important single point is that toxicity experiments are by their nature intended to detect unexpected effects. Unexpected effects are often only evident to the prepared mind of an expert observer and this is one element of an experiment that should never be omitted.

The intimate association of pathologists with toxicity experiments, for obvious reasons, has led to some unsatisfactory attitudes in the evaluation of the experiments with which they are concerned. One suspects that this is because pathologists' training has classically been concerned with the precise diagnosis of human lesions and little with the functional assessment of the lesion and even less with its predictive significance for individuals of different species in different circumstances from those in which the lesions studied actually arose. For much human pathology the job in hand can be satisfactorily completed by a careful study of a single section conventionally stained and examined in a light microscope; indeed, the pathologist's opportunity may be confined to this classic situation. This is not the case in the pathological observation of toxicity experiments. In these circumstances a diagnosis of a lesion is merely the beginning of a process of assessment of its significance that may, and should, involve not only the skills of the modern experimental pathologist in histochemistry, electron microscopy and other specialized techniques, but also experts from other disciplines such as pharmacology and biochemistry. Only the most complete picture of the meaning of the lesion detected by the pathologist can serve as a satisfactory basis for the prediction of likely human effects from effects discovered in toxicity experiments.

This latter process is, of course, the purpose of all toxicity experiments and is the toxicologist's most difficult task. Much has been written about the basis for this prediction and many of the precepts that guide it are obvious. Thus, if a compound has been given in adequate doses to a large number of different species of animals and all have shown a particular toxic effect, it is not unreasonable to predict that such an effect will be encountered in man. Unfortunately, the converse is not true. That is to say, if the compound has been given to a number of species and none has shown a significant effect, it does not necessarily follow that human beings, when exposed to the compound, will not show some serious toxic effect.

However, these clear-cut and simple cases, where all the species used in toxicity experiments give homogeneous and consistent results, are far from being the rule. More commonly toxic effects of one sort or another will be found in some but not all the species used in toxicity experiments. These discordant results pose the real problems in the interpretation of toxicity experiments in the prediction of likely effects in man and in deciding upon a proper course of action. Again, some conclusions are obvious. A serious effect found even in only one species should disqualify a trivial compound intended for a trivial condition or purpose from further study in man. There is a tendency, however, to extend this obvious precept to one that while appealing is not obvious and is certainly retrogressive. It is often suggested that any significant effect found in any species should disqualify any compound from further study in man. Such a doctrine, of course, makes life easy for the toxicologist and for regulatory agencies, since all risk and responsibility is removed from those making the judgement. It is the case, however, that virtually every drug commonly used in human beings can be shown in appropriate experiments in animals on some occasions in some species to produce adverse effects such that, if they had been discovered prior to the use of the drug and the experiments had been assessed on the simple precept enumerated above, would have disqualified the drug from further use and removed a valuable agent from the therapeutic armamentarium. Such a sweeping generalization cannot, therefore, be sensibly used as a basis of judgement.

Certainly in all cases where adverse effects are detected in toxicity experiments the nature of the effect must be assessed against the need for the drug and the seriousness of the condition in which it is used. Indeed, this precept has a validity beyond the field of therapeutics since it must also be true of feed additives, pesticides, and industrial chemicals. Certainly, too, caution and prudence should govern this analysis but neither should be carried to the point where all action is vitiated.

With compounds sufficiently important, both in their intended use and commercially to justify the expense, it will often be possible to determine the mechanism by which they produce a disturbing effect found in the toxicity experiment. This mechanism of action may suggest whether the effect is likely to be encountered in man or not. Even where such an approach fails, consideration of the nature of the effect detected in experiments may suggest that should such an effect occur in man it could be detected before catastrophic damage had occurred. With important compounds, in these circumstances, it would be justifiable to mount well controlled and cautiously conducted experiments in human beings to determine whether or not the adverse effect would occur in that species. Logic suggests that these human beings are certainly no more at risk, and possibly even less at risk, than those first receiving drugs that have been without adverse effects in toxicity experiments since, as I have pointed out above, even in these circumstances the possibility of an adverse effect occurring in man remains, but in such circumstances, of course, there is no guidance to the investigator as to what that unexpected effect might be. It is possible to summarize this situation by saying that the interpretation of toxicity experiments requires not only deep technical knowledge but also prudence in the investigator, but that cowardice, like ignorance, vitiates the experiments.

It is appropriate to say something of toxicity experiments in man. There is, of course, general repugnance to the idea that human beings may be used to assess the toxicity of drugs and other environmental chemicals. If such chemicals are to be brought into use and widely distributed the alternative is not whether human beings should be used in toxicity experiments or not but rather whether human beings should be used in small numbers in controlled toxicity experiments or whether large populations should be exposed to chemicals, knowledge about which is confined to their effects on other animal species. In these circumstances, it is clear that the rational course, before any new chemical, whether drug, pesticide, or food additive, is added to the human environment, is for cautious, closely controlled and observed trials to be carried out in groups of human beings. To these groups every observational aid of modern medicine should be applied. Certainly such toxicity experiments in man will not detect important effects of rare occurrence. Properly conducted, however, they will detect those effects that are likely to occur in the majority of a population exposed to the agent. The legal and ethical considerations in arranging and conducting such studies are outside the scope of this book, as are the techniques involved. It is plain, however, that such observations in man are merely a rational extension of the studies of toxicity conducted on lower animals and that no matter how comprehensive these laboratory studies have been no chemical has been completely studied for its potential toxicity to man until such human studies have been carried out.

CHAPTER 2

The Provision of Laboratory Animals

H. HURNI

INTRODUCTION

In animal experiments in general, and particularly in chronic toxicity tests, the variability of individual parameters and hence the evaluation and reproducibility of the results depend to a large extent on the quality of the animals used. Reduced variability not only increases the accuracy of results but decreases the number of animals needed, which for ethical reasons is an important consideration.

Although of prime importance in toxicity testing, laboratory animals cost very little in relation to the total costs of chronic experiments; thus, if better animals cost even 100% more, the cost of the experiment will increase relatively little. This moderate increase is justified when one considers the added time and expense of repeated tests which the use of poor quality animals may necessitate.

What characterizes suitable laboratory animals? The answer is plain: they respond uniformly to extrinsic stimuli. All requirements are implicitly covered by this statement. In order to maintain uniformity of response, one must first recognize all factors which modify the response pattern of the animal, i.e. which determine the dramatype (Ellis, 1967). Only then can we endeavour to keep them constant.

Table 2.1 lists groups of factors which affect the laboratory animal and its reactions. Included are not only genotype and environment but also intrinsic factors under the heading 'life cycle', e.g. age, sexual maturity, and health. It is useful in the preliminaries of an experiment to distinguish between the active and the passive phases. The duration of the passive phase, which includes recovery and adaptation, depends on the mode of active preparations for the experiment.

11

Table 2.1   Factors affecting animal reactions (after Hurni, 1969).

Genotype			
	Physiological status		age
			maturity
			oestrous cycle
			pregnancy
			lactation
	Environment	Microclimate	season
		Macroclimate	temperature
			humidity
			barometric pressure
			atmospheric constituents
			air circulation
			electric charges
			light intensity
			light spectrum
			light cycles
		Diet	constituents
			quantity
			mode of application
		Drinking	water quality
			water quantity
			mode of application
		Caging	size
			material
			shape
		Bedding	source
			quantity
			frequency of changes
		Handling	physical contacts
			noise
			commotion
			personnel qualities, e.g.
			training, temperament,
			replacement, etc.
	Health		deficiencies
			spontaneous and acquired
			immunity
			clinical and latent infections
Phenotype			
	Preliminaries for experiments		transfer
			regrouping
			altered surroundings
			adaptation
			recovery
Dramatype			
	(actual test animal)		
	Preliminary test		
	Test		

Breeder (bracket spanning from Genotype through Phenotype)

Investigator (bracket spanning from Phenotype through Dramatype)

Two examples will illustrate how strongly various factors can influence the outcome of simple experiments. On the instigation of a study group of the European Society for the Study of Drug Toxicity, several independent laboratories performed routine determinations of the acute LD_{50} for hexobarbitone and phenobarbitone. The results varied from 'no difference' to 'significantly higher toxicity of phenobarbitone' (Wien *et al.*, 1963).

In a similar experiment carried out simultaneously in several institutes, the acute toxicity of four common household chemicals was determined (Griffith, 1964). Not only did absolute LD_{50} values of any one product vary greatly between investigators, but also the relative toxicities of the four products. The results of these experiments warn against uncritical confidence in the parameters used for measuring drug activities.

INFLUENCE OF VARIOUS FACTORS UPON EXPERIMENTAL ANIMALS

The Genotype

The wide variation of responses to extrinsic stimuli exhibited by different animal species is so obvious that it need not be further discussed here. Similar variations are shown even by closely related breeds, strains, or lines within a species. Examples of variation of sex response in different mice strains are presented below:

Response	Author
Resistance to experimental tubercle bacillus infection	Pierce *et al.*, 1947 Grumbach, 1949 Donovick *et al.*, 1949
Resistance to specific viruses, bacteria or protozoa	Bonnod, 1967
Susceptibility to leukaemia, mammary tumours	Mouriquand & Mouriquand, 1964
Susceptibility towards toxic effects of histamine	Brown, 1962

Collins & Lott (1968) showed a strain and sex specificity in the response of rats to the toxicity of pentobarbital sodium. As a rule, however, the genetic sex of the animal does not affect the course of the experiment unless hormonal factors exert an influence. Thus, in various experimental infections no differences in resistance were found between male and female (Hurni *et al.*, 1951; Roger & Roger, 1963).

Difference in response to various influences by closely related animals can be attributed to hereditary metabolic differences between families, breeds, or strains (Meier, 1963).

Homozygous animals generally respond with greater sensitivity than do heterozygotes (Bonnod, 1967). Prior to this Porter *et al.* (1963) have already recommended the use of animals from inbred strains for nutrition experiments.

Sabourdy (1961) attributes an estimated 25% variability in animal experiments to genotypic variations, and 75% to environmental influences.

Life Cycles

This heading incorporates those influences occurring more or less unavoidably in the course of an animal's life, such as ageing, sexual maturity and mating, and for females pregnancy and the rearing of young.

The effects of these factors on the animals' reactions have rarely been investigated. The age of the animal is often inadequately considered, although differences in the success of experimental infections and in toxicity levels of substances such as vitamin D_2 have been demonstrated between old and young animals.

Although we presume continuous immunization to take place during ageing (e.g. against bacterial components in the feed—silent protection), the increasing resistance to infection frequently associated with ageing cannot be fully explained by this mechanism. Examples of age-dependent responses are tabulated below.

Furthermore, the hormonal changes connected with sexual maturity are undoubtedly associated with physiological changes which may modify the results of investigations if they are not properly considered. For example, resistance to infection with *Bacillus anthracis* is age-dependent in male rats of Fischer and NIH strains, but not in females of these strains (Klein *et al.*, 1961).

	Response	Author
Mice, rats	Susceptibility to viruses, e.g. mouse hepatitis, Coxsackie, mouse-adapted foot-and-mouth disease	Ciacco, 1963
Rats	Susceptibility to *Eperythrozoon coccoides*	Raffyi *et al.*, 1964
Chick	Susceptibility to bacterial endotoxins	Smith & Thomas, 1956
	Susceptibility to Vibrio cholerae	Finkelstein & Ramm, 1961
Pigs	Susceptibility to Toxoplasma gondii	Folkers, 1964

Examples of age-dependent responses

Hormonal changes of pregnancy and lactation may also affect susceptibility to infection. In the mouse, for example, pregnancy reduced the resistance to infection by Coxsackie and mouse poliomyelitis virus and in lactating mice a rise in susceptibility to foot-and-mouth virus is positively correlated with the number of pups (Campbell, 1964).

Environmental Factors

Many observations on effects of the environment have been made incidentally during experiments focusing on other problems and are thus widely scattered through the literature. Specific experiments dealing with our problem are still relatively few; laboratory animal science is after all a recent discipline.

Other factors which, in conjunction with the genotype determine the phenotype, have been relatively well investigated; these include macro- and micro-climate (climatic conditions in animal house and in the cage) (Weihe, 1964; Chevillard *et al.*, 1967, and Flynn, 1967); intensity, quality, periodicity and duration of light (Halberg *et al.*, 1960; Aschoff, 1964; Young, 1965; Porter, 1967); noise (Fox, 1965; Iturian & Fink, 1968); size, construction, shape of cages (Mundy & Porter, 1969); type of bedding and frequency of its change (Artsay, 1966; Porter, 1967; Iturian & Fink, 1968b).

Up to now it has not been sufficiently appreciated that the study of climate involves not only temperature and air changes per hour and air speed, but also air composition, ionization, and barometric pressure. Ozone for example, which has long been known to have toxic effects, has recently been shown (Purvis *et al.*, 1961) as an atmospheric contaminant that lowers the resistance to respiratory infections. Ionization, i.e. positive or negative atmospheric charges, also influence various physiological processes. For instance: a negatively charged atmosphere not only reduces the germ content of the air but also favourably affects breathing and blood flow in the tissues; as shown by Tschischewsky in 1934.

Temperature as a climatic factor has been much more intensively investigated. Temperature changes can disturb results, especially in experimental infections. Cold appreciably shortens the survival time of mice following infection with *Salmonella typhimurium, Staphylococcus aureus* (Previte & Berry, 1962), and *Pseudomonas aeruginosa* (Hackett *et al.*, 1968). Clark & Shepard (1962) showed that propagation of various mycobacteria in mice depends upon the ambient temperature. 20° C ambient temperature supported optimal propagation of *Mycobacterium marinum*. The duration of one generation of the same strain of bacteria in fish, amphibia, and reptiles was found to be 0·8 days at 30° C, 1·9 day at 20° C, and indefinite at 10° C. In experiments on phagocytosis, Kaufmann & Northey (1965) established that hypothermia in rabbits increased activity of leucocytes towards *Diplococcus pneumoniae*. Miraglia & Berry (1962) reduced the LD_{50} of an avirulent strain of *S. typhimurium* in mice a hundredfold by lowering the ambient temperature from 25° to 5° C. The work of Chen *et al.* (1943) and Chance (1957) showed that temperature increases in the environment raised the acute toxicity in mice of various substances. Nomura *et al.* (1967) established the least acute toxicity around 20° C; they found furthermore that substances which are considered harmless under most conditions, e.g. vitamin A, may suddenly act teratogenically when the ambient temperature is raised. According to Porter (1967) the ambient temperature acts on the blood pressure in mice.

The influence of dietary factors on experiments has repeatedly been investigated. The increased sensitivity to diphtheria toxin in guinea pigs in winter, for example, has been ascribed to the lack of greenstuffs during this season (Fauchet & Picard, 1965). Food of varying composition can lead to wide differences in the mode of reaction of experimental animals; for instance, non-specific resistance tends to depend on it (Schneider, 1962). This can conveniently be demonstrated in the course of experimental infections.

Effects of different diets on the results of experimental tuberculosis have been found (Dubos, 1947; Hurni *et al.*, 1951; Costello & Hedgecock, 1961; Layton & Youmans, 1965) and as shown in Table 2.2, the diet not only determines the extent of lung tuberculosis in the mouse but also the course it follows, i.e. whether the relatively mild productive form or the more serious necrotic-exudative form will result.

Table 2.2 Differences in resistance to infections in mice on different diets (groups of 20 mice, infected with the same strain of tubercle bacilli, duration of experiments: 28 days) (after Hurni *et al.*, 1951).

Condition	Maize–potato diet	Balanced diet
Histology determined proliferation stages in the lungs (max.=4)	3·0	2·2
Incidence of necrotic changes	30%	0%
Surviving at 28 days	13 animals	17 animals
Weight changes of survivors, compared with initial weight	−22·7%	−5·9%

Similar results were obtained by Eisman *et al.* (1961) with *Mycobacterium leprae* infections. Kretschmar & Haakh (1964) showed that the rate of spontaneous recovery from *Plasmodium berghei* infections in mice depends on the milk content of the diet. Increased dietary iron supports and accelerates experimental listeriosis in the mouse, since it promotes growth of the bacterium both *in vitro* and *in vivo* (Sword, 1965). Ross & Bras (1965) showed that the caloric and albumin content of the diet affects the tumour incidence in rats. The susceptibility of mice to Friend leukaemia virus depends on their nutritional state (Sidwell *et al.*, 1965).

The diet can directly affect drug action in experimental infections. Thus, it is virtually impossible to demonstrate a bacteriostatic action of a sulphonamide if the food has a high *p*-aminobenzoic acid content. The food composition can also affect the results of toxicity experiments. Food with a high meat content alters the effects of drugs on cardiazole cramp, while oatmeal inhibits gammahexane cramps (Herken, 1951). Changes in diet (and also in handling) could cause short-term changes in the rate of growth in mice (Porter and Festing, 1969).

Effects of the Experimental Preliminaries on the Results

On arrival in the laboratory animals will usually have been moved, often just from one room to another. On occasions they will have been moved from one hemisphere to another, in a cargo plane with badly-controlled pressure cabins, perhaps from summer into winter. Upon arrival changes in food and caging, and rearrangement into altered social groups produces additional disturbance. These events process the phenotype and lead to the experimental animal, described as the dramatype (Ellis, 1967).

The effect of environmental changes on the experimental results is generally underestimated. Heinecke (1967) showed that the transportation of mice in their breeding cages even from one building to the next influences the blood status, especially by decreasing erythrocytes, increasing leucocytes and shortening the clotting time which lasts 4–6 days. Air travel leads to similar changes lasting 4–6 weeks. Transport of mice from Bern (540 m above sea level) to the Scientific Research Station on the Jungfraujoch (3,450 m) altered the titre of actively acquired antibodies, which only returned to control levels after 4 weeks (Weihe & Hurni, 1962). Transferring mice from low to higher altitudes has, furthermore, an effect on the non-specific resistance to infection. It happened that three different mouse strains used in our studies reacted differently: Jax mice showed a significant reduction in non-specific resistance compared to the controls in Bern; 'Swiss-Washington' mice showed no changes; and 'Charles-River' mice showed an increase. The changes reached their peaks on the day following the displacement. The responses of different mouse strains to the same stress can thus markedly differ from each other.

Even altered handling, such as results from a change of technician, may markedly affect an animal's behaviour and its reactions (Hurni, 1969a).

Transport of animals is normally followed by regrouping. Caging singly or in groups affects toxicity experiments. Hatch *et al.* (1965) who caged Wistar rats from one batch of a local colony singly and those from another batch in groups of 10 (Table 2.3), observed an

Table 2.3 LD$_{50}$ of isoprotenerol for Wistar rats caged in groups or singly (Hatch *et al.*, 1965).

Housing	Duration (weeks)	Number	LD$_{50}$ (mg/kg)
Singly	3	24	815
In groups	3	24	815
Singly	8	24	118
In groups	8	24	815
Singly	12	24	< 50

astonishing increase in toxicity with the duration of isolation. Nineteen days after returning to groups of 10, the LD$_{50}$ in rats kept isolated for over 3 months had fallen to control levels; clearly, a reversible reaction to isolation stress had developed. Puppies kept in groups tend towards hyperactivity (Fox, 1965) and dogs in groups show higher learning ability than solitary animals (Cosnier, 1967); the same is true for rats. The incidence of infantile diarrhoea in mice due to natural infection was—among other factors—influenced by the population density in the cage (Allen *et al.*, 1962).

Lemonde (1967) showed that the incidence of leukaemia in mouse strain AKR was strongly influenced by social factors and conditions of husbandry (Table 2.4).

Table 2.4 Effect of fighting, fasting and infection on the incidence of spontaneous leukaemia in AKR inbred mice (after Lemonde, 1967).

Treatment	Percentage spontaneous leukaemia
Controls, individually caged	95
Fighting (5 or 6 in a cage)	
losers	91
winners	83
Fasting (every third day), singly	*ca.* 95
Fasting and fighting	80
BCG infection	
males	50
females	78
Fasting and fighting and BCG infection	
males	0
females	50

Individual factors can potentiate each other, even where one of them alone is without effect, as demonstrated by the interference of grouping with a conflict situation. Population density increases animal activity (Bronson, 1967), and consequently the weight of the adrenals. Isolated rats which receive an electric shock when they attempt to take food or water develop more gastric ulcers than rats caged in pairs or in groups of 10 (Ader, 1967); comparable results were obtained by Albert (1967). When strange male mice were caged with recently mated females, only 5% females remained pregnant; in the majority of females implantation of the fertilized eggs was inhibited (Bronson, 1967).

Not only the population density, but also cage equipment exerts appreciable influence, as Bennett *et al.* (1964) found in rat experiments: rats having an exercise wheel at their disposal had larger brains than controls without a wheel; the two groups also showed differences in learning ability, in body and organ weight, and in biochemical and histological features of the brain.

Stain marks put on the animals are partly ingested and can have unwanted effects. Thus, rats marked with picric acid excrete the dye in the urine.

Soave and Boyle (1965) concluded from a comparison of well-adapted and conditioned dogs from a recent batch, that adaptation up to 4 months greatly reduces the variability of haemoglobin and blood corpuscle counts.

Effect of Animal Health on the Outcome of Experiments

Health, together with environmental influences that determine the phenotype, have a decisive influence on the response of the drama-type. This is true during preparation of the animal for the experiment as well as in the experiment itself. A normal animal is regarded as healthy when it is free from any potentially pathogenic micro- or macro-organisms.

Reliable laboratory animals should be free of pathogens not only during a particular phase of investigations, but throughout their lifetime. It is obvious that acute intercurrent infections leading to the death of the animal falsify the outcome of the experiment and demand that it be repeated. Hidden, latent infections, which can be activated by stress must likewise be excluded (Sacquet, 1962). However, even past infections may leave disturbing traces, e.g.

through cross-immunity or interference. Infection with the virus of lymphocytic choriomeningitis protected mice of the BALB/c strain against subsequent infection with Rauscher mouse leukaemia (Barski & Youn, 1964). Infection with the protozoan genus Leishmania increases the resistance of mice to subsequent infection with *Mycobacterium tuberculosis* (Konopka *et al.*, 1961). This has been interpreted as a case of rather unexpected cross-immunity. Eperythrozoon infections in mice, on the other hand, increase the susceptibility to subsequent attack by mouse hepatitis (Seamer *et al.*, 1961). Infection with herpes virus protects hamsters against polyoma infection (Barski, 1963).

A preceding infection and the resulting acquired immunity can, however, affect later experiments in a quite unexpected manner. As Gueralt & Quevillon (1965) showed, a previous infection with *Bordetella pertussis* increased sensitivity of the chick to histamine. Brown and Wallace (1968) observed the same effect in mice. Infection of mice with *Listeria monocytogenes* leads to disturbed iron metabolism (Wilder & Sword, 1965). During the course of the infection, rats experimentally infected with *Mycobacterium tuberculosis* showed increased requirement for the vitamins A, D_2, and B_1 (Hurni, 1954).

Past infections may, through persistent histologic lesions, simulate toxicity in long-term studies. Similarly, tissue lesions or high mortality may result from activation of a latent infection by a toxic stress which by itself would not have a drastic effect. Misinterpretation of such 'simulated toxicity' may even have economic consequences, as witnessed in reports by Gilmartin (1961) and Thomas & Ferrebee (1961).

Even more frequent are the episodes when latent infections become acute as a result of decreased resistance brought about by experimental stress. Hammond (1963) has described such an event: daily treatment with streptomycin lowered the mortality of X-irradiated mice from 75% to 10%; when the experiment was later repeated, the antibiotic treatment had no effect and investigation revealed that in the interim period the mouse colony had been latently infected with the streptomycin-resistant *Pseudomonas aeruginosa* through drinking water. Latent Bordetella infection in a rat colony led to acute, fatal pneumonia when, during a period of unusual cold, the fresh air intake to the animal house was reduced and the resulting accumulation of ammonia acted as a stress and

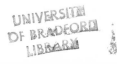

lowered resistance (Hurni, 1964). The influence of animal health on the experimental results is so important that the efforts to exclude or to minimize infections have markedly promoted laboratory animal science during the past 15 years.

STABILIZATION AND STANDARDIZATION OF INFLUENCING FACTORS

All factors which influence results must be kept constant if consecutive experiments carried out in a laboratory over a long period are to be comparable. If results are to be exchanged between institutes, these factors must be standardized as far as possible.

Standard terms and definitions are a prerequisite for the standardization of factors. Unless they are generally accepted and have the same unambiguous meaning in different languages, communications are handicapped in a field which comprises as many disciplines as does laboratory animal science (Sabourdy, 1963, 1965; Loosli & Hurni, 1969).

Stabilization of Hereditary Factors

It is relatively easy to keep the genotype reasonably constant. To this end two fundamentally differing breeding methods have proved particularly useful: (i) strict inbreeding of strains, and (ii) 'outbreeding' (Loosli, 1964).

International convention has defined inbred strains: only strict breeding of brother × sister or of offspring × parent is acceptable and must have been continued during at least 20 generations (Staats, 1968). Individual members of an inbred strain are virtually as homogeneous genetically as are identical twins. Specific and desirable features remain genetically fixed in inbred strains. Most inbred strains were developed with rats or mice since these rodents have rapid generation time. Although over 200 inbred strains of mice alone have been developed, the search for new, desirable properties goes on, as appears from a comparison of the 2nd and 3rd editions of *Standardized Nomenclature for Mice* (Committee on Standardized Genetic Nomenclature for Mice, 1960, 1964). The same source of reference identifies DBA as the oldest inbred mouse strain: it was established in 1909 by Little and shows a high incidence of spontaneous mammary tumours in addition to a particular coat pigmentation.

Inbred strains are altered by mutations occurring with characteristic incidence. Therefore, inbred strains which have been separated during many generations are no longer truly isogenic. Tissues, especially skin, no longer 'take' when transplanted, this being a test for genetic homogeneity of sublines (Brown, 1965; Petrányi & Kállai, 1967). Mutational and selective differences are often considerable, both in inbred strains and in closed colonies: this was shown by Jöchle (1961) in comparative tests on the induction of mammary carcinoma in Sprague-Dawley rats by methylcholantrene, using two lines that had been separated during several years. In order to avoid such genetic divergence and to attain true standardization, inbred strains must be propagated no longer than three to five generations from a particular breeding stock. New breeding pairs of the strain should then be obtained from a recognized 'primary type colony'. It is one of the tasks of ICLA (International Committee on Laboratory Animals), in co-operation with WHO and other international organizations, to appoint such centres.

The alternative breeding method is designated 'outbreeding' as opposed to 'inbreeding' (Loosli, 1964), or more specifically 'random breeding'. This system avoids inbreeding in a closed colony through observing rules of probability. The goal of random breeding is to preserve an unaltered pool of hereditary factors in a population from generation to generation. Inbreeding leads to a loss of alleles from the pool and eventually to homozygosity. However, introduction of new genetic factors through crossing would disrupt the genetic continuity as well. For this reason it is imperative to maintain closed colonies and to refrain from introducing 'fresh blood'.

The success of the outbreeding precautions in closed colonies depends on population size. In small colonies the degree of inbreeding increases rapidly, and alleles are lost correspondingly (Falconer, 1960). Adequate measures of hygienic control, on the other hand, tend to require small colonies. This is especially true of germ-free reference stocks in isolators where space is limited.

In this conflicting situation, a compromise has been found in the production of F_2 hybrids from two to four inbred strains (Loosli, 1969a). F_1 hybrids from two inbred strains are genotypically and phenotypically uniform, but are none the less heterozygous as the gene complement of these hybrids is derived from two different

2—M.T.

strains. Sib-mating or crossing F_1 hybrids leads to a segregating F_2 with extensive genotypic variability. No care is required to maintain their variability unaltered through consecutive generations, since it is reconstituted from inbred strains which have no heterozygosity to lose and therefore are relatively stable.

In hybrids, heterosis takes the place of the inbreeding depression which is typical of homozygous strains. The vitality and fertility of hybrids equals that of good outbred stocks. Characteristics of F_2 hybrids appear frequently unrelated to those of the parent strains (Loosli, 1969b), so that standards of performance have to be established empirically for new hybrids. Since F_2 hybrids are easier to breed in standard quality and perform adequately in experiments, they are for the most part superior to outbred stocks. It is advisable to use the F_2 method for the production of mice and rats in particular.

Table 2.5 Terminology of Breeding Methods (after Loosli & Hurni, 1969)

Source	Breeder				Dealer
Production type	Closed colony			Open colony	Street gang
Mating system	Inbreeding	Outbreeding pedigreed rotated randomized		Pedigreed Selected	(catch-as-catch-can)
	Hybridization of inbred strains	Crossing of uniform F_1 hybrids			
	Chance breeding without system				
Goal of breeding	Fixation of			Rising quality	
	Homozygosity	Heterozygosity			
	Phenotypic uniformity	Reproducible variability			
Animal standard	Inbred strains	Outbred stocks		Breeds	Mongrels
	Uniform F_1 hybrids	F_2 hybrids			

Table 2.5 summarizes the principal goals of the major breeding methods. Animals purchased from an outside source should also be of genetically defined origin.

Stabilization of Life Cycles

Investigators often use animals of which they know nothing but weight and sex, i.e. characteristics which they determine or measure themselves. The body weight, however, depends not only on age and sex of the animal but also on feed, number of animals per cage, micro-climate and many other factors, including the manner of handling by the attendants. Thus, mice of the same strain weighing 20 g may vary from 3 to 7 weeks of age. The experimenter should insist on precise indication of the age of his animal and, when repeating experiments, use animals of the same age. Early segregation of the sexes is of course mandatory, since otherwise errors can arise through unexpected pregnancy.

Stabilization and Standardization of Environmental Factors

This is primarily a problem of technology and organization. Prior to the construction of breeding or experimental rooms, the desired optimal conditions must be established. The type of cage to be used, fixed versus mobile cage racks, and the number of animals per room are key decisions, for they determine the room size and the capacity of the air conditioning plant. In our experience it is convenient to place the cages on mobile racks with castors. Cage dimensions for different animal species are so related that different cage racks, regardless of the cage type which they carry, always cover the same floor space. In this way an animal room can be adapted to different animals provided the air conditioning plant has been designed to match the maximum requirement for mice.

A constant micro-climate is supported by solid cage bottoms rather than wire mesh. Plastic as a cage material further contributes to constant conditions, since it dissipates the animals' body heat more slowly than metal. The air conditioning should operate evenly and without draughts throughout the room. Its capacity is generally indicated by the number of air changes in the room per hour. It is not usually designed to meet the requirements of the animals, i.e. their oxygen consumption and heat and humidity release, but rather adjusted to ensure comfort of the personnel, i.e. to free the room of odours. For this reason 15–23 air changes are specified, which means not only larger plant but also higher operation costs. In order to stabilize the air condition in modern, usually windowless rooms, while simultaneously increasing the comfort by increased oxidation of odour particles and germs, negative charging of the air on entry into the room appears advantageous (Habicht, 1965). By means of special discharge tubes an excess of 2,000 negative ions per cubic centimetre is produced in the air. This simulates the electrostatic conditions found outdoors during sunshine at 1,000 m above sea level.

Illumination of the animal rooms should not be too bright, especially for small rodents; 300–500 lux is sufficient for mice and rats. The intensity must be adequate for the personnel to make the necessary observations and write the records. Daylight cycles should be automatically controlled to suit the particular animal species. Rats and mice, being nocturnal animals, require not more than 10 hours light per day, while 14 hours daylight is preferable for cats.

For bedding in the cages wood shavings are recommended (Porter, 1967). A considerable contribution towards stabilization of the environment is made by using sterilized pine shavings exclusively. Hardwood shavings such as oak which are rich in tannic acid lead to constipation in small rodents, since the animals invariably chew some bedding. Woods which are particularly rich in resin may have bactericidal effect and hence influence results. Dusty bedding is frequently charged with causing lung infection, especially in rats. In our laboratories, we have even found the average litter size at birth reduced by about 30% when rats were bred on dusty shavings. Smith *et al.* (1968) reported mortality increased by more than 40% in suckling rats due to dust.

It is difficult to keep the diet constant over long periods and to standardize it between regions. Porter *et al.* (1963) compared effects of three samples of a standard diet for mice, produced by three different manufacturers within the same region according to the same formula, and observed considerable growth differences in the young (Table 2.6).

In order to produce a diet of constant quality from natural constituents, the individual components must be standardized. This could be achieved by blending individual ingredients such as wheat from crops of different years and origin, but no manufacturer of

Table 2.6 Feeding experiment with LAC grey strain of mice using a standard diet produced by three different manufacturers (after Porter *et al.*, 1963).

	Standard diet, produced by		
	A	B	C
Litter weight (g) on weaning at 19 days (average of four generations)	222·3	207·8	299·0
Average individual weights of young at 19 days:			
1st generation	8·5	8·4	10·0
2nd generation	9·0	8·4	10·0
3rd generation	8·6	8·4	10·0
4th generation	9·6	8·9	9·6

diets has yet been persuaded to try this procedure. Efforts are being made to attain the goal more quickly and to achieve better results by the use of standard diets made up of purified compounds or small-molecular breakdown products of natural substances (Drepper, 1967). Water-soluble diets are particularly promising, since not only can they be filtered to achieve sterility without physico-chemical degradation, but can even be rendered antigen-free for particular purposes (Wostmann *et al.*, 1967). At present such diet mixtures or solutions are expensive, and the success obtained through them is limited (West *et al.*, 1962; Levenson & Tennant, 1963).

A further obstacle in the desired standardization is the contact of attendants with the animals, particularly in animals which are difficult to breed and maintain, e.g. Meriones or certain inbred strains of mice, where a change of attendants leads to slowed production lasting from several weeks to several months. Increased and improved training of attendants may reduce the effects of this factor; however, it certainly should be borne in mind in comparative experiments.

Noise control presents similar difficulties, since the effect of noise on the animal tends to be under-estimated. Also many sources of sound, including the human voice, are virtually unavoidable in an animal house and the animals must become accustomed to them. This protects the animals against stress resulting from sudden noise, and it is conveniently achieved by exposing the animals to continuous radio broadcasts in which human voices appear at frequent intervals.

Standardization of Experimental Preliminaries

In order to reduce to a minimum all influences in the active preliminary phase, and to shorten or eliminate the resulting passive phase of recovery and adaptation, each experimenter would have to breed his own animals. This would eliminate transportation and changes of most environmental factors including diet. Change of cages and regrouping could be done in the breeding room.

Recovery and adaptation are delayed in animals from outside sources. The speed of adaptation depends on the animal species and on the degree of stresses induced by transportation and environmental changes. Under the most favourable conditions involving short transportation and an essentially steady environment, the recovery time is at least 4–6 days for mice (Heinecke, 1967) or 4 weeks for dogs (Hess, 1966).

Establishing Adequate Health

If one succeeds in obtaining healthy animals that are free from all undesired acute or latent infections, and if they remain adequately protected against infections through the experiment, a constant health factor is largely ensured, since it is principally the specific infections which affect the course of experiments. This requirement appears easy but its realization is very demanding.

It is difficult also to define specific pathogens among many microorganisms. Under extreme environmental conditions or other stress factors, the natural resistance to infection can be lowered so that normally harmless germs may become pathogenic and lead to fatal infections.

The problem is overcome by the use of germ-free animals (Gustafsson, 1948, 1949; Reyniers et al., 1946; Pleasants, 1959; Luckey, 1963). In practice, however, the method is cumbersome and, in spite of the development of plastic isolators, expensive (Trexler & Barry, 1958; Trexler, 1959). Furthermore, many reactions of germ-free animals differ fundamentally from reactions of conventional controls, these differences are due mainly to the fact that germ-free animals have never experienced contact with micro-organisms.

Morphological divergence is morphologically conspicuous in the respiratory system and the digestive tract (Gordon, 1965a). Germ-free rodents have an enlarged caecum, and intestinal water resorp-

28

tion is diminished (Csaky, 1965). Digestive breakdown is slowed in the intestinal tract, and enzymes and bioactive substances are increased in the faeces (Gustafsson & Lanke, 1960; Phillips *et al.*, 1961; Lachapelle, 1963; Lepovsky *et al.*, 1964). On the other hand, the faeces of germ-free animals lack substances produced by microbiological degradation, such as coprostonal (Evrard, 1965) and breakdown products of bile (Midtvedt, 1965). Further significant differences appear in the urine (Gustafsson, 1965). The urine of germ-free rats has a higher pH; excretion of citrate and calcium is higher than in conventional animals, whereas phosphate excretion is decreased. Following contamination of the intestinal tract of germ-free rats with a conventional flora, the various parameters reach values typical of conventional rats within 8 days.

Germ-free animals grow more quickly than conventional controls on identical diets (Coates *et al.*, 1963; Doft, 1965; Eyssen, 1965; Forbes & Park, 1959). Absorption of amino acids proceeds twice as fast in germ-free mice (Phillips & Newcomb, 1965). Blood volume and heart weight are lower (Gordon *et al.*, 1963), and the arterial blood pressure is higher in germ-free animals than in conventional controls. Haemoglobin content and dry weight of blood are higher, cardiac output is lower in germ-free rats.

Since the stimulation due to live micro-organisms is lacking, germ-free animals have underdeveloped immunological defence mechanisms (Bauer, 1965). They are free of many localized, ever-present minor infections, and hence from persistent inflammations in various organs, especially in the respiratory and digestive tracts, which are typical of conventional life (Gordon, 1965b).

In consequence, germ-free mice live on average 50% (males) or 30% (females) longer than conventional controls of the same Swiss-Webster strain. It is interesting that germ-free males live on average longer than females, while the opposite holds true for conventional animals.

The types of tumours, both induced and spontaneous, and their localization are the same in germ-free and in conventional animals (Ward, 1961; Pollard *et al.*, 1964). Liver cirrhosis due to choline deficiency, however, develops more rapidly in germ-free animals (Levenson & Tennant, 1965). The liver is lighter in germ-free mice (Quevanviller *et al.*, 1964). The gamma-globulin content of germ-free mice is considerably lower than that of conventional mice (Lachapelle & Phillips, 1965). Agglutinin and properdin are missing from the serum of germ-free animals. The complement titre is un-affected, and so essentially is phagocytosis, although the dissolving phase of the latter appears slow in germ-free animals (Wostmann, 1964, 1965).

The differences between germ-free and conventional animals are often predictable, and they are advantageous or even indispensible in certain experiments (Levenson *et al.*, 1959; Pleasants, 1965). As a rule, however, particularly if animal experiments serve as a basis for the prediction of human reactions, such differences may be undesirable or may modify the results thus leading to erroneous conclusions. A positive advance has been made through an elegant compromise combining the advantages of both germ-free and con-ventional animals, i.e. absence of infectious diseases and normal physiological reactions, the so-called Specific Pathogen Free (SPF) animals (Lane-Petter, 1962).

The SPF Concept

The term SPF was coined during a meeting organized by the Sub-committee for Production of the Institute of Laboratory Animal Resources (USA) attended by 25 scientists and animal breeders in June 1957 (Cumming, 1962). The discussion centred on the produc-tion of animals of a defined disease 'status'. The participants agreed unanimously to use the term 'specific pathogen free' as it adequately reflects the desired state of health of the animals. SPF animals are thus free of pathogenic micro-organisms and parasites normally found in the particular animal species (Foster, 1959). Several new terms have been proposed as substitutes for 'SPF'. 'COBS' stands for 'caesarean-originated, barrier-sustained' (Foster, 1962b), and defines the hygienic derivation of the animals, but says nothing about their actual state of health. Like COBS, terms such as 'clean animals' or 'healthy animals', fail to stipulate that the state of health of the animals must be regularly checked. It is only logical to ask what a specific pathogen is. Of course micro-organisms and para-sites which affect animals of reduced natural resistance, caused by extreme environmental conditions, are not typical pathogens. It appears advisable to have an International Committee setting up lists that specify the organisms to be considered specific pathogens in each species of laboratory animals, despite the opposition raised by some breeders against this proposal (Baker, 1967; Hurni, 1967).

Not only rats and mice but also guinea-pigs, rabbits, cats, and possibly even dogs and monkeys are bred under SPF-conditions, and the intensive use of these animals is expected to bring to light new specific infections. Lists of specific pathogens would therefore

Table 2.7   Microbiological and parasitological checking list for SPF-animals.

	Mice	Rats	Guinea pigs	Rabbits	Cats
Corynebacterium murisepticum	×				
Corynebacterium kutscheri	×				
Diplococcus pneumoniae	×	×	×	×	
Staphylococcus haemolyticus	×	×	×	×	×
Streptococcus haemolyticus	×	×	×	×	×
Bordetella bronchiseptica	×	×	×	×	×
Haemophilus parainfluenzae					×
Haemophilus influenzae-murium	×				
Klebsiella pneumoniae	×		×	×	
Neisseria	×	×	×	×	×
Pasteurella multocida	×	×	×	×	
Pasteurella pseudotuberculosis	×	×	×	×	×
Pseudomonas aeruginosa	×	×	×	×	×
Salmonella	×	×	×	×	×
Streptobacillus moniliformis	×	×			
Mycoplasma (PPLO)	×	×	×	×	×
Dermatophytes	×	×	×	×	×
Endoparasites	×	×	×	×	×
Ectoparasites	×	×	×	×	×
Bartonellaceae	×	×			
Leptospira icterohaemorrhagiae		×			
Toxoplasma	×	×	×	×	×
Mouse pox (Ectromelia)	×				
Mouse hepatitis	×				
Kilham's rat virus		×			
Lymphocytic choriomeningitis	×	×	×		
Pneumonia virus of mice	×				
Polyoma	×				
Reo-3 virus	×				
Sendai virus	×	×			
Mouse encephalomyelitis (Theiler's disease)	×				
K-Virus	×				
Mouse adeno virus	×				
Toolan's virus		×			
Diarrheal disease and intestinal virus infection	×				

need to be revised regularly. Animals in each SPF stock should be tested at definite intervals for freedom from these infections. The tests should be carried out routinely, preferably histologically (Meister *et al.*, 1967), and where the findings deviate from normal, they should be supplemented by specific microbiological techniques (Pollard, 1965; Wagner, 1959, 1965; Werderitch & Pollard, 1963; Gledhill, 1968). A list of pathogens that are not acceptable in SPF colonies of major species has been compiled in Table 2.7. (Ohder, 1969).

Derivation of SPF Animals from a Healthy Nucleus

SPF animals are obtained from the original stock in two steps. First suitable breeding stock must be rendered SPF through hygienic techniques, including specific therapy. Using this stock as a nucleus

Table 2.8   Terminology of hygiene (after Loosli & Hurni, 1969).

Method of derivation	Aseptic hysterectomy		Selection	Chemotherapy	Tradi-tional
Intestinal flora established	By addition		By subtraction		By chance
Precautions in production	Barriers		No barriers		
	Isolator	Pathogen barriers			

Microbiological state:
  No demon-strable germs
  All germs identified
	Germfree axenic Associated or contami-nated (mono-, di-, poly-)				

Tested for absence of specified germs	SPF (clean, healthy, etc.)	SPF (healthy)	SPF (healthy)	Decon-tami-nated	
Unqualified state					Conven-tional

the second step is to build up a production colony from regularly reproducing nucleus animals. Obviously appropriate conditions must be maintained to ensure a constant SPF state. Various methods have been used to attain the SPF state in the first step. A summary of hygienic specifications is presented in Table 2.8.

The simplest method is selection: healthy animals whose offspring must satisfy SPF requirements, are selected from a convenional population of experimental animals. Selective derivation of animals which are free of latent infections is difficult, but this process leads to the elimination of parasites, e.g. round worm in dogs (Griesemer & Gibson, 1963). The second method may be designated as decontamination; by means of chemotherapy, immunization, or a combination of both, conventional animals are freed of the undesirable infections (van der Waay, 1965). The results obtained by this technique are equally unreliable.

The most dependable procedure relies on germ-free derived animals, i.e. aseptic hysterectomy followed by artificial rearing. This method of obtaining and raising breeding animals has already been described for many species: e.g. mice and rats (Nelson & Collins, 1961; Davey, 1959; Foster, 1958, 1959; Graham & Feenstra, 1958); guinea-pigs (Gilstedt, 1936; Calhoon & Matthews, 1964; Hämmerli & Hurni, 1969); rabbits (Bernard, 1962; Hämmerli & Hurni, 1969; Broadfoot, 1969); dogs (Wagner, 1959; Reece *et al.*, 1968); cats (Rohovsky *et al.*, 1966; Hämmerli & Hurni, 1969); sheep (Grace *et al.*, 1959); pigs (Young & Underdahl, 1953).

Although a whole range of viruses, bacteria, fungi, protozoa, and multicellular parasites has been transmitted experimentally across the placenta (Flamm, 1959), infections of the foetus are in practice rarely encountered after hysterectomy. Mycoplasma has been isolated from conventional rat ovaries and uterus with a high incidence, e.g. (Graham, 1963), but these organisms were not found in young obtained by hysterectomy (Wagner, 1959; Werderitsch & Pollard, 1963). On the other hand, viruses were demonstrated in several germ-free strains of mice (Pollard, 1965). Van Hoosier *et al.* (1966) found that in a sample of nine inbred mouse strains seven out of nine virus infections were eliminated by means of hysterectomy. The rate of infection with the viruses that remained detectable, Reovirus type 3 and Theiler's encephalomyelitis virus, dropped from 37% and 33% respectively, to 3% each.

In germ-free rats of Wistar, Fisher, and Sprague-Dawley origin, Pollard (1965) found no virus infections, while Ashe *et al.* (1965) demonstrated an as yet unidentified virus in Sprague-Dawley rats.

The only parasites so far detected in germ-free animals are the worms *Toxocara canis* and *Ancylostoma caninum* in dogs (Wagner, 1959); the infection occurred *in utero*, by active migration of the larvae which interestingly carried no bacterial infection with them. Other transplacental passages of parasites are not known (Bell, 1968).

The rearing of the hysterectomy-derived young is achieved either by hand or by fostering. Both methods can be performed under sterile or non-sterile conditions. During non-sterile hand-rearing the animals acquire a randomly composed intestinal flora derived mostly from man (Wheater, 1967). This may lead to the intestinal tract being overgrown with incidental and unphysiological saprophytes (Balish & Phillips, 1963), which often leads to heavy losses of animals. The same problem arises when adult germ-free animals are transferred to SPF conditions. Hence it is advisable to associate the germ-free animals with a minimal intestinal flora assembled from pure cultures of a few specific micro-organisms. This intermediate stage of defined bacterial association or gnotobiosis facilitates the adjustment of the germ-free animals to SPF conditions (Baker, 1967). Unfortunately the method is not useful in young animals raised in a conventional environment, since a synthetic intestinal flora will not as a rule become established in a gut already accidentally infected.

No general agreement has been reached on the composition of a minimal intestinal flora for particular species. Little is known even of the specific composition of various conventional floras, since their analysis is still hampered by technical difficulties (Dickinson & Raibaud, 1965). Attempts to reconstitute the flora of germ-free mice from single, isolated germs has met with little success, since all necessary types of bacteria have not yet been isolated. Various species of bacterioides and clostridia along with lactobaccilli appear to be part of the normal intestinal flora of mice, and lead to a reduced caecal size (Skelly, 1963; Hagen *et al.*, 1968). Even less is known about the intestinal flora of other experimental animals.

A minimal intestinal flora frequently used in rodents consists of strains of lactobacilli, bacterioides, and enterococci. Our experiments with cats suggest a minimal flora of lactobacilli, *Streptococcus faecalis*, and *Clostridium difficile*.

The dynamic state of an intestinal flora is subject to interaction between the many microbes and it is affected by dietary factors and host conditions. Mice whose intestinal flora consists mainly of lactobacilli are much less sensitive to endotoxins from gram-negative bacteria than are mice showing mainly enterococci and gram-negative bacteria with lactobacilli in the faeces (Schaedler & Dubos, 1962). The composition of the bacterial flora of the mouse depends largely on the diet (Dubos & Schaedler, 1962). Semi-synthetic diets and purified proteins greatly reduce the number of lactobacilli, and consequently the resistance to infection. The elements of an intestinal flora vary further between sections of the gut and between mice of different age (Schaedler & Dubos, 1965).

Experiments by Kenworthy (1965) have demonstrated the importance of the intestinal flora for non-rodents. In germ-free pigs, monocontamination with a so-called pathogenic *E. coli* has no apparent effect. If the animal is then supplied with a 'non-pathogenic' strain of *E. coli*, enteritis results and is further aggravated by addition of a 'total flora'.

Production of SPF Animals

Producing all SPF animals by hysterectomy would be far too expensive. For this reason a small breeding stock only is derived by hysterectomy, and is then expanded by normal breeding. Of course the breeding rooms, cages, bedding, diet, water, air, i.e. the entire environment, must be controlled to ensure continuation of an unaltered state of health of the animals. This means that any possibility of infection with specific pathogens must be guarded against. The 'clean' zone must be protected from the infectious outside world by a barrier and everything that is brought into this zone must be sterilized where possible, or at least disinfected in a suitable manner.

The barrier separating the outside world and the SPF zone assumes critical importance. In spite of all precautions to separate the SPF zone from the infectious surrounding, there always remains a possibility that specific pathogenic germs may penetrate the barrier, produce an epidemic and necessitate the eradication of the entire stock. As an added precaution, in our unit we decided to keep groups of animals derived by hysterectomy in isolators where they are either germ-free or as gnotobiotics. By using these animals the SPF production colony can always be supplemented or, in case of emergencies, built up anew.

Between the extremes of keeping each animal family in an isolator under aseptic conditions, and safeguarding a room of conventional design with a double door acting as a lock, any intermediate solution is conceivable. The efforts spent on barrier installations depend on the estimated risk of infection and on financial capacity. A sensible, practical solution is bound to be a compromise between the two extremes. It must be remembered in this connection that a chain of barrier installations is as effective as the weakest link. Obviously the personnel are the most difficult to render non-infectious, for they cannot be effectively disinfected (Züger, 1969).

The ideal method would be to equip the animal attendants with skindiving equipment and to send them through a disinfecting dip tank into the animal house where they would remain isolated from the animals by their skindiving suits (Reyniers, 1946). This inconvenient, time-consuming and troublesome procedure is not suited to the handling of large numbers of animals. As a compromise it has become customary for the personnel to undress on the conventional side of the lock, pass through a shower to the clean side and there put on sterile clothing. Speers *et al.* (1965) have demonstrated increased shedding of bacteria from the surface of human skin into the atmosphere 1–3 hours following a shower. Although the shower fails to provide effective disinfection, it assures general cleanliness, and reminds personnel of the particular precautions that must be strictly adhered to on the clean side of a barrier. For this reason the shower appears justified. The wearing of gloves and face masks serves both as an individual barrier and as a constant reminder. Bacteriological screening of

Fig. 2.1 Flexible plastic isolator, Tierfarm type (Hurni, 1969). Left: air inlet with filter cartridge; centre: rubber gauntlets for manipulations inside the isolator; right: lock for chemical sterilization, air exhaust valve. Isolators afford maximum protection from infections. Unfortunately they are uneconomical for mass production of laboratory animals.

Fig. 2.2 Large-scale barriers against infections: an SPF breeding unit of Tierfarm AG. The concrete shell without windows is airtight, it takes the place of a giant plastic bag. Dark superstructures on the roof shelter sterile ducts which distribute bedding and food pellets.

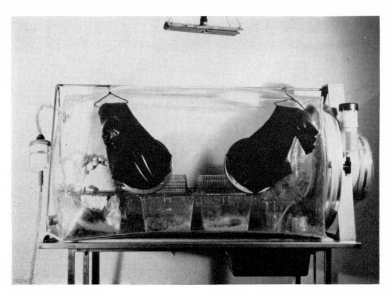

Fig. 2.1 See facing page.

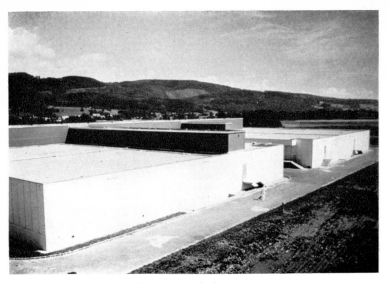

Fig. 2.2 See facing page.

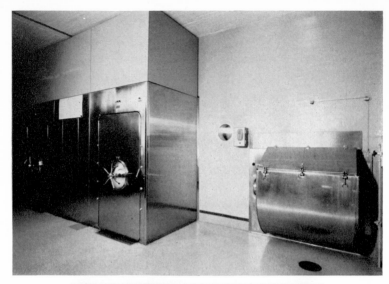

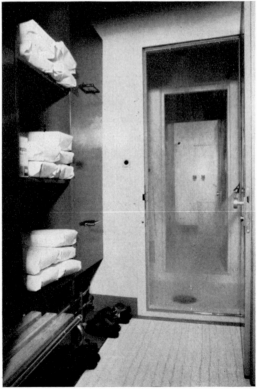

Captions: see facing page.

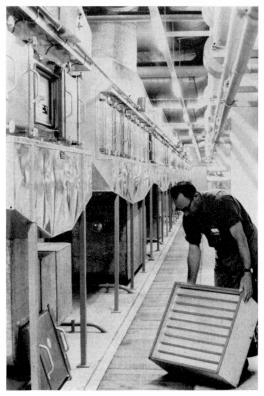

Fig. 2.5 Large-scale barriers against infections: sterilizing filters in the air conditioning plant of the SPF units of Tierfarm AG. Like isolator filters, they retain particles exceeding 0·3 μ. The resulting air is free not only of bacteria but even of viruses, because the latter are apparently attached to larger dust particles.

Fig. 2.3 (*Left top*)   Large-scale barriers against infection: Each breeding unit of Tierfarm AG is fitted with a double-door steam autoclave (left) and a dip tank (right), both analogous to an isolator's chemical lock. The autoclave has a rapid cooling device, for it also serves as delivery hatch for laboratory stock.

Fig. 2.4 (*Left bottom*)   Large-scale barriers against infections at Tierfarm AG: breeding rooms cannot be operated from gauntlets, personnel must enter the rooms. View from the SPF dressing room through the shower cell towards the outer stripping room. The doors were opened to take the picture; in operation they are electronically interlocked and open alternatingly. Lockers in the left foreground contain personal, sterile laundry packs consisting of underwear, overall, socks, cap, gloves, and face mask. Plastic sandals are soaked in disinfectant overnight.

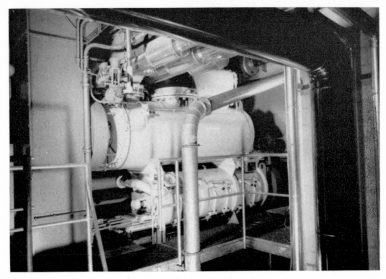

Fig. 2.6 See facing page.

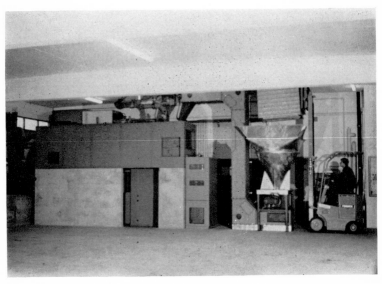

Fig. 2.7 See facing page.

personnel does not prevent the entry of infection since, owing to the diagnostic methods used in bacteriology, temporary shedders of undesired micro-organisms can only be detected retrospectively. For these reasons every technical and organizational possibility must be exploited to economize personnel and to reduce or avoid traffic between rooms and to the central service facilities. Particularly important are automatic sterilization and transportation of food and bedding to the animal rooms, and the removal of soiled bedding from the rooms (Davey, 1959; Foster, 1959, 1962a; Hurni, 1964; Heine, 1964). Despite the refinement of mechanical installations, adequate training and supervision of personnel is indispensable (Lane-Petter, 1967). See Figs 2.1 to 2.7 (following p. 36).

As an additional precaution against undesirable infections during breeding and experiments, the use of 'filter-caps' over each cage has been recommended (Kraft, 1961; Schneider & Collins, 1966). The caps greatly diminish the risk of infection reaching the cage, and dust is retained in the cage. It should, however, be borne in mind that the filters restrict the exchange of gas and heat, and that fewer animals should be kept in each cage (Simmons *et al.*, 1968). Their use is indicated mainly for small rodents and in experiments utilizing SPF animals in inadequately protected animal houses and laboratories.

CONCLUSIONS

The provision of laboratory animals has become more difficult and more expensive. To serious investigators it is no longer satisfactory

---

Fig. 2.6 Large-scale barriers against infections: an automated steam autoclave, the horizontal cylinder in the centre, is the bedding sterilizer of Tierfarm AG. Pulsating vacuum facilitates steam penetration and thus reduces autoclaving time. Following sterilization during 3 min at 150°C, the bedding is shuttled to an attached vacuum drier underneath.

Fig. 2.7 Large-scale barriers against infection: the food pellets for SPF animals have to be thoroughly pasteurized. In this condition the diet is free of specified pathogens yet sufficiently rich in vitamins. To achieve this, Tierfarm AG utilizes a high-frequency range. From the loading funnel (right), the pellets are conveyed between the electrodes where they are heated to 130°C within 1 min. Sterile hot air maintains the temperature during eight additional minutes. The pellet is then forwarded to the cooling tunnel (left), where sterile cold air reduces the pellet temperature to 50°C within 30 sec.

to utilize the cheapest animals that are obtainable from various sources, and about which nothing is known except what can be determined in the laboratory, i.e. weight and sex. A growing number of scientific journals refuse to publish experimental work in which the animal used is not adequately defined. The animals must be of known genetic origin and in a satisfactory state of health. The latter requirement is best met by SPF animals. Acute toxicity tests using SPF animals can even be carried out in clean conventional rooms. In a difficult situation 'filter-caps' on the cages will reduce the risk of infection. On no account must conventional and SPF animals be housed together during the experiment.

In order to keep the period of passive preliminaries of the experiment, i.e. the adaptation and recovery time, as short as possible, breeding rooms and laboratory are best kept under the same roof. This eliminates disturbances of the animals due to transportation, and it keeps changes in the environment to a minimum.

Geographic and chronologic separation seem to introduce insurmountable obstacles into the standardization of animal experiments. In fact we have not found a convincing solution even to an apparently simple problem, namely the diet. Another problem of growing importance, handling of the animals, has not met with adequate attention either. On the other hand, the development of SPF animals has suddenly made the standardization of animal health possible. One set of predominant factors influencing animal experiments within a particular institute is now under control, and hence a certain reproducibility of results over extended periods is assured.

REFERENCES

ADER R. (1967) The influence of psychological factors on disease susceptibility in animals. *Husbandry of Laboratory Animals*, pp. 219–38. London & New York, Academic Press.

ALBERT Z. (1967) Effect of number of animals per cage on the development of spontaneous neoplasms. *Husbandry of Laboratory Animals*, pp. 275–84. London & New York, Academic Press.

ALLEN R.C., WESTMORE P.W. & HOAG W.G. (1962) Factors effecting the incidence of infantile diarrhoea in mice. *Bact. Proc.* **M147,** 99.

ARTSAY H. (1966) A preliminary study of the habitat preferences of white mice in a laboratory environment. *Anim. Welfare Inst. Rep.* **15,** No. 1.

ASCHOFF J. (1964) Die Bedeutung der Tagesperiodik für Tierhaltung und Tierexperiment. *Int. Z. Vitamin Forsch.* Beiheft, 9, 43–65.

ASHE W.K., SCHERP H.W. & FITZGERALD R.J. (1965) A transmissible cytopathic agent from salivary glands of gnotobiotic and conventional rats. *Bact. Proc.* **V41**, 104.

BAKER D.E.J. (1967) Gnotobiotics applied to the standardization of laboratory mice. *Symp. Series immunobiol. Standard* **5**, 31–42. Basel & New York, Karger.

BALISH E. & PHILLIPS A. (1963) Bacterial effects on multiplication, morphogenesis and infectivity of Candida albicans in the alimentary tract. *Bact. Proc.* **M51**, 67.

BARSKI G. (1963) Interférence entre les virus d'herpès et de polyome chez le hamster adulte in vivo. *C. r. Acad. Sci.* **356**, 5459–5462.

BARSKI G. & YOUN J.K. (1964) Interférence entre la chorioméningite lymphocytaire et la leucémie de souris de Rauscher. *C. r. Acad. Sci.* **259**, 4191–4.

BAUER H. (1965) Morphology and function of lymphatic tissue. Paper presented at the NATO Advanced Study Institute, held at Elvetham Hall, Hartley Wintney, Hampshire, England, August 24th–September 2nd.

BELL D.P. (1968) Disease in a caesarian-derived albino rat colony and in a conventional colony. *Lab. Anim.* **2**, 1–17.

BENNET E.L., DIAMOND M.C., ROSENZWEIG M.R. & KRED D. (1964) Chemical and anatomical plasticity of the brain. *Science* **146**, 610–19.

BERNARD E. (1962) Methods and problems concerned with hand-rearing of rabbits. *J. Anim. Techn. Ass.* **13**, 35–40.

BONNOD J. (1967) Immunité génétique et prédisposition à la maladie par espèce et par lignée. *Symp. series immunibiol. Standard* **5**, 73–82. Basel & New York, Karger.

BROADFOOT J. (1969) Hand-rearing rabbits. *J. Inst. Anim. Tech.* **20**, 91–9.

BRONSON F.H. (1967) Effects of social stimulation on adrenal and reproductive physiology of rodents. *Husbandry of Laboratory Animals*, pp. 513–44. London & New York, Academic Press.

BROWN A.M. (1962) Differential characteristics in uniform strains of mice. *Nature* **195**, 204–5.

BROWN. A.M. (1965) Skin grafting for the determination of histocompatibility in mice. *3rd Intern. ICLA Symposium on the Husbandry of Laboratory Animals,* Dun Laoghaire.

BROWN A.M. & WALLACE M.E. (1968) Genetic control of the reaction to histamine in mice after sensitization with pertussis vaccine. *Lab. Anim.* **2**, 63–74.

CALHOON J.R. & MATTHEWS P.J. (1964) A method for initiating a colony of specific pathogen free guinea pigs. *Lab. Anim. Care* **14**, 388–94.

CAMPBELL C.H. (1964) Relation of physiologic condition to variations in susceptibility of mother mice to foot-and-mouth disease virus. *J. Immun.* **92**, 858–63.

CHANCE M.R.A. (1957) The contribution of environment to uniformity. *L.A.C. Coll. Papers* **6**, 59–73.

CHEN K.K., ANDERSON R.C. & STELDT F.A. (1943) Environmental temperature and drug action in mice. *J. Pharmac. Exp. Ther.* **79**, 127–32.

CHEVILLARD L., BERTIN R. & CADOT M. (1967) The influence of rearing temperature on some physiological characteristics of usual laboratory animals (Homeotherms). *Husbandry of Laboratory Animals*, pp. 395–446. London & New York, Academic Press.

CIACCO G. (1963) Adaptation d'une souche de virus aphteux du groupe A à la souris de 24 à 40 jours et au rat de 17 à 18 jours. *Ann. Inst. Pasteur* **105**, 447–9.

CLARK H.F. & SHEPARD C.C. (1962) Effect of environmental temperature on the growth of Mycobacterium marinum in homothermic and poikithermic animals. *Bact. Proc.* **M55**, 76.

COATES M.E., FULLER R., HARRISON G.G., LEV M. & SUFFOLK S.F. (1963) A comparison of chicks in the Gustafsson germfree apparatus and in a conventional environment, with and without dietary supplements of penicillin. *Brit. J. Nutr.* **17**, 141–50.

COLLINS T.B. jr. & LOTT D.E. (1968) Stock and sex specificity in the response of rats to pentobarbital sodium. *Lab. Anim. Care,* **18**, 192–4.

COMMITTEE ON STANDARDIZED GENETIC NOMENCLATURE FOR MICE (1960) Standardized nomenclature for inbred strains of mice. Second listing. *Cancer Res.* **20**, 145–69.

COSNIER J. (1967) The role of certain early environmental conditions on the psychophysiological development of animals. *Husbandry of Laboratory Animals*, pp. 493–512. London & New York, Academic Press.

COSTELLO R.L. & HEDGECOCK L.W. (1961) The effect of dietary vanadium on resistance of the mouse to tuberculosis. *Bact. Proc.* **M128**, 134.

CSAKY T.Z. (1965) Humoral regulation of intestinal water transport in normal and in germfree rats. NATO Advanced Study Institute, held at Elvetham Hall, Hartley Wintney, Hampshire, England, August 24th–September 2nd.

CUMMING C.N.W. (1958) Report on a meeting held at the New York Academy of Sciences, concerning specific-pathogen-free animals. *Proc. Anim. Care Panel* **8**, 84–9.

CUMMING C.N.W. (1962) The commercial production of rats under SPF conditions. *J. Anim. Techn. Ass.* **12**, 75–81.

CUMMING C.N.W. (1967) Large-scale production of mice and rats in a controlled environment. *Husbandry of Laboratory Animals*, pp. 51–60. London & New York, Academic Press.

DAVEY D.G. (1959) Establishing and maintaining a colony of specific pathogen free mice, rats, and guinea-pigs. LAC Collected Papers, **8**, 17–34.

DICKINSON A.B. & RAIBAUD P. (1965) The microflora of the alimentary tract of the rat. Paper presented at the NATO Advanced Study Institute, held at Elvetham Hall, Hartley Wintney, Hampshire, England, August 24th–September 2nd.

DOFT F.S. (1965) Nutrition and metabolism, vitamins and amino acids. Paper presented at the NATO Advanced Study Institute, held at Elvetham Hall, Hartley Wintney, Hampshire, England, August 24th–September 2nd.

DONOVICK R., McKEE C.M., JAMBOR W.P. & RAKE G. (1949) The use of the mouse in a standardized test for antituberculosis activity of compounds of natural or synthetic origin. *Am. Rev. Tuberc.* **60,** 109–20.

DREPPER D.K. (1967) Production of diets for SPF and germ-free animals with special regard to injury of the protein value following sterilization. *Husbandry of Laboratory Animals,* pp. 207–16. London & New York, Academic Press.

DUBOS R.J. (1947) The experimental analysis of tuberculous infections. *Experientia* **3,** 45–52.

DUBOS R.J. & SCHAEDLER R.W. (1962) The effect of diet on the fecal bacterial flora of mice and on their resistance to infection. *J. Exp. Med.* **115,** 1161.

EISMAN P.C., GEFTIC S.G. & BARKULIS S.S. (1961) Multiplication of Mycobacterium leprae in rats maintained on a pro-oxidant diet. Effect of antileprosy drugs. *Bact. Proc.* **M130,** 134.

ELLIS T.M. (1967) Environmental influences on drug responses in laboratory animals. *Husbandry of Laboratory Animals,* pp. 569–88. London & New York, Academic Press.

EVRARD E. (1965) The influence of intestinal bacteria on faecal lipids and faecal sterols. Paper presented at the NATO Advanced Study Institute, held at Elvetham Hall, Hartley Wintney, Hampshire, England, August 24th–September 2nd.

EYSSEEN H. (1965) Effects of intestinal bacteria on growth and nutrient absorption. Paper presented at the NATO Advanced Study Institute, held at Elvetham Hall, Hartley Wintney, Hampshire, England, August 24th–September 2nd.

FALCONER D.S. (1960) *Introduction to Quantitive Genetics.* Edinburgh & London, Oliver & Boyd.

FAUCHET S. & PICARD F. (1965) Contrôle des vaccins diphtériques et tétaniques. *Rev. Immun.* **29,** 49–69.

FINKELSTEIN R.A. & RAMM G.M. (1961) Effect of age on susceptibility to cholera in embryonated eggs. *Bact. Proc.* **M63,** 118.

FLAMM H. (1959) *Die pränatalen Infektionen des Menschen.* Stuttgart, Georg Thieme.

FLYNN R.J. (1967) Note on ringtail in rats. *Husbandry of Laboratory Animals,* pp. 285–88. London & New York, Academic Press.

FOLKERS C. (1964) Toxoplasmosis in pigs. The influence of age on the pathogenicity of T. gondii for pigs. *Vet. Rec.* **76,** 747–49.

FOSTER H.L. (1958) Large scale production of rats free of commonly occurring pathogens and parasites. *Proc. Anim. Care Panel,* **8,** 92–100.

FOSTER H.L. (1959) Housing of disease-free vertebrates. *Ann. N.Y. Acad. Sci.* **78,** 80–8.

FOSTER H.L. (1962a) Establishment and operation of S.P.F. colonies. *The problem of Laboratory Animal Disease,* pp. 249–59. London & New York, Academic Press.

FOSTER H.L. (1962b) 'COBS' animals (Caesarean-originated, barrier-sustained animals). *Charles Riv. Dig.* **1,** No. 2 (July).

FORBES M. & PARK J.T. (1959) Growth of germfree and conventional chicks: Effect of diet, dietary penicillin and bacterial environment. *J. Nutr.* **67**, 69–84.

FOX M.W. (1965) Environmental factors influencing stereotyped and allelomimetic behaviour in animals, *Lab. Anim. Care* **15**, 363–70.

GILMARTIN J.E. (1961) The establishment of a dog breeding kennel for pharmaceutical research. *Proc. Anim. Care Panel* **11**, 222–9.

GLEDHILL A.W. (1968) Control of some viruses and other filtrable agents of mice. *Z. Versuchstierk.* **10**, 3–16.

GLIMSTEDT G. (1936) Bakterienfreie Meerschweinchen. Aufzucht, Lebensfähigkeit und Wachstum, nebst Untersuchungen über das lymphatische Gewebe. *Acta path. microbiol. scand. Suppl.* **30**, 1–295.

GORDON H.A. (1965a) Anomalies of germfree life. Paper presented at the NATO Advanced Study Institute, held at Elvetham Hall, Hartley Wintney, Hampshire, England, August 24th–September 2nd.

GORDON H.A. (1965b) Ageing studies in germfree animals. Paper presented at the NATO Advanced Study Institute, held at Elvetham Hall, Hartley Wintney, Hampshire, England, August 24th–September 2nd.

GORDON H.A., WOSTMAN B.S. & BRUCKNER & KARDOS E. (1963) Effects of microbial flora on cardiac output and other elements of blood circulation. *Proc. Soc. Exp. Biol. Med.* **114**, 301–4.

GOWEN J.W. (1962) Genetic factors in disease, in *The Problems of Laboratory Animal Disease*, ed. Harris R.J.C., pp. 83–98. London & New York, Academic Press.

GRACE O.D., UNDERDALL N.R. & YOUNG G.A. (1959) Procurement of lambs by hysterectomy and their isolation. *J. Vet. Res.* **20**, 239–41.

GRAHAM W.R. (1963) Recovery of a pleuropneumonia-like organism (P.P.L.O.) from the genitalia of the female albino rat. *Lab. Anim. Care* **13**, 719–24.

GRAHAM W.R. & FEENSTRA E.S. (1958) A program for the development of pathogen-free laboratory animals. *Proc. Anim. Care Panel* **8**, 54–66.

GRIESEMER R.A. & GIBSON J.P. (1963) The establishment of an ascarid-free Beagle dog colony. *J. Amer. Vet. Med. Ass.* **143**, 965–7.

GRIFFITH J.F. (1964) Interlaboratory variations in the determination of acute oral LD50. *Toxic. Appl. Pharmac.* **6**, 726–30.

GRUMBACH A. (1949) Der erbliche Einfluss auf Lebensdauer, Organlokalisation und Manifestation im Tuberkuloseversuch. *Schweiz. Z. Path. Bakt.* **12**, 614–27.

GUERAULT A. & QUEVILLON M. (1965) Influence of Bordetella pertussis on histaminsensitivity of chicks. *Bact. Proc.* **M74**, 52.

GUSTAFSSON B.E. (1959) Germfree rearing of rats. A preliminary report. *Acta anat.* **2**, 370–85.

GUSTAFSSON B.E. (1959) Lightweight stainless steel systems for rearing germfree animals. *Ann. N.Y. Acad. Sci.* **78**, 17–28.

GUSTAFSSON B.E. (1965) Nutrition and metabolism: minerals. Paper presented at the NATO Advanced Study Institute, held at Elvetham Hall, Hartley Wintney, Hampshire, England, August 24th–September 2nd.

GUSTAFSSON B.E. (1966) Endosymbiosis and its importance for gnotobiotic and SPF animals. Paper presented at the 4th Scientific Meeting of Gesellschaft für Versuchstierkunde, Kopenhagen, April 21–23.

GUSTAFSSON B.E. & LANKE L.S. (1960) Bilirubin and urobilins in germfree, ex-germfree and conventional rats. *J. Exp. Med.* **112**, 975–81.

HABICHT J.C. (1965) Luftionisation, die Erzeugung biologischer Frischluft in geschlossenen Räumen. *Techn. Rdsch.* No. 8, 27, and 29.

HACKETT J.A.E., DAVIS A.J. & NATSIOS G.A. (1968) The effect of cold stress and Pseudomonas aeruginosa gavage on the survival of three-week-old Swiss mice. *Lab. Anim. Care,* **18**, 94–6.

HAGEN CH.A., BARBERA P.W., BLAIR W.H., SHEFNER A.M. & POILEY S.M. (1968) Similarity of intestinal microflora of BDF conventional mice from different sources and of different ages. *Lab. Anim. Care,* **18**, 550–6.

HALBERG F., JOHNSON E.A., BROWN B.W. & BITTNER J.J. (1960) Suscepti-bility rhythm to E. coli endotoxin and bioassay. *Proc. Soc. Exp. Biol. Med.* **103**, 142–4.

HÄMMERLI MARGRITH & HURNI JOHANNA (1969) Aufzuchtmethoden für Gnotobionten. *Bibl. Microbiol.* **7**, 59–62.

HAMMOND C.W. (1963) Pseudomonas aeruginosa infection and its effects on radiobiological research. *Lab. Anim. Care* **13**, 6–10.

HATCH A., BALAZS T., WIBERG G.S. & GRICE H.C. (1965) The importance of avoiding mental suffering in laboratory animals. *Anim. Welfare Inst. Rep.* **14**, No. 3.

HEINE W. (1964) Zur Planung von Einrichtungen für die Zucht und Haltung von Versuchstieren. *Z. Versuchstierk.* **5**, 1–20.

HEINECKE H. (1967) The experimental environment and its influence on the blood picture of laboratory animals. *Husbandry of Laboratory Animals,* pp. 447–58, London & New York, Academic Press.

HERKEN H. (1951) Eingriff am Nervensystem mit Hexachlorcyclohexan. *Arzneimittelforsch.* **1**, 356–59.

HESS R. (1966) Personal communication.

VAN HOOSIER G.L., TRENTIN J.J., SHIELDS J., STEPHENS K., STENBACK W.A. & PARKER J.C. (1966) Effect of caesarean-derivation, gnotobiotic foster nursing and barrier maintenance of an inbred mouse colony on enzootic virus status. *Lab. Anim. Care* **16**, 119–28.

HURNI H., HIRT R. & RAGAZ L. (1951) Die Wirkung von PAS (p-Aminosali-cylsäure) und PAS-Derivaten auf die experimentelle Mäusetuberkulose. *Schweiz. Z. Path. Bakt.* **14**, 17–33.

HURNI H. (1954) Unpublished results.

HURNI H. (1964) Zucht und Haltung von Laboratoriumstieren. *Int. Z. VitaminForsch.* Beiheft 9. 15–26.

HURNI H. (1967) SPF-Animals. *Symp. Series immunobiol. Standard* **5**, 43–52. Basel & New York.

HURNI H. (1969a) Einflüsse von Umweltfaktoren auf das Versuchstier. *Bibl. Microbiol.* **7**, 22–41.

HURNI H. (1969b) Bauart und Betrieb eines Isolators. *Bibl. Microbiol.* **7**, 54–8.

44 *Methods in Toxicology*

Jöchle W. (1961) Zur experimentellen Erzeugung von Mammatumoren bei Ratten. *Naturwissenschaften* **48**, 481–2.

Iturian W.B. & Fink G.B. (1968a) Comparison of bedding material: habitat preference of pregnant mice and reproductive performance. *Lab. Anim. Care* 18, 160–4.

Iturian W.B. & Fink G.B. (1968b) Effect of noise in the animal house on seizure susceptibility and growth of mice. *Lab. Anim. Care* 18, 557–60.

Kaufmann H.M. & Northey W.T. (1965) Effect of hypothermia on phago-cytosis by rabbit leukocytes of Diplococcus pneumoniae. *Bact. Proc.* M175, 68–9.

Kenworthy R. (1965) The significance of Escherichia coli in conventional and gnotobiotic pigs. Paper presented at the NATO Advanced Study Institute, held at Elvetham Hall, Hartley Wintney, Hampshire, England, August 24th–September 2nd.

Klein F., Fernelius A.L., Taylor M.J., Lincoln M.A. & Mahlandt B.G. (1961) Factors affecting resistance of the rat to Bacillus anthracis spores. *Bact. Proc.* M65, 118.

Konopka E.A., Goble F.C. & Lewis L. (1961) Effects of prior infection with Leishmania donovani on the course of experimental tuberculosis in mice. *Bact. Proc.* M129, 134.

Kraft L.M. (1962) Two viruses causing diarrhoea in infant mice. *The Problem of Laboratory Animal Disease*, pp. 115–30. London & New York, Academic Press.

Kretschmar W. & Haakh U. (1964) Die Abhängigkeit des Verlaufs der Nagetiermalaria (Plasmodium berghei) in der Maus von exogen Faktoren und der Wahl des Mäusestammes. II. Beunruhigung und Ernährung der Mäuse. *Z. Versuchstierk.* **4**, 32–45.

Lachapelle R.C. (1963) Bacterial effects on monoamine oxidase and sero-toxin in the chick. *Bact. Proc.* M54, 68.

Lachapelle R.C. & Phillips A.W. (1965) Serum Proteins in germ-free and conventional mice. *Bact. Proc.* M47, 47.

Lane-Petter W. (1962) Trends in the use of laboratory animals. *ICSU Rev.* **4**, 92–7.

Lane-Petter W. (1967) Selection, training and control of staff. *Husbandry of Laboratory Animals*, pp. 61–76. London & New York, Academic Press.

Layton H.W. & Youmans G.P. (1965) Nutritional effects upon the host-parasite relationship in tuberculosis. *Bact. Proc.* M98, 56.

Lemonde P. (1967) Influence of various environmental factors on neoplastic diseases. *Husbandry of Laboratory Animals*, pp. 255–74. London & New York, Academic Press.

Lepkovsky S., Wagner M., Furuta F., Ozone K. & Koike T. (1964) The proteases, amylase and lipase of the intestinal contents of germ-free and conventional chickens. *Poult. Sci.* **43**, 722–6.

Levenson St.M., Mason R.P., Huber T.E., Horowitz R.E. & Einheber A. (1959) Germfree animals in surgical research. *Anim. Surg.* **150**, 713–30.

Levenson St.M. & Tennant B. (1963) Germfree research: Metabolic and nutritional studies. *Proc. 16th Int. Congr. Zoo. Washington* 3, 148–54.

LOOSLI R. (1964) Der Genotyp als variabler Faktor im Tierversuch. *Int. Z. VitaminForsch.* Beiheft 9, 27–42.

LOOSLI R. (1969a) Stabilisierung genetischer Faktoren im Tierversuch. *Bibl. Microbiol.* **7**, 9–21.

LOOSLI R. (1969b) Beobachtungen an der Hybridmaus Tif MF2, verglichen mit den Elternstämmen. Meeting Soc. Lab. Animal Sci., Nijmegen.

LOOSLI R. & HURNI H. (1969) Das Versuchstier: Begriffe und Definitionen. *Bibl. Microbiol.* **7**, 3–8.

LUCKEY T.C. (1963) *Germfree Life and Gnotobiology*, p. 512. London & New York, Academic Press.

MEIER H. (1963) *Experimental pharmacogenetics*, p. 213. London & New York, Academic Press.

MEISTER G., HOBIK H.P. & METZGER K.G. (1967) Comparative bacteriological and pathological investigations on commercially available SPF-animals. *Husbandry of Laboratory Animals*, pp. 387–99. New York & London, Academic Press.

MIDTVEDT T. (1965) The isolation of intestinal bacteria with effect upon bile acids. Paper presented at the NATO Advanced Study Institute, held at Elvetham Hall, Hartley Wintney, Hampshire, England, August 24th–September 2nd.

MIRAGLIA G. J. & BERRY L.J. (1962) Secondary bacterial involvement following primary experimental infections in mice at 25° and 50°. *Bact. Proc.* **M37**, 72.

MOURIQUAND C. & MOURIQUAND J. (1964) Action cancérigène d'extraits acellulaires de tumeurs de souris PS, sur différentes souches de souris. *Ann. Inst. Pasteur* **106**, 553–60.

MUNDY L.A. & PORTER G. (1969) Some effects of physical environment on rats. *J. inst. Anim. Technol.* **20**, 78–81.

NELSON J.B. & COLLINS G.R. (1961) The establishment and maintenance of a specific-pathogen-free colony of Swiss mice. *Proc. Anim. Care Panel* **11**, 65–72.

NOMURA T., YAMAUCHIC C. & TAKAHASHI H. (1967) Influence of environmental temperature on physiological functions of the laboratory mouse. *Husbandry of Laboratory Animals*, pp. 459–70. London & New York, Academic Press.

OHDER H. (1969) Mikrobiologische Probleme in der Versuchstierzucht. *Bibl. Microbiol.* **7**, 42–53.

PETRÁNYI G. & KÁLLAI L. (1967) A technique of skin grafting in rats and rabbits. *Husbandry of Laboratory Animals*, pp. 43–50. London & New York, Academic Press.

PHILLIPS A.W., NEWCOMB H.R., SMITH J.E. & LACHAPELLE R.G. (1961) Serotonin in the small intestine of conventional and germfree chicks. *Nature* **192**, 380.

PHILLIPS A.W. & NEWCOMB H.R. (1965) Absorption of amino acids in germfree and conventional mice. *Bact. Proc.* **M149**, 64.

PIERCE C., DUBOS R.J. & MIDDLEBROOK G. (1947) Infection of mice with mammalian tubercle bacili grown in Tween-Albumin. *J. Exp. Med.* **86**, 159–173.

PLEASANTS J.R. (1959) Rearing germfree, cesarean-born rats, mice and rabbits through weaning. *Ann. N.Y. Acad. Sci.* **78**, 116–26

PLEASANTS J.R. (1965) General characterisation of germfree life. Paper presented at the NATO Advanced Study Institute, held at Elvetham Hall, Hartley Wintney, Hampshire, England, August 24th–September 2nd.

POLLARD M. (1965) Testing for viruses in germfree animals. Paper presented at the NATO Advanced Study Institute, held at Elvetham Hall, Hartley Wintney, Hampshire, England, August 24th–September 2nd.

POLLARD M., MATSUZAWA T. & SALOMON J.C. (1964) Induction of neoplasms in germfree rodents by 3-methylcholantrene. *J. Nat. Cancer Inst.* **33**, 93–9.

PORTER G. (1967) Assessment of environmental influence on the biological responses of the animal. *Husbandry of Laboratory Animals,* pp. 29–42. London & New York, Academic Press.

PORTER G., LANE-PETTER W. & HORNE N. (1963) Assessment of diets for mice. *Z. Versuchstierk.* **2**, 75–91.

PORTER G. & FESTING M. (1969) Effects of daily handling and other factors on weight gain of mice from birth to six weeks of age. *Lab. Anim.* **3**, 7–16.

PREVITE J.J. & BERRY L.J. (1962) Virulence and infection following acute exposure to cold. *Bact. Proc.* **M38**, 72.

PURBIS M.R., MILLER S. & EHRLICH R. (1961) Effect of ozone, an atmospheric pollutant, on resistance to respiratory infections. *Bact. Proc.* **M166**, 143.

QUEVANVILLER A., LAROCHE M.-J., COTTART A., SACQUET E. & CHARLIER E. (1964) Activités anesthésique et métabolique comparées de l'hexobarbital chez la souris aseptique (germ-free) et classique (conventional). *Ann. Pharm. France* **22**, 339–44.

RAFFYI A. & VERGAMMEN-GRANDJEAN P.H. (1964) Sur la morphologie et la transmission d'Eperythrozoon coccoïdes. *Ann. Inst. Pasteur* **106**, 38–42.

REECE W.O., HOFSTAD M.S. & SWENSON M.J. (1968) Establishment and maintenance of a Beagle dog colony. *Lab. Anim. Care* **18**, 509–12.

REINERT H. & SMITH G.K.A. (1966) Establishment of an experimental cat breeding colony. *Nature* **209**, 1005–8.

REYNIERS J.A. (1946) Germfree life applied to nutrition studies. *Lobund Rep.* **1**, 87–120.

REYNIERS J.A., TREXLER P.C. & ERVIN R.F. (1946) Rearing germ-free albino rats. *Lobund Rep.* **1**, 1–84.

ROGER F. & ROGER A. (1963) Etudes sur le pouvoir pathogène expérimental du virus de la chorioméningite lymphocytaire. IV. Niveau de mortalité des souris après inoculation souscutanée plantaire. *Ann. Inst. Pasteur* **105**, 476–85.

ROHOVSKY M.W., GRIESEMER R.A. & WOLFE L.G. (1966) The germfree cat. *Lab. Anim. Care* **16**, 52–9.

ROSS M.H. & BRAS G. (1965) Tumor incidence patterns and nutrition in the rat. *J. Nutrit.* **87**, 245–60.

SABOURDY M.A. (1961) Techniques with germ-free animals. Paper presented at the Lecture tour, organized by ICLA with the support of UNESCO and IAEA. Sept.–Oct.

SABOURDY M.A. (1963) Definitions of terms. *ICLA Bull.* no. 12, March 1963.

SABOURDY M.A. (1965) The need for specification in laboratory animals: suggested terms and definitions. *Food Cosmet. Toxicol.* **3**, 9–19.

SACQUET E. (1962) Les infections inapparentes des animaux de laboratoire, *The Problems of Laboratory Animal Disease,* ed. HARRIS R.J.C., pp. 57–71. London & New York, Academic Press.

SCHAEDLER R.W. & DUBOS R.J. (1962) The fecal flora of various strains of mice. Its bearing on their susceptibility to endotoxin. *J. Exp. Med.* **115**, 1149.

SCHAEDLER R.W. & DUBOS R.J. (1965) Reconstitution of the autochthonory flora in germfree mice. Paper presented at the NATO Advanced Study Institute, held at Elvetham Hall, Hartley Wintney, Hampshire, England, August 25th–September 2nd.

SCHNEIDER H.A. (1962) Natural resistance to disease. *The Problems of Laboratory Animal Disease,* ed. HARRIS, R.J.C., pp. 73–82, London & New York, Academic Press.

SCHNEIDER H.A. & COLLINS G.R. (1966) Successful prevention of infantile diarrhoea of mice during an epizootic by means of a new filter cage unopened from birth to weaning. *Lab. Anim. Care* **16**, 60–71.

SEAMER J., GLEDHILL A.W., BARLOW J.L. & HOTCHIN J. (1961) Effect of Eperythrozoon coccoides upon lymphocytic choriomeningitis in mice. *J. Immunol.* **86**, 512.

SIDWELL R.W., DIXON G.J., SELLERS S.M., MAXWELL C.F. & SCHABEL F.M. (1965) Effect of host weight loss on friend leukemia virus infections in Swiss, DBA/2, BALB/c mice. *Proc. Soc. Exp. Biol. Med.* **119**, 1141–7.

SIMMONS M.L., ROBIC D.M., JONES J.B. & SERRANO L.J. (1968) Effect of a filter cover on temperature and humidity in a mouse cage. *Lab. Anim.* **2**, 113–20.

SKELLY B. (1963) Effect of intestinal bacteria upon cecal size of gnotobiotic mice. *Bact. Proc.* **M50**, 67.

SMITH R.T. & THOMAS L. (1956) The lethal effect of endotoxins on the chick embryo. *J. exp. Med.* **104**, 217–31.

SMITH P.C., STANTON J.S., BUCHANAN R.D. & TANLICHAROENYOS P. (1968) Intestinal obstruction and death in suckling rats due to sawdust bedding. *Lab. Anim. Care* **18**, 224–8.

SOAVE O.A. & BOYLE C.C. (1965) A comparison of the hemograms of conditioned and non-conditioned laboratory dogs. *Lab. Anim. Care* **15**, 359–62.

SPEERS R., BERNARD H., O'GRADY F. & SCHOOTER R.A. (1965) Increased dispersal of skin bacteria into the air after shower-baths. *Lancet* **1965**, 478–80.

STAATS, JOAN (1968) Standardized nomenclature for inbred strains of mice, fourth listing. *Cancer Res.* **28**, 391–420.

SWORD C.P. (1965) Influence of iron on experimental infections of mice with Listeria monocytogenes. *Bact. Proc.* **M169**, 67.

THOMAS E.D. & FERREBEE J.W. (1961) Disease-free dogs for medical research. *Proc. Anim. Care Panel* **11**, 230–3.

TREXLER P.C. (1959) The use of plastics in the design of isolator systems. *Ann. N.Y. Acad. Sci.* **78**, 29–36.

TREXLER P.C. & BARRY E.D. (1958) Development of inexpensive germ-free animal rearing equipment. *Proc. Anim. Care Panel* **8**, 75–8.

TSCHISCHEWSKY A.L. (1934) Die Wege des Eindringens von Luftionen in den Organismus und die physiologische Wirkung von Luftionen. *Acta med. scand.* **83,** 219–72.

VAN DER WAAI D. (1965) Bacteriological decontamination of mice. Paper presented at the NATO Advanced Study Institute, held at Elvetham Hall, Hartley Wintney, Hampshire, England, August 24th–September 2nd.

WAGNER M. (1959) Determination of germ-free status. *Ann. N.Y. Acad. Sci.* **78,** 89–101.

WAGNER M. (1965) Bacteriological and mycological testing procedures. Paper presented at the NATO Advanced Study Institute, held at the Elvetham Hall, Hartley Wintney, Hampshire, England, August 24th–September 2nd.

WARD T.G. (1961) Spontaneous tumors in germfree mammals. *Fed. Proc.* **20,** 150.

WEIHE W.H. (1964) Der Einfluss der Temperatur als Faktor der physikalischen Umwelt auf den Stoffwechsel der Ratte. *Int. Z. VitaminForsch.* Beiheft 9, 89–113.

WEIHE W.H. & HURNI H. (1962) The resistance of three inbred strains of immunized and non-immunized mice to E. coli infection at low and high altitude. Paper presented at the Symposium on the physiological effects of high altitude, Interlaken.

WERDERITS E.J. & POLLARD M. (1963) Examination of germfree rats and mice for PPLO. *Bact. Proc.* **M48,** 66.

WEST L.M., HILL G.A. & MARCUS S. (1962) Relation between low levels of exposure to ionizing radiations and occurrence of spontaneous infection diseases in mice. *Bact. Proc.* **M40,** 73.

WHEATER D.W.F. (1967) The bacterial flora of an SPF-colony of mice, rats and guinea pigs. *Husbandry of Laboratory Animals,* pp. 343–60. London & New York, Academic Press.

WIEN R., HURNI H., LAMMERS W. & LOOSLI R. (1963) Progress report, presented at the Meeting of the European Society for the Study of Drug Toxicity. Leyden, 29th June.

WILDER M. & SWORD C.P. (1965) Biochemical changes in mice infected with Listeria monocytogenes. *Bact. Proc.* **M170,** 68.

WOSTMANN B.S. (1964) Germfree animals: Standards for Production. Paper presented at the Ann. Meeting Ass. Appl. Gnotobiotics, June 1964, East Lansing.

WOSTMANN B.S., PLEASANTS J.R. & REDDY B.S. (1967) Water-soluble, non-antigenic diets. *Husbandry of Laboratory Animals,* pp. 187–206. London & New York, Academic Press.

WOSTMANN B.S. (1965) Immune functions in germfree and ex-germfree life. Paper presented at the NATO Advanced Study Institute, held at Elvetham Hall, Hartley Wintney, Hampshire, England, August 24th–September 2nd.

YOUNG D.A.B. (1965) A photoperiodic influence on the growth in rats. *J. exp. Zool.* **160,** 241–6.

YOUNG G.A. & UNDERDALL N.R. (1953) Isolation units for growing baby pigs without Colostrum. *J. Vet. Res.* **14,** 571–4.

ZÜGER A. (1969) Personal-Hygiene, *Bibl. Microbiol.* **7,** 63–8.

CHAPTER 3

Measurement of Acute Toxicity

T. BALAZS

THE OBJECTIVES OF THE MEASUREMENT OF ACUTE TOXICITY

Acute toxicity is a term that signifies the toxic effects produced by a single dose of a compound. It is investigated in experimental animals in the course of the safety evaluation of chemicals intended for use as household products, food additives, cosmetics, drugs, biocides, etc.

Knowledge of the acute toxicity of a compound is of great importance when either the case of an accidental poisoning with a chemical or the therapeutic trial of a drug is considered. The results of acute toxicity tests are also used for planning chronic toxicity studies. Acute toxicity tests might reveal effects which cannot be detected in multiple-dose tests due to the lower doses administered in the latter, or to tolerance.

The investigation consists of a series of bioassays in which quantitative relationships are established between the administration of a compound and the appearance of toxic effects. The primary objective is usually to determine the lethal dose in one or two species—usually in rodents. A secondary objective of the acute toxicity test is the assessment of induced syndromes as well as the estimation of doses producing specific toxic effects.

The intended use of the compound greatly influences the scope of the acute toxicity test. For example, the extensive investigation of the acute toxicity of a dye which might be used in a cosmetic in an infinitesimal dose compared to the lethal dose appears to be superfluous. On the other hand, the acute toxicity of a compound which might be used in amounts close to the toxic dose should be extensively investigated. It should be appreciated that the scope of the

49

measurement of acute toxicity depends upon the over-all plan of the safety evaluation of a chemical.

THE TECHNIQUES OF MEASUREMENT OF ACUTE TOXICITY*

Principles

In the measurement of acute toxicity two types of dose–response relationships are involved: the graded or quantitative, and the all-or-none or quantal responses. The range of dosage and the method of statistical analysis are usually different for the two kinds of response. Therefore, most investigators plan the assay for one kind of response. Initially this is usually the quantal one. However, examinations can be performed in the quantal assay to investigate the occurrence of specific toxic effects of a quantitative nature. Information gained from these examinations can aid in the determination of the clinical and pathological syndrome and can indicate the necessity for carrying out quantitative assays for specific toxic effects.

Linear relationship usually exists between the logarithms of the doses and the toxic responses; therefore, doses are usually chosen so that the logarithm of the dose increases by equal increments. The route of administration depends upon the intended use of the chemical; however, oral and intravenous administrations are desirable in at least one species.

Because of the availability of uniform strains of mice and rats, ease of housing, size, relatively low cost, and profusion of published toxicologic data on these two species, they are the animals of choice for the measurement of acute toxicity. However, other species should also be considered.

Measurement in Rodents

(a) SELECTION OF DOSES

Usually, a pilot test is carried out to determine a range of doses which is estimated to cause 10–90% deaths in the final test. The selection of doses on a body weight basis in 0·6 log intervals is

* The technique recommended by the author does not represent a standard method of any laboratory.

practical for the first exploratory step (Davidow & Hagan, 1955). However, to avoid logarithmic transformation of doses, the antilog of the selected log interval provides the factor for the dose ratios; e.g. antilog of 0·6=4. Thus, if the first dose level chosen is an equivalent of 50 mg/kg, the next doses are 200 and 800 mg/kg. Each of these doses is given to four animals. On the basis of mortality, higher or lower doses may be similarly selected, or intermediate doses may be selected at 0·2 log intervals (factor 1·6).

The range of doses selected for the final assay is delineated by the highest dose that did not cause death, and the lowest dose that caused death in every animal. This range is usually divided into four or five equal logarithmic intervals depending upon its magnitude. In this manner the selection of dose levels producing increasing mortalities of 10–90% is usually accomplished. This is necessary for the determination of the median lethal dose (LD_{50}).

(b) PREPARATION AND DOSAGE

It is desirable to hold the animals in the laboratory for at least a week before use to allow for their adaptation to the environment and to ascertain their physical well-being. Animals of similar body weight (not more than 10% difference), selected 1 day before dosing, are identified and assigned randomly to the various groups. Ten animals are chosen for each dose level, and a similar number, treated with the vehicle only, serve as control. Each animal is caged individually.

The compound is prepared in such a way that its chemical character does not change during the period of administration, while it is kept at room temperature. A solution of the same concentration for all doses selected can be used for parenteral routes if the volume is within the appropriate range. (See *Factors Inherent to the Administration of a Compound.*) For oral dosing a standard volume is given, thus solutions of different concentrations are prepared for each dose level. The amount of compound injected intravenously should be at a constant rate for each dose level. Suspensions are usually not given by this route. For the techniques of administration by the various routes see Moreland (1965).

(c) EXAMINATIONS

Following administration of a compound, animals are observed for the appearance of signs of toxicity. The incidence and time of appearance of such signs are recorded separately for each animal. The preparation of tables for the recording of the toxic signs facilitates the routine performance of the test. Standardized observational screening procedures have been described (Campbell and Richter, 1967). A guide-line for physical examination is presented in Table 3.1. Body weight and food intake are measured at appropriate intervals or at least prior to dosing and at the termination of the observation period.

It is not customary to perform clinical pathologic tests in the measurement of acute lethality in rodents. It is more appropriate to conduct such tests in separate studies as a quantitative assay. Nevertheless, some of these tests are included herein, because occasionally their application may be considered even in the course of the primary, quantal test.

Clinical pathologic tests can be used to detect the presence of damage to a specific or target organ. It is sufficient to examine a few animals of a representative dose group and controls in a quantal assay. Since the development of detectable hepatic, renal, or hematopoietic damage often takes 1 to 2 days, clinical pathologic tests are best performed on the third day. Urine is collected and blood samples are taken if the condition of the animal permits. Not more than one drop of blood (from the tail veins) is taken. This is sufficient to carry out the tests outlined below, if half of the animals at one dose level are used for one of the tests (e.g., a haematocrit and blood smear) and the other half for the second test (e.g., a hepatic test).

For the detection of haematoxicity, a haematocrit and a stained blood smear are examined. The haematocrit reflects the factors affecting the production and disposition of circulating cells as well as changes in the fluid phase (e.g., haemoconcentration). Plasma colour is indicative of haemolysis, icterus, or lipaemia. The examination of a uniformly prepared, stained blood smear reveals not only morphologic changes of the red blood cells, but also major changes in haemoglobin concentration and in the leukocyte and thrombocyte counts.

For the detection of hepatotoxicity, the measurement of plasma glutamic pyruvic transaminase or arginase level is recommended. Arginase determination is more practical, since, using a micromethod, only one drop of whole blood is required. These enzyme

Table 3.1 Physical examinations in acute toxicity tests in rodents.

Organ system	Observation and examination	Common signs of toxicity
CNS and somatomotor	Behaviour	Change in attitude to observer, unusual vocalization, restlessness, sedation
	Movements	Twitch, tremor, ataxia, catatonia, paralysis, convulsion, forced movements
	Reactivity to various stimuli	Irritability, passivity, anaesthesia, hyperaesthesia
	Cerebral and spinal reflexes	Sluggishness, absence
	Muscle tone	Rigidity, flaccidity
Autonomic nervous system	Pupil size	Myosis, mydriasis
	Secretion	Salivation, lacrimation
Respiratory	Nostrils	Discharge
	Character and rate of breathing	Bradypnoea, dyspnoea, Cheyne–Stokes breathing, Kussmaul breathing
Cardiovasular	Palpation of cardiac region	Thrill, bradycardia, arrhythmia, stronger or weaker beat
Gastrointestinal	Events	Diarrhoea, constipation
	Abdominal shape	Flatulence, contraction
	Faeces consistency and colour	Unformed, black or clay coloured
Genitourinary	Vulva, mammary glands	Swelling
	Penis	Prolapse
	Perineal region	Soiled
Skin and fur	Colour, turgor, integrity	Reddening, flaccid skinfold, eruptions, piloerection
Mucous membranes	Conjunctiva, mouth	Discharge, congestion, haemorrhage cyanosis, jaundice
Eye	Eyelids	Ptosis
	Eyeball	Exophthalmus, nystagmus
	Transparency	Opacities
Others	Rectal or paw skin temperature	Subnormal, increased
	Injection site	Swelling
	General condition	Abnormal posture, emaciation

levels increase if necrotic change is present (Balazs *et al.*, 1961). By the analysis of urine for bilirubin, functional changes of the liver may be detected. However, negative findings in these tests do not exclude the presence of liver injury.

For the detection of nephrotoxicity, urine volume is measured and urinalysis is performed. In small volumes of samples, concentrations of protein, glucose and the pH are estimated, and occult blood is detected with reagent strips. The measurement of urine glutamic oxalacetic transaminase content is suitable for the quantitation of renal tubular necrosis (Balazs *et al.*, 1963). Results of urinalysis may reveal systemic toxic effects, such as diabetes, porphyrinuria, acidosis, alkalosis, etc.

Additional clinical chemistry measurements that would provide useful information depend upon the clinical signs as well as the biochemical pharmacologic effects of the compound.

Post-mortem examination of animals dying several hours after dosing can ascertain that death was not due to faulty intubation and may contribute to the establishment of the pathologic syndrome. Alterations in the colour of blood, haemorrhages, excess fluid in body cavities, lung oedema, congestion of liver and of the mesenteric vessels or gastrointestinal mucous membrane might be seen at this time. Specific gross pathologic changes (e.g., degenerative changes of the parenchymatous organs) are not generally detected prior to the second or third day.

It is particularly desirable to carry out pathologic examination on the carcasses of animals dying several days after dosing. Useful information can be obtained by necropsying a representative number of animals at the end of an acute toxicity study. Weights and water content of the parenchymatous organs are measured in some laboratories (Boyd, 1968).

(d) DURATION OF THE TEST

When deaths occur solely within the first 24 hours and no delayed toxic effects are detected, the test is terminated one week after dosing. However, if the general condition of the animals is not satisfactory, or delayed toxic effects are detected, the test period is prolonged. Some laboratories terminate the test routinely at the end of 2 weeks to comply with requirements of established standards (e.g., Federal Hazardous Substances Act of the USA).

Measurement in Non-rodents

The objective of this test is to detect species differences to the toxic effects of the compound in the range of lethal doses. The dog is the first choice of a non-rodent species since data can usually be utilized in chronic toxicity studies with this species. Also it is desirable to choose a species in which, as in man, emesis readily occurs.

The measurement of acute toxicity in the dog, or other species, such as the monkey, is somewhat different from that in rodents. The median lethal dose is not ordinarily determined, but the approximate lethal dose is estimated and the character of the induced toxic syndrome is established. It is not necessary to use purebred animals in such an experiment; mongrel dogs are satisfactory.

Information on the toxicity of a compound in rodents prior to the acute toxicity measurement in dogs enables one to estimate that dose which gives the anticipated toxic effect. The effect of the initial dose in a single animal indicates the second dose level. The subsequent dosage is given to another dog according to the geometric progression as indicated by the results of the acute toxicity measurement in rodents (staircase technique). Animals are observed for several days for delayed toxic effects.

Another method of measuring acute toxicity in dogs consists of initially dosing two animals with identical doses. The dosing is repeated in one animal at intervals indicated by the rate of the development of toxic effects in the test with rodents (pyramid technique). By this method the acute toxicity of compounds that have a rapid effect and a slow rate of detoxification can be estimated.

An advantage of the measurement of acute toxicity in dogs lies in the availability of adequate clinical diagnostic procedures in this species. These can be utilized for the assessment of toxic effects at sublethal dose levels. Liver and kidney function tests, electrocardiographic and haematologic examinations can be carried out a few days after dosing. Post-mortem examination is desirable.

Measurement of Prenatal and Neonatal Acute Toxicity

To measure acute toxicity in the embryo, both avian and mammalian species have been used. In the former, the compound is injected into the yolk sac of fertile eggs prior to incubation (McLaughlin *et al.*, 1963). In the mammalian species, the test is performed by treatment of pregnant animals in various stages of gestation, so that both embryonic and foetal toxicity can be examined. In the embryo, an acute toxicity test is often confined to the assessment of the interference of a sub-lethal dose; in the foetus it might include also the examination of effects on selected organs. For this purpose, several animals are sacrificed at birth and tissues are examined histologically. In both tests the number and weight of newborn animals are recorded and their development is followed for one week in the neonatal period. Teratologic studies complement this assay.

In the measurement of acute toxicity in newborn or suckling animals, littermates are chosen for each dose level. Five to six animals of one litter are left together. The mother is removed during the period of dosing which is done orally. The design of the acute toxicity study is similar to that in adult animals. Since clinical pathologic tests are not usually performed in young rodents, a number of animals on the highest dose levels are sacrificed during the first week for histopathologic studies of selected organs. The development of the remaining animals is followed to sexual maturity, which is represented by the time of vaginal opening or the descent of the testicles.

It is difficult to divorce an inherent sensitivity of the newborn from exogenous factors of the experiment, which can influence mortality (e.g., lack of sucking, and of maternal care of the newborn during the effect of the compound).

The calculation of the dose on the basis of body surface might be appropriate when toxicity in the newborn and in adult animals is to be compared.

Measurement of Acute Dermal Toxicity

Dermal acute toxicity tests are performed with chemicals to which the skin might be exposed intentionally or by accident. The method of Draize (1955) is used for this measurement. This consists of a single exposure to the agent which is kept in contact with the skin (on at least 10% of the body surface) for periods up to 24 hours by means of a rubber sleeve. The sleeve should fit tightly over the entire abdomen and back which have been clipped prior to the test. Solution is introduced under the sleeve and evenly distributed; dry powder is moistened with isotonic saline to prepare a paste, which is applied on the area, and covered with cotton gauze. A wire screen may be used instead of the rubber sleeve in testing materials that adhere readily to the skin. The screen is padded and raised approximately 2 cm from the exposed skin. At the end of exposure, the sleeve or screen is removed, and the skin is wiped dry with paper towelling.

The albino rabbit, 2–3 kg body weight, is the animal of choice in dermal toxicity tests. As with other tests, a range-finding test is necessary to obtain the lethal dose levels. Four to six animals are used for each dose level in the final test. Clinical and pathologic examinations carried out in dermal toxicity tests are identical with those described for the tests of other routes. In addition, the local dermal effect is examined. The period of observation is usually 2 weeks. (The subject has been reviewed by Barnes, 1968.)

Measurement of Acute Inhalation Toxicity*

[see also Chapter 6]

In acute inhalation toxicity studies, an atmosphere containing the test substance is generated and experimental animals are exposed to air containing the material. Test animals may be exposed in a static or a dynamic air-flow chamber. A static chamber is simply a closed container into which the animals are placed and the test material is introduced. It can be useful when working with a small quantity of material or for exposures of short (few minutes) duration, but the concentration will vary with time as the animals absorb the material. A static chamber has another serious disadvantage. The respiratory rate of the animals, and hence their absorption of the test material, may change as carbon dioxide builds up in the unit. Dynamic flow chambers have a constant flow of air, which passes through the test material into the chamber. With adequate flow-rates, the losses by absorption, adsorption, and other causes are kept low, and a build-up of excessive heat and moisture is prevented.

Convenient, practical devices for exposing a limited number of small laboratory animals can be made from 5 gal. battery jars.

* The author is grateful to Dr G.J. Levinskas for writing the section on acute inhalation toxicity; to Dr J.F. Noble for generous advice in the course of the review of the manuscript; and to Mrs D. Lennon for editorial assistance.

Spiegl *et al.* (1953) have described a system in which the jar is
mounted horizontally on a wooden rack with a front board which
serves as a closure for the jar and an instrument-mounting panel.
Alternatively, the jar may be positioned vertically with a glass or
plastic top ground to fit the cylinder (Fraser *et al.*, 1959). The cover
should have openings for the air inlet and exhaust and a sampling
port. In its simplest form, air from an essentially oil-free compressed-air line (or a pump if a compressed-air line is lacking) is
introduced into two channels by a 'T' tube. Each arm of the 'T'
tube is equipped with a calibrated flowmeter and a valve for
regulating the flow of air through it. One flowmeter is adjusted to
measure the air being bubbled through the test material, while the
other regulates the amount of the make-up air. The two air streams
are mixed and led into the exposure chamber. Control of the chamber concentration is achieved by regulating the relative rates of flow
of the agent-laden and make-up air. The exhaust port of the
chamber is led into a well-ventilated hood. If the test material
presents a high degree of hazard, the exhaust air should be passed
through a suitable absorbent before it is vented into the hood.

Procedures for generating the test atmospheres and their complexity will vary with the nature of the material under study. Gases
may be metered from cylinders under pressure. A simple bubbler
can be used for liquids with an appreciable vapour pressure (Spiegl
et al., 1953). The Vaponephrine nebulizer can be used to generate
mists and fogs of liquids with low or negligible vapour pressures
(Fraser *et al.*, 1959). References to the special problems encountered
in generating test atmospheres of liquid–liquid or liquid–solid mixtures and dusts or powders are found in the articles of Fraser *et al.*
(1959) and Lehman *et al.* (1964). If particulates are sufficiently large,
i.e., greater than 20μ in diameter, they fail to reach the terminal
bronchioles and thus present a negligible inhalation hazard in acute
exposure. Even particles larger than 2μ are removed prior to the
alveoli. Thus particle size should be less than 2μ for alveolar
absorption (Kanig, 1963).

The concentration of the test substance in the chamber air and
the duration of the exposure should be specified. Chamber concentrations are expressed in terms of milligrams of compound per cubic
meter of air (mg/m^3), although gases may be expressed in terms of
parts by volume per million parts of air (p.p.m.). Tables for the
interconversion of these concentration units may be found in books

on industrial hygiene and toxicology. Chamber concentrations may be described as nominal or analytical. Nominal concentrations are those calculated from the amount of the material dispersed and the volume of air into which it is dispersed. Analytical concentrations are the actual levels of the air-borne contaminant as determined by measurement. Silver (1946) has detailed many of the factors which may cause analytical values to be less than the nominal concentrations. Whenever possible, chamber concentrations should be determined by analysis with due regard for the accuracy of the analytical method and the sampling procedure used.

If a series of animals is exposed to varying concentrations of the test material, a median lethal concentration (LS_{50}) can be determined which is analogous to the LD_{50}. The LC_{50} is that air concentration of the material that is expected to kill 50 per cent of an exposed group of test animals. Obviously, the duration of the exposure to each concentration should be constant. A 4 hour exposure, followed by a 14 day observation period, frequently is used to determine the LC_{50}. Examinations carried out in this period are similar to those suggested for other routes of administration.

Unlike exposures by other routes, in which the measurement of the administered dose is simple, there is no simple way to measure the dose received by animals in inhalation experiments. Dose measurement is complicated since the concentration of the material in the ambient air is not a measure of the amount absorbed into the bloodstream, which in turn, depends upon the duration of the exposure. To determine the actual dose absorbed, the levels of the agent in the inspired and the expired air would have to be determined. The difference between these concentrations would represent absorption. Weston and Karel (1946), working with phosgene, have described a procedure for measuring the retained dose of an inhaled substance.

EVALUATION OF DATA

Qualitative Interpretation

To appraise the results, a systematic tabulation of the data is helpful. A separate listing of each animal shows how the different findings are combined in any individual. This may reveal the occurrence of two distinct syndromes at one dose level; for example, in acute toxicity studies with acetyl salicylic acid, early deaths are due to convulsions and respiratory failure, whereas delayed deaths are due to cardiovascular shock (Boyd, 1959). Another example may be observed in oral acute toxicity studies with hexachlorophene in rabbits. Gastrointestinal effects are observed during the first day and sacral paralysis a few days thereafter (Balazs, 1968—unpublished). Since some of the clinical signs are not specific, their interpretation is often difficult. However, the complexity of signs, the syndrome, characterizes the induced condition. For example, death on the first day is usually caused by cardiovascular or respiratory failure. There are similar toxic signs such as cyanosis, dyspnoea and convulsions due to anoxia in each condition. However, in cardiovascular failure, prostration and specific cardiac signs (marked changes in rate or rhythm) are prominent. In primary respiratory failure, deaths are fulminant and the heart beat continues after cessation of respiration. The sequence of toxic signs, as well as their occurrence at various dose levels, aids in their interpretation. For example, convulsions might be due to a direct CNS effect or to anoxia. If they occur without dyspnoea in the prodromal stage, or with no death loss at the low end of the dose range, a primary CNS effect is suggested.

The onset and duration of signs of toxicity might suggest whether a pharmacologic action or organic damage has developed. For example, paralysis from a pharmacologic effect usually manifests itself rapidly but normally does not last more than 1 day. However, the occurrence of paralysis due to organic damage is usually delayed. Similarly, it takes 1–2 days for signs of hepatic or renal insufficiency to develop. Thus, deaths attributable to these conditions do not occur on the first day. Pharmacologic effects of a compound may be known from other investigations and may aid in the interpretation of toxic signs that are related to pharmacologic action. In some instances an antagonist of the compound may be used to resolve this problem. The use of a protective agent may also help to reveal specific toxic effects when mortality supervenes due to the pharmacologic effect (e.g., hypoglycaemia). Decreased body weight gain should be considered a sign of toxicity. The return of the normal weight gain suggests recovery.

The interpretation of clinical pathologic test results cannot be divorced from clinical findings. For example, starvation is known to influence the weight and water content of several organs (Peters & Boyd, 1965); it induces leukopenia (Zbinden, 1963); reduces the ability of rats to concentrate urine (Bauman *et al.*, 1964); and reduces water intake. The latter may cause dehydration which affects the concentration of plasma constituents. Organ damage may be present without causing functional disturbances (Balazs & Grice, 1963) and functional disturbances may be present without histologically-detectable tissue injury; e.g., elevated serum bilirubin due to prevention of glucuronide formation (Golberg, 1959).

The increase of certain serum enzyme values does not arbitrarily reflect organ damage, since stress has been shown to increase serum glutamic-oxalacetic transaminase activity (Pearl *et al.*, 1966). In the interpretation of clinical chemical test results, the peculiarities of the species should be considered. For example, proteinuria in rats and bilirubinuria in dogs occur in normal animals. It is desirable to examine whether the compound under investigation interferes with the reaction of the clinical chemical tests.

In the interpretation of post-mortem findings, the lesions of spontaneous diseases of laboratory animals should not be mistaken for toxic effects. Though a compound may activate a latent pathologic condition, the stage of the lesion indicates whether it can be attributed to such an action. Particular attention should be given to possible local irritative effect of the compound, because this effect could induce a syndrome which might have been avoided had a different route of administration been used. In the appraisal of the clinical chemical and pathologic data, it should be considered that the possibility exists that more refined measurements will disclose hitherto undetected effects.

Several chemically-induced untoward reactions occur in man that cannot be revealed in animal experiments. It is possible to observe only physical signs in speechless animals, not symptoms. Thus headache, heartburn, tinnitus, vertigo, blurred vision, etc. cannot be detected.

Statistical Calculation

When quantal responses are measured each animal contributes only a positive or negative response to the total information. The number of positive reactions provides information for any dose level. By the use of statistical analyses, the dose level that can be expected to cause an effect in 50% of the animals under the conditions of the assay can be determined. It is also desirable to determine the

reliability of this value (e.g., standard error), which provides information on the limits of variation. An appraisal of the statistical
method of the quantal assays has been presented by Miller (1950).
The most common parameter calculated is the dose that is expected
to cause death in 50% of the animals (LD_{50}). Estimation of the LD_{50}
from the results of the range-finding experiment is often desirable,
since this may provide a yardstick for selecting doses for pharmacologic studies. A calculation based on the principle of moving
averages might be applicable to these data (Weil, 1952). Similarly,
the calculation of LD_{50} from data where the true nature of the dose-
response curve cannot be ascertained can be accomplished by this
method. Weil (1952) elaborated tables that can be used for this
calculation, provided a constant number of animals is used on each
dosage level, and the dosage levels are spaced in a geometric progression. For data of the main assay in rodents approximating
normal frequency distribution, the methods derived from the probit
analysis are most often used in calculation of the doses affecting
50% of the animals. A practical procedure for LD_{50} calculation
and estimation of its standard error is the method of Miller and
Tainter (1944). The data (between 10 to 90% effect) are plotted on
a logarithmic percentage-probability paper. If a straight line fits
the plotted points satisfactorily, the LD_{50} is represented by the
dosage value at 50% (probit 5), and is read directly from the
graph paper. The standard error is estimated by the formula: (Doses
$84\%-16\%)/\sqrt{2N}$. The doses of 84% and 16% (2 probits range)
are read from the graph. N represents the number of animals con-
tributing to the values plotted. The widely used method of Litchfield
and Wilcoxon (1949) is derived also from probit analysis. In this
method, 0 to 100% effects can be included, the heterogeneity of the
data can be recognized, and corrected confidence limits can be
given in such cases. The calculation is carried out by a system of
nomographs included in the method.

The numerous factors that have been shown to influence the result
of this assay indicate that the LD_{50} is a function of the test procedure
as well as of the toxic character of the compound. A recent report on
inter-laboratory variations in LD_{50} of four chemicals demonstrated
two- to threefold differences in the data from six laboratories (Griffith, 1964). It has been shown that even when the acute toxicity of
drugs is measured under standardized conditions, LD_{50} values vary
significantly (Allmark, 1951). Though explanations can be offered

for the variations, it appears that values obtained from a simultaneous determination of LD_{50} (with a standard compound), or LD_{50} and ED_{50} provide more reliable indices than comparison of values obtained at different times. The study of Allmark (1951) indicates that, in a comparative measurement, simultaneous administration of the compounds according to a definite procedure (pair treatment) is necessary to obtain reliable data. The standard compound chosen for a comparative study should be one within the same pharmacologic class, which provides a slope of the dose-effect curve parallel to that of the compound being investigated. Since an expression of mortality data in terms of MLD (minimum lethal dose), LD_0, or LD_{100} has no precise meaning, the LD_{50} and the standard error best describe the lethal dose level. Similarly other quantal responses (e.g., appearance of toxic signs or a gross pathologic change) can be calculated and designated as convulsive dose 50, hepatotoxic dose 50, etc. If distinct syndromes are detected, LD_{50}'s should be calculated for 24 hours as well as for delayed mortalities. Sometimes it is of interest to calculate doses other than the median, LD_1, LD_{95}, etc. which can be done by the Litchfield & Wilcoxon (1949) method.

Measurement of acute toxicity can also provide other quantitative data. The dose level that induces either some specified response or a significantly different response from the control can be determined. Statistical analysis of quantitative data usually requires the application of least squares regression methods although, in some cases, a short-cut method, such as Wilcoxon's test (1945), based on rank numbers of determining the significance of differences between groups, may be useful. This test does not assume a normal distribution of the variability, and is considered to be insensitive to a gross error of observation. Tables of probabilities are provided with the method.

Data on acute toxicity can give information also on the variability of responses of the test population. It might be reflected by the slope of the dose-effect line, which is the reciprocal of the standard deviation. A linear dose-response curve indicates a normal distribution of variability. Deviation from linearity (skewed probit plots) suggests a lack of uniformity of the tested population. Data of the quantitative responses might be more sensitive than those of quantal responses to confirm a bimodal distribution (Kalow, 1965).

In studying the acute toxicity of chemical combinations, it is of interest to determine whether their joint effect is greater or less than would be expected on the basis of their separate effects. Statistical tests are available for the evaluation of these data (Finney, 1964).

The Transfer of Data from Animals to Man

The estimation of toxic dose levels in man based on the values from an acute toxicity test in animals is also of interest. Several drugs elicit toxicologic effects of similar intensity in animals and man when the dose is calculated on a mg/kg basis. The doses of chemicals which interfere with processes related to basal metabolism are similar in animals and man when calculated on the basis of body surface.

Such a relationship was found in a quantitative comparison of acute toxicity of anticancer agents (Freirech *et al.*, 1966). Estimation of the human dose on the basis of surface area indicates a smaller toxic dose than on the basis of weight. Thus this approach is considered wise in the estimation of the toxic dose in man (Paget & Barnes, 1964).

The differences in the intensity of the toxic effect between animals and man are best compared on the basis of drug levels in the plasma (Brodie, 1966). If these levels are determined following the administration of pharmacologic or toxic doses in animals and pharmacologic doses in man, an estimation of the toxic dose in man can be made.

If the toxic syndrome is similar in various species, it is reasonable to assume a carry-over of effects to man, so far as the character of acute toxicity is concerned.

FACTORS THAT INFLUENCE ACUTE TOXICITY

A toxic effect is usually attained only when the stimulus to a significant biologic mechanism reaches a certain value. The stimulus supposedly is proportional to the quantity of agent-receptor complex formed at a certain moment, which is dependent upon the concentration of the agent at the receptor site (Ariëns and Simonis, 1964). The absorption, storage, metabolism, and elimination processes influence the effective concentration of the agent at the receptor sites. Thus the differences in the rate or intensity of these processes betweeen species, individuals, and even under various conditions contribute to the variations in toxicologic responses. Recognition of the factors that influence this variability permit a standardization of measurement, and therefore, a greater precision. The exploration of the significance of these factors in the measurement of acute toxicity of a particular compound leads to a greater accuracy of these measurements.

Species, Strain and Individual Variation

Species differences are frequently found in acute toxicity studies. Constitutional characteristics of a species, such as the inability of rodents to vomit or qualitative differences in pathways of detoxification might result in qualitative differences of toxicologic responses. The quantitative differences are largely attributed to the unequal rate of the pharmacokinetic process (particularly the metabolism of the compound) in the various species (Brodie, 1964). The species chosen for an acute toxicity study of a drug is usually one in which the desirable pharmacologic effect of the compound manifests itself. However, another species, which does not show this effect, may also be of interest, since a toxic effect due to a different metabolic pathway may also be revealed. Another consideration is the selection of the species from different orders within the mammalian class, such as a rodent (mouse or rat), a carnivore (dog or cat), and a primate. For convenience, the first choice of species is usually a rodent, and for intravenous tests, the mouse. In studies of chemicals intended for use in animals, acute toxicity is measured not only in experimental animals but also in the species in which the product will be used. However, in studies of chemicals destined for man, only experimental animals can be used. Therefore, the use of more than one species appears to be in order when one wishes to foresee effects in man from data of animal experiments.

Although various strains of laboratory animals have not been developed for toxicologic interest (e.g., dissimilarities of drug-metabolizing systems), significant differences have been detected in acute toxicity measurements when various inbred strains of mice are used comparatively (Chance, 1947; Brown, 1964). Different rates of drug metabolism in inbred rat strains have also been demonstrated (Quinn *et al.*, 1958; Siegert *et al.*, 1964). Genetically determined individual variation in the rate of drug metabolism has been observed in several species (Siegert *et al.*, 1964; Werner, 1965; Balazs & Kupfer, 1966). A toxic effect might occur only in individuals genetically deficient in an enzyme system. Examples of this phenomenon have been reviewed by Kalow (1962). Evidence has been presented that the use of inbred strains does not assure a smaller variation than the use of a random bred population (Gaddum, 1953; Balazs & Fabian, 1958). Moreover, the reactivity of a particular inbred strain for a specific drug might be at an extreme level (Brown, 1964). The advantage of using animals from a single colony lies in the chance of increasing the reproducibility of experimental data.

Sex, Age, and Weight-dependent Variation

The sex of an animal often has an influence on the acute toxicity of chemicals. Minor differences have been attributed to a lower fat-free body weight in females. Hurst (1958) reviewed some examples of sex differences and their mechanism. Major differences are shown to be under direct endocrine influence. The nephrotoxic effect of chloroform in the male mouse can be reduced by oestrogen treatment and by castration; androgen treatment in the female mouse induces susceptibility to this effect (Culliford & Hewitt, 1957). Ethionine induces fatty infiltration in the liver of the female and in castrated male rats; testosterone protects both (Farber *et al.*, 1951). A protein-sparing effect of this hormone is thought to be responsible for the protection. In other instances, the effect of sex hormones on the enzymatic biotransformation of a compound might be responsible for the sex differences. The rapid metabolic rate *in vivo* and *in vitro* (liver microsomal preparations) of hexobarbitone in male rats is lowered by a pretreatment with estradiol. The low metabolism of this drug is enhanced in females after their treatment with testosterone (Quinn *et al.*, 1958). The rate of metabolism is reflected in the sleeping time. These examples of sex differences are not evident in immature animals. It is desirable to measure acute toxicity in both male and female animals of two species.

Age-dependent variations in acute toxicity have been reviewed by Done (1964). The ratios of the LD_{50}'s in adults to those in newborn animals vary from 0·002 to more than 16, for drugs of various pharmacologic classes. There appears to be some consistency in this relationship within some pharmacologic classes; for example, a low neonatal sensitivity to CNS stimulants has been demonstrated (Setnikar & Magistretti, 1964). Several factors are responsible for the different sensitivities of newborn animals. First, the lack of drug-metabolizing enzymes should be considered. For example, in rabbits the hepatic microsomal enzyme system starts to develop about the end of the first week after birth, and reaches an appreciable level in two to three weeks (Fouts & Hart, 1965). Increased membrane permeability (e.g., of the skin and blood-brain barrier), as well as low renal and hepatic clearances have also been considered in the different toxicologic responses of neonatal animals. The transition from the newborn to the adult toxicologic response is not a smooth progression inasmuch as wide fluctuations have been noted with some drugs from one day of age to weaning (Done, 1964). Neonatal animals of various species are used as models for predictive, neonatal, human toxicity tests. In this stage of development perhaps more similarities exist between the various species than at a later stage. Alterations of drug activities have also been found in senescent animals (Man, 1965; Petty & Karler, 1965). A decreased rate of drug metabolism and excretion could be responsible for this phenomenon.

Acute toxicity tests are usually carried out in young adult animals (e.g., not less than 6–8 week-old rodents). If the compound is destined to be used in neonates, its acute toxicity is determined also in newborn animals.

A disproportionate increase in drug toxicity (in terms of dose per kilogram of body weight) in experimental animals of high body weight is not uncommon (Chance, 1947; Rona *et al.*, 1959; Pallotta *et al.*, 1962). The lethal doses of some compounds are proportional to the 2/3 power of body weight (Jacobsen & Larsen, 1951; Nyhan, 1961), which approximates the metabolically active weight. Nevertheless, for simplicity in measurement of acute toxicity, dosage is determined on the basis of body weight. However, the animals selected are usually young adults; hence they represent a characteristic weight for the species.

Environmental Factors

Several climatic factors are known to influence acute toxicity. The effect of temperature on the LD_{50} of 58 chemicals was investigated in rats housed at three different environmental temperatures, 8°, 26°, or 36°C (Keplinger *et al.*, 1959). Fifty-five compounds were most toxic at 36°C, and least toxic at 26°C. Among several climatic factors (light, temperature, relative humidity, etc.) only relative humidity influences the acute toxicity of nicotine bitartrate in rats as demonstrated by lower LD_{50}'s which are obtained when the relative humidity is higher than 80% (Selisko *et al.*, 1963). A warm, humid environment is known to enhance dermal absorption (Stoughton, 1965) as well as to affect the results in certain inhalation toxicity studies (Lehman *et al.*, 1964). Differences in altitude or barometric pressure do not appear to affect the acute toxicity of strychnine sulphate in mice (Swoap, 1955). However, the sensitivity of rats to metabolic stimulators, such as dinitrophenol or thyroid powder, increases when the oxygen tension of the inspired air is reduced (Tainter, 1934). Seasonal variation in the acute toxicity of a biguanide hypoglycemic drug in mice has been reported (Sterne & Hirsch, 1964). The light from ultraviolet lamps has been shown to elicit erythema and liver necrosis in mice dosed with 8-methoxypsoralen (Hakin *et al.*, 1961).

Diurnal variations have been detected in the acute toxicity of several compounds, e.g. methopyrapone, alcohol, and nikethamide in mice (Carlsson & Serin, 1950; Haus & Halberg, 1959; Ertel *et al.*, 1964). Rodents are more active, eat, drink, defaecate, and urinate more frequently at night than during the day. Their metabolic processes, including drug metabolism, follow this pattern, and might be responsible for the circadian (approximately 24 hours) system phase-dependent variations. Acute toxicity tests are most satisfactorily carried out in rooms with controlled temperature, humidity, and cycle of lighting.

The significance of the number of animals in a cage has been shown by the increased acute toxicity of several CNS stimulants in grouped vs individually caged mice (Greenblatt & Osterberg, 1961). It has been postulated that among other factors, the sudden crowding-induced anxiety is a critical factor in this phenomenon (Swinyard *et al.*, 1961). Prolonged isolation of the mouse has been shown to increase the toxicity of CNS agents (Consolo *et al.*, 1965). Long-term isolation of rats induces behavioural changes and sensitizes the rats to cardiotoxic effects of a catecholamine (Balazs *et al.*, 1962a).

The significance of cage construction has been shown in acute toxicity tests with respiratory depressants in rats. When, during distress, the nose is pressed against a sheet metal surface, animals suffocate, but this is avoided by housing the animals in wire-mesh cages (Winter & Flataker, 1962).

Several substances to which animals may be exposed, such as insecticides and feed additives, might stimulate drug metabolism (Hart & Fouts, 1963); therefore exposure to chemicals should be avoided in animals destined for use in acute toxicity tests.

The Feed and Feeding

The composition of the feed can affect the results of acute toxicity tests. High fat diets sensitize animals to, while high carbohydrate and high protein diets provide protection from, the hepatotoxic effects of chloroform (Goldschmidt *et al.*, 1939). High protein diets also protect against the hepatotoxicity of thoacetamide (McLean *et al.*, 1965). The effects of protein-rich diet are probably due to the presence of lipotropic factors in the protein (e.g., methionine, cysteine). Homocysteine protects the liver from the hepatotoxic effect of allyl alcohol in rats (Balazs *et al.*, 1962b).

It is of toxicologic interest that the activity of hepatic drug-metabolizing enzyme systems decreases in mice kept on a low protein diet (Lee *et al.*, 1966). Vitamin C deficiency has been shown to affect the rate of drug metabolism in guinea pigs (Axelrod, 1960).

A change from one laboratory diet to another has been shown to cause a fifteen-fold increase in the resistance of one strain of rats to thiourea (Dieke & Richter, 1945). Altered reactions were observed in acute toxicity tests in animals kept on synthetic diets (Surthin & Yagi, 1958; Boyd *et al.*, 1965). Some food ingredient might induce a toxic reaction during a drug treatment. For example, sympatho-mimetic effects due to the interaction of monoamine oxidase inhibitors and cheese of high tyramine content have been demonstrated (Natoff, 1964). These findings indicate that it is necessary to provide a standard and nutritionally adequate diet in toxicity studies. However, the study of acute toxicity in animals with some nutritional deficiency (e.g. protein) is of considerable interest.

A chemical interaction between a compound and gastro-intestinal content, as well as retarded absorption of the compound in animals fed prior to intubation, is frequently encountered in oral toxicity tests (Webster *et al.*, 1957; Worden & Harper, 1964). Therefore, to assure a more uniform absorption it is customary to withhold the feed for 16–18 hours prior to intubation. However, starvation-induced catabolic effects may also influence the results of acute toxicity. A marked depletion of the liver glycogen in rats and mice is found after 2 hours of fasting, and blood glucose levels decrease after 8 hours (Block, 1961). It has also been shown that a decrease in the activity of drug-metabolizing enzymes follows glycogen depletion (Dixon *et al.*, 1961). Since the upper gastrointestinal canal is emptied within 4 to 5 hours, withholding feed for such a period appears to be sufficient. Nevertheless for practical reasons, overnight starvation is a common practice. In this case feed is provided following intubation. Water is offered *ad libitum* prior to and following dosage.

Factors Inherent to the Administration of a Compound

The vehicle used in acute toxicity tests should be compatible with the compound, and should possess no toxicologic effects at the dose given. Though the absorption of a compound depends primarily upon its lipoid solubility, dissociation constant, and particle size, the vehicle might influence this process. For example, gastrointestinal absorption is enhanced by surface-active agents (Eickholt and White, 1960). Some vehicles facilitate penetration of a compound into the follicular canal or even through the epidermis (Barr, 1962).

A compound might be dissolved readily in water, by gentle heating, or by changing the pH of ionizable substances. Among the non-aqueous solvents, vegetable oils and polyethylene glycols are probably the most pharmacologically inert. The laxative effect of oils restricts their volume in oral intubation. Vegetable oil is suitable for the oral or intramuscular route, polyethylene glycol 300 for oral, subcutaneous, or intravenous routes. The solubility of water-insoluble compounds often increases exponentially with increasing concentrations of solvent in water. Thus, to reduce the dose, the non-aqueous solvent might be used in as high as a 30–40% concentration. The dose of such a solvent should not exceed $\frac{1}{5}$ of its LD_{50} and its intravenous administration should be very slow (not more than 1 ml/min). The compatibility of this solution with plasma should be examined *in vitro*. The toxicity of a drug dissolved in a non-aqueous solvent might be different from the toxicity of the same drug dispersed in an aqueous system.

Colloidal solutions, emulsions, and suspensions are also used in acute toxicity tests. Polysorbate 80 USP might be used to prepare a colloidal solution except for intravenous use in the dog, since it has a histamine-like effect in this species. Emulsions have been used intravenously in the dog. These consist of 15–20% vegetable oil, an emulsifying agent, such as lecithin and water or saline (Davidow and Hagan, 1955). If a compound is prepared as a suspension, micropulverization is desirable to produce uniform particles (Nash, 1965). Starch, acacia, or tragacanth and carboxymethylcellulose are used as suspending agents. (Carboxymethylcellulose given parenterally could interfere with the function of the reticuloendothelial system.) These agents are protective colloids that are adsorbed to the drug particles. The particle size of a compound exercises a critical effect on the site of deposition and absorption from the respiratory tract.

The volume of even the most inert vehicle influences the acute toxicity of a compound. The intravenous LD_{50} of distilled water in the mouse is 44 ml/kg, and that of isotonic saline is 68 ml/kg (Kampmann and Frey, 1964). Thus, the intravenous injection of 1 ml of hypotonic solution might be lethal to the mouse because of the toxicity of the vehicle. The acute oral toxicity of twelve compounds examined increased with the degree of dilution with water (Ferguson, 1962). An increase in the rate of gastric passage and intestinal absorption could be responsible for the higher toxicity of dilute solutions (Moore *et al.*, 1960). However, if the local irritating property of a compound is responsible for high toxicity, this could be reduced in dilute solutions.

The volume of material administered orally should not exceed 2–3% of the body weight, and the volume of rapid intravenous injections should be limited to 0·1–0·5 ml for rodents, and 2 ml for larger laboratory animals. If larger volumes are to be given subcutaneously or intramuscularly, the total dose should be divided and injected in several sites to facilitate absorption of the material. An overwhelming volume should be avoided even in intravenous infusions in toxicity studies because excessive hydration can alter the renal clearance of the compound.

For parenteral administration, the osmolarity and pH of a solution should also be considered. Distilled water, 1 ml/kg, intravenously injected into rats, induces bradycardia and hypotension (Carlini and Jurkiewicz, 1966). The intravenous acute toxicity of tetracyclines is higher in hypotonic solutions than in isotonic saline (Maffi *et al.*, 1957). Since slightly hypertonic solutions are tolerated better than hypotonic solutions in intramuscular and subcutaneous injections, the use of isotonic saline diluent is desirable for these routes. For most parenteral routes a pH range of 5–8 is satisfactory, provided the solution has no significant buffer capacity (Woodard, 1965). For intravenous injections, a wide range of pH is suitable if the rate of injection is slow. Oral administration of solutions with a low pH is tolerated if the titratable acidity does not exceed the equivalent of 0·1 N HCl (Woodard, 1965). Extreme changes from physiological osmolarity and pH might induce severe local or systemic reactions.

Compounds may be administered in dry form orally (in capsules). Absorption is usually slower in this form than in solution. The feed has served as a vehicle in a species that is difficult to intubate, or under special circumstances (e.g., when the toxicity of biocides in farm animals is examined). However, it must be determined that the compound does not change in the presence of moisture and feed constituents and it must be consumed in a short period (less than an hour). In the acute toxicity test of pharmaceuticals, it is desirable to use the same vehicle as will be used in the final product.

Route and Rate of Administration

Generally, toxicity is greatest by the route that carries the compound to the bloodstream most rapidly. However, a compound could be more toxic orally than parenterally if an active product is formed in the gastrointestinal tract. The gastrointestinal absorption of a drug is most variable. The difference between oral and parenteral LD_{50}'s gives some indication as to the extent of absorption of a compound. Although the route of administration in acute toxicity tests depends upon the eventual use of a compound, measurement of acute toxicity by intravenous administration in at least one species is always desirable. Often the toxicity best manifests itself by this route. Intraperitoneal injection, a common practice in the mouse and rat, may induce a specific shock reaction as manifested by decreased body temperature (Gloxhuber, 1964). Since the peritoneum is sensitive to irritants, other routes should be explored before selecting this route of administration.

The site of injection might influence the effect of a compound. Subcutaneous injection on the dorsal or ventral sites produces different LD_{50}'s of strychnine sulphate (Balazs, 1957—unpublished data), and of ammonium chloride in mice (Lallouette *et al.*, 1960). Variations in mortality rates due to the administration of drugs into different veins have been reported (Craver *et al.*, 1950). Regional variations have been found in dermal absorption (Stoughton, 1965). Thus the site of administration should be constant in an assay.

The intravenous toxic dose is greatly influenced by the rate of injection. A slow rate of infusion might equilibrate with the rate of detoxification of the compound and not induce a toxic response. The rate of disposal of a rapidly acting compound might be estimated on this basis (Cahill *et al.*, 1965). A rapid rate of infusion might also give misleading results; for example, the lethal dose of dihydroouabain in the guinea pig is 5 mg/kg at the rate of infusion of 1 mg/kg/min and about 30 mg/kg at 10 mg/kg/min. At the higher rate, more of the glycoside is infused than could be effective (Bach and Reither, 1964). Similar paradoxical results are obtained in rapid infusions of high concentrations of pentylenetetrazol and sodium cyanide in mice (Richter, 1958). This problem should be kept in mind, especially when the estimation of the intravenous lethal dose is attempted in dogs or in cats using only a few animals.

Changes in the Internal Environment

Several physiologic or pathophysiologic conditions have been found to influence acute toxicologic effects. Physical activity increases the sensitivity to cholinesterase inhibitors in the rats (Punte *et al.*, 1958). The acute toxicity of a catecholamine increases in stressed and in obese rats (Balazs *et al.*, 1962a, c). Drug toxicity is often influenced by the hormonal state of the animal. It has been stated that toxicity generally increases in a hyperthyroid state (Zbinden, 1963). Stimulation of the pituitary adrenal axis increases the activity of drug-metabolizing enzymes (Bousquet *et al.*, 1965) which are depressed in alloxan-diabetic rats (Dixon *et al.*, 1961).

Since fever increases renal and hepatic blood flow, removal of drugs that are dependent upon renal blood flow for excretion might be enhanced in this condition (Rantz *et al.*, 1944). Gastrointestinal diseases (achlorhydria, increased motility, etc.) can influence absorption (Smyth, 1964). Hydration, hyperaemia, or abrasion of the skin greatly enhances dermal absorption (Stoughton, 1965).

Degenerative changes in the metabolic and excretory organs delay drug metabolism and excretion and influence drug toxicity (Kunin, 1964; Gibson & Becker, 1966). Inflamed tissue might modify drug distribution (Heathcote & Nassau, 1951) as does a slight change in the pH of body fluids. Changing the pH of renal tubular fluid may alter the renal excretion rate by changing tubular reabsorption of the compound (Peters, 1963).

Changes in metabolism or body composition during pregnancy (King & Becker, 1963) and lactation, as well as following major surgery, could influence toxicologic responses.

The normal bacterial flora might play a role in acute toxicity tests when a facultative pathogenic microbe becomes activated by the decreased resistance of the host due to glucocorticoids or nitrogen mustard (White & Claflin, 1963; Tonelli, 1966).

Alteration of drug toxicity induced by a compound given prior to the one under investigation is of great importance. As has been mentioned previously, a compound may induce an increased synthesis of liver microsomal enzymes and influence the metabolism of another. The effect of drug-induced enzyme induction on the acute toxicity of drugs in the rat has been demonstrated (Burns *et al.*, 1965). Inhibition of drug metabolism, displacement of protein binding of a drug, or inhibition of its renal clearance can also be accomplished by chemicals. Any one of these greatly enhances drug toxicity.

Acute toxicity tests should be carried out in healthy animals. However, it is also desirable to evaluate acute toxicity in animals prepared by various procedures that result in a predictable functional change. The significance of this change on the toxicity of a compound may be a valuable addition to the data of acute toxicity. Similarly, the simultaneous administration of several drugs in therapy indicates that it is necessary to measure acute toxicity in animals treated with drugs that are often given concomitantly to patients. The measurement of acute toxicity of drug combinations is a common practice.

CONCLUSION

Measurement of the LD_{50} alone is no substitute for acute toxicity studies since the assessment of the toxic syndrome is of importance.

The multitude of factors influencing the data of an acute toxicity test makes it imperative that experimental conditions be specified in detail when reporting results. When acute toxicities of various compounds are to be compared, or factors affecting acute toxicities are to be explored, the measurements should be made under identical conditions.

One should be cautious in drawing general conclusions solely from the data of acute toxicity tests. Though these tests reveal toxic effects that interfere with the vital functions within the period of observation, it should always be expected that some toxic effect remains undetected because of limitations of examinations and the numerous factors that influence the results. The measurement of acute toxicity represents only a small portion of the safety evaluation of chemicals.

REFERENCES

ALLMARK M.G. (1951) A collaborative study on the acute toxicity testing of several drugs. *J. Am. Pharm. Ass.* **40**, 27–31.

ARIËNS A.J. & SIMONIS A.M. (1964) A molecular basis for drug action. *J. Pharm. Pharmac.* **16**, 137–57.

AXELROD J. (1960) Biochemical factors in the activation and inactivation of drugs. *Naunyn-Schmiedebergs Arch. exp. Path. Pharmak.* **238**, 26–35.

BACH E.J. & REITER M. (1964) The difference in velocity between the lethal and inotropic action of dihydrodigoxin. *Naunyn-Schmiedebergs Arch. exp. Path. Pharmak.* **248**, 437–49.

BALAZS T. & FABIAN GY. (1958) Laboratoriumi allatok genetikai ellenorzesenek alapelveirol hazai egertorzsek vizsgalataval kapcsolatban. *Kisérl. Orvostud.* **10**, 510–17.

BALAZS T., MURRAY T.K., MCLAUGHLAN J.M. & GRICE H.C. (1961) Hepatic tests in toxicity studies on rats. *Toxic. appl. Pharmac.* **3**, 71–9.

BALAZS T., MURPHY J.B. & GRICE H.C. (1962a) The influence of environmental changes on the cardiotoxicity of isoprenaline in rats. *J. Pharm. Pharmac.* **14**, 750–75.

BALAZS T., AIRTH J.M. & GRICE H.C. (1962b) The use of the serum glutamic pyruvic transaminase test for the evaluation of hepatic necrotropic compounds in rats. *Can. J. Biochem. Physiol.* **40**, 1–6.

BALAZS T., SAHASRABUDHE M.R. & GRICE H.C. (1962c) The influence of excess body fat on the cardiotoxicity of isoproterenol in rats. *Toxic. appl.. Pharmac.* **4**, 613–20.

BALAZS T. & GRICE H.C. (1963) The relationship between liver necrosis and pentobarbital sleeping time in rats. *Toxic. appl. Pharmac.* **5**, 387–91.

BALAZS T., HATCH A., ZAWIDZKA Z. & GRICE H.C. (1963) Renal tests in toxicity studies on rats. *Toxic. appl. Pharmac.* **5,** 661–74.

BALAZS T. & KUPFER D. (1966) Adrenocortical function test: Estimation of cortisol production rate in the guinea pig. *Toxic. appl. Pharmac.* **8,** 152–8.

BARNES J.M. (1968) Percutaneous toxicity, in *Modern Trends in Toxicology,* eds BOYLAND E. & GOULDING R. London, Butterworths.

BARR M. (1962). Percutaneous absorption. *J. Pharm. Sci.* **51,** 395–409.

BAUMAN J.W., GUYOT-JEANNIN C.A. & DOBROWOLSKI J. (1964) Nutritional state and urine concentrating ability in the rat. *J. Endocr.* **30,** 147–8.

BLOCK B.P. (1961) The effect of fasting, cold stress and ACTH administration on the blood sugar and liver glycogen levels of normal and adrenalecto-mised rats and mice. *J. Pharm. Pharmac.* **13,** 479–84.

BOUSQUET W.F., RUPE B.D. & MIYA T.S. (1965). Endocrine modification of drug responses in the rat. *J. Pharmac. exp. Ther.* **147,** 376–9.

BOYD E.M. (1959) The acute oral toxicity of acetyl salicylic acid. *Toxic. appl. Pharmac.* **1,** 229–39.

BOYD E.M., MULROONEY D.A., PITMAN C.A. & ABEL M. (1965) Benzyl peni-cillin toxicity in animals on a synthetic high sucrose diet. *Can. J. Physiol. Pharmac.* **43,** 47–54.

BOYD E.M. (1968) Predictive drug toxicity: Assessment of drug safety before human use. *Can. Med. Ass. J.* **98,** 278–93.

BRODIE B.B. (1964) Distribution and fate of drugs; therapeutic implications, in *Absorption and Distribution of Drugs,* ed BINNS T.B., pp. 199–251. Baltimore, Williams & Wilkins Co.

BRODIE B.B. (1966) The mechanism of adverse reactions, in *Mechanism of Drug Toxicity,* ed. RASKOVA H., Vol. 4, pp. 23–46. Proceedings of the LD_{50}'s from different laboratories comparable. *A.M.A. Arch. ind. Hyg.* Pergamon Press.

BROWN A.M. (1964) Strain and sex differences in response to drugs, in *Evaluation of Drug Activities: Pharmacometrics,* eds. LAURENCE D.R. & BACHARACH A.L., pp. 111–23. London & New York, Academic Press.

BURNS J.J., CUCINEL S.A., KOSTER R. & CONNEY A.H. (1965) Application of drug metabolism to drug toxicity studies. *Ann. N.Y. Acad. Sci.* **123,** 273–86.

CAHILL J.F., ALDOUS J.G. & WENNING A.S. (1965) The relation between acute toxicity and critical rate of disposal of several local anesthetics. *Can. J. Physiol. Pharmac.* **43,** 343–9.

CAMPBELL P.E.S. & RICHTER W. (1967) An observation method estimating toxicity and drug actions in mice applied to 68 reference drugs. *Acta Pharmac. Toxic.* **25,** 345–63.

CARLINI E.A. & JURKIEWICZ A. (1966) Hypotensive response to intravenous injection of distilled water in the rat. *Arch. int. Pharmacodyn.* **159,** 317–26.

CARLSSON A. & SERIN F. (1950) The toxicity of nikethamide at different times of the day. *Acta Pharmac. Toxic.* **6,** 187–93.

CHANCE M.R.A. (1947) Factors influencing the toxicity of sympathomimetic amines to solitary mice. *J. Pharmac. exp. Ther.* **89,** 289–96.

CONSOLO S., GARATTINI S. & VALZELLI L. (1965) Sensitivity of aggressive mice to centrally acting drugs. *J. Pharm. Pharmac.* **17**, 594.

CRAVER B.N., BARRETT W.A. & EARL A.E. (1950) Some requisites to making LD$_{50}$'s from different laboratories comparable. *A.M.A. Arch. ind. Hyg. Occup. Med.* **2**, 280–3.

CULLIFORD D. & HEWITT H.B. (1957) The influence of sex hormone status on the susceptibility of mice to chloroform-induced necrosis of the renal tubules. *J. Endocr.* **14**, 381–93.

DAVIDOW B. & HAGAN E.C. (1955) 'Acute toxicity', in Procedures for the Appraisal of the Toxicity of Chemicals in Foods, Drugs and Cosmetics. *Fd Drug Cosmetic Law J.* 685–94.

DIEKE S.H. & RICHTER C.P. (1945) Acute toxicity of thiourea to rats in relation to age, diet, strain and species variation. *J. Pharmac. exp. Ther.* **83**, 195–202.

DIXON R.L., HART L.G. & FOUTS J.R. (1961) The metabolism of drugs by liver microsomes from alloxan-diabetic rats. *J. Pharmac. exp. Ther.* **133**, 7–11.

DONE A.K. (1964) Developmental pharmacology. *Clin. Pharmac. Ther.* **5**, 432–79.

DRAIZE J.H. (1955) 'Dermal toxicity', in Procedures for the Appraisal of the Toxicity of Chemicals in Foods, Drugs and Cosmetics. *Fd Drug Cosmetic Law J.* 722–32.

EICKHOLT T.H. & WHITE W.F. (1960) The toxicity and absorption enhancing ability of surfactants. *Drug Stand.* **28**, 154–61.

ERTEL R.J., HALBERG F. & UNGAR F. (1964) Circadian system phase-dependent toxicity and other effects of methopyrapone (Su 4885) in the mouse. *J. Pharmac. exp. Ther.* **146**, 395–9.

FARBER E., KOCH-WESER D. & POPPER H. (1951) The influence of sex and of testosterone upon fatty liver due to ethionine. *Endocrinology* **48**, 205–12.

FERGUSON H.C. (1962) Dilution of dose and acute oral toxicity. *Toxic. appl. Pharmac.* **4**, 759–62.

FINNEY D.J. (1964) *Statistical Method in Biological Assay*, 2nd Edition. New York, Hafner Publishing Co.

FOUTS J.R. & HART L.G. (1965) Hepatic drug metabolism during the perinatal period. *Ann. N.Y. Acad. Sci.* **123**, 245–51.

FRASER D.A., BALES R.E., LIPPMAN M. & STOKINGER H.E. (1959) *Exposure chambers for research in animal inhalation.* Public Health Monograph No. 57. Superintendent of Documents, U.S. Government Printing Office, Washington 25, D.C.

FREIREICH E.J., GEHAN E.A., RALL D.P., SCHMIDT L.H. & SKIPPER H.E. (1966) Quantitative comparison of toxicity of anticancer agents in mouse, rat, hamster, dog, monkey and man. *Cancer Chemotherap. Report* **50**, 219–44.

GADDUM J.H. (1953) Bioassay and mathematics. *Pharmac. Rev.* **5**, 87–134.

GIBSON J.E. and BECKER B.A. (1966) Acute lethality of cardiac glycosides in anuric and cholestatic mice. *Fed. Proc.* **25**, 555.

GLOXHUBER CHR. (1964) Körpertemperatursenkung als Folge intraperitonealer Injektionen bei Ratten. *Naunyn-Schmiedebergs Arch. exp. Path. Pharmak.* **246**, 88–9.

GOLBERG L. (1959) Discussion, in *Quantitative Methods in Human Pharmacology and Therapeutics,* ed. LAURENCE D.R., p. 197. New York, Pergamon Press.

GOLDSCHMIDT S., VARS H.M. & RAVDIN I.S. (1939) Influence of the foodstuffs upon the susceptibility of the liver to injury by chloroform, and the probable mechanism of their action. *J. Clin. Invest.* **18**, 277–89.

GRIFFITH J.F. (1964) Interlaboratory variations in the determination of acute oral LD$_{50}$. *Toxic. appl. Pharmac.* **6**, 726–30.

GREENBLATT E.N. & OSTERBERG A.C. (1961) Correlations of activating and lethal effects of excitatory drugs in grouped and isolated mice. *J. Pharmac. exp. Ther.* **131**, 117–19.

HAKIN K.E., FREEMAN R.G., GRIFFIN A.G. & KNOX J.M. (1961) Experimental toxicologic studies on 8-methoxypsoralen in animals exposed to the long ultraviolet. *J. Pharmac. exp. Ther.* **131**, 394–9.

HART L.G. & FOUTS J.R. (1963) Effects of acute and chronic DDT administration on hepatic microsomal drug metabolism in the rat. *Proc. Soc. exp. Biol. Med.* **114**, 388–92.

HAUS E. & HALBERG F. (1959) 24-Hour rhythm in susceptibility of C mice to a toxic dose of ethanol. *J. appl. Physiol.* **14**, 878–80.

HEATHCOTE A.G.S. & NASSAU E. (1951) Concentration of penicillin in the lungs. Effects of two penicillin esters in chronic pulmonary infections. *The Lancet* **i**, 1255–7.

HURST E.W. (1958) Sexual differences in the toxicity and therapeutic action of chemical substances, in *The Evaluation of Drug toxicity,* eds. WALPOLE A.L. & SPINKS A., pp. 12–22. Boston, Little, Brown & Co.

JACOBSEN E. & LARSEN V. (1951) Experiences with the bioassay of digitalis on guinea pigs. *Acta Pharmac. Toxic.* **7**, 35–50.

KALOW W. (1962) Pharmacogenetics. *Heredity and the Response to Drugs.* Philadelphia, W.B. Saunders Co.

KALOW W. (1965) Dose-response relationships and genetic variation. *Ann. N.Y. Acad. Sci.* **123**, 212–18.

KAMPMANN E. & FREY H.H. (1964) Von kleinen Laboratoriumstieren bei intravenöser Zufuhr tolerierte Flüssigheitsmengen und Einfluss des Injektions volumens auf enige Arzneimittelwirkungen. *Naunyn-Schmiedebergs Arch exp. Path. Pharmak.* **246**, 89–90.

KANIG J.L. (1963) Pharmaceutical aerosols. *J. Pharm. Sci.* **52**, 513–33.

KEPLINGER M.L., LANIER G.E. & DEICHMANN W.B. (1959) Effects of environmental temperature on the acute toxicity of a number of compounds in rats. *Toxic. appl. Pharmac.* **1**, 156–61.

KING J.E. & BECKER R.F. (1963) Sex differences in the response of rats to pentobarbital sodium. I. Males, nonpregnant females, and pregnant females. *Am. J. Obstet. Gynec.* **86**, 856–74.

KUNIN C.M. (1964) Pharmacology of the antimicrobials. *Mod. Treat.* **1**, 829–848.

LALLOUETTE P., BOURDERON G. & GEGUIN J.C. (1960) Experimental factors influencing acute poisoning with ammonium chloride in mice. *Compt. Rend.* **251**, 288–9.

LEE N.H., HOSPADOR M. & MANTHEI R.W. (1966) Hexobarbital metabolism in mice on a low protein diet. *Fed. Proc.* **25**, 531.

LEHMAN A.J., FASSETT D.W., GERARDE H.W., STOKINGER H.E. & ZAPP J.W. (1964) Principles and procedures for evaluating the toxicity of household substances. Publication 1138. National Academy of Sciences, National Research Council, Washington, D.C.

LITCHFIELD J.T. & WILCOXON F. (1949) A simplified method of evaluating dose-effect experiments. *J. Pharmac. exp. Ther.* **96**, 99–113.

MAFFII G., SEMENZA F. & SONCIN E. (1957) Saline solution as a factor affecting the toxicity of intravenously injected tetracyclines in mice. *J. Pharm. Pharmac.* **9**, 105–12.

MANN D. E. (1965). Biological aging and its modification of drug activity. *J. Pharm. Sci.* **54**, 499–510.

MCLAUGHLIN J., MARLIAC J.P., VERRETT M.J., MUTCHLER M.K. & FITZHUGH O.G. (1963) The injection of chemicals into the yolk sac of fertile eggs prior to incubation as a toxicity test. *Toxic. appl. Pharmac.* **5**, 760–71.

MCLEAN A.E.M., MCLEAN E. & JUDAH J.D. (1965) Cellular necrosis in the liver induced and modified by drugs, in *International Review of Experimental Pathology,* eds. RICHTER G.W. & EPSTEIN M.A., pp. 127–52. New York & London, Academic Press.

MILLER L.C. (1950) Biological assays involving quantal responses. *Ann. N.Y. Acad. Sci.* **52**, 903–19.

MILLER L.C. & TAINTER M.L. (1944) Estimation of the ED$_{50}$ and its error by means of logarithmic-probit graph paper. *Proc. Soc. exp. Biol. Med.* **57**, 261–4.

MOORE P.F., YIM G.K.W. & MIYA T.A. (1960) Effect of concentration on oral toxicity of drugs. *Fed. Proc.* **19**, 390.

MORELAND A.F. (1965) Collection and withdrawal of body fluids and infusion techniques, in *Methods of Animal Experimentation,* ed. GAY W.I., pp. 1–40. New York & London, Academic Press.

NASH R.A. (1965) The pharmaceutical suspension. *Drug Cosmetic Ind.* **97**, 843–951.

NATOFF I. L. (1964) Toxic manifestations of foodstuffs during drug therapy. *Proc. Eur. Soc. for the Study of Drug Toxicity* **4**, 158–66 (International Congress Series No. 81). Excerpta Medica Foundation, Amsterdam.

NYHAN W.L. (1961) Toxicity of drugs in the neonatal period. *J. Pediat.* **59**, 1–20.

PAGET G.E. & BARNES J.M. (1964) Toxicity Tests, in *Evaluation of Drug Activities: Pharmacometrics,* eds. LAURENCE D.R. & BACHARACH A.L., pp. 135–66. London & New York, Academic Press.

PALLOTTA A.J., KELLY M.G., RALL D.P. & WARD J.W. (1962) Toxicology of acetoxycycloheximide as a function of sex and body weight. *J. Pharmac. exp. Ther.* **136**, 400–5.

PEARL W., BALAZS T. & BUYSKE D.A. (1966) The effect of stress on serum transaminase activity in the rat. *Life Sci.* **5**, 67–74.

PETERS J.M. & BOYD E.M. (1965) Organ weights and water levels in albino rats following fortnight starvation. *Toxic. appl. Pharmac.* **7**, 33.

PETERS L. (1963) Urinary excretion of drugs, in *Proceedings of the First International Pharmacological Meeting 10,* ed. LINDGREN P., pp. 137. New York, MacMillan Company.

PETTY W.C. & KARLER R. (1965) The influence of aging on the activity of anticonvulsant drugs. *J. Pharmac. exp. Ther.* **150**, 443–7.

PUNTE C.L., OWENS E.J., KRACKOW E.H. & COOPER P.L. (1958) Influence of physical activity on the toxicity of aerosols and vapors. *A.M.A. Arch. ind. Hlth* **17**, 34–7.

QUINN G.P., AXELROD J. & BRODIE B.B. (1958) Species strain and sex differences in metabolism of hexobarbitone, amidopyrine, antipyrine and aniline. *Biochem. Pharmac.* **1**, 152–9.

RANTZ L.A., KIRBY W.M.M. & RANDALL E. (1944) The absorption and excretion of penicillin following continuous intravenous and subcutaneous administration. *J. clin. Invest.* **23**, 789–94.

RICHTER A.W. (1958) Estimation of the i.v. mean lethal dose for mice by a constant infusion titration. *Acta Pharmac. Toxic.* **15**, 37–42.

RONA G., CHAPPEL C.I., BALAZS T. & GAUDRY R. (1959) The effect of breed, age, and sex on myocardial necrosis produced by isoproterenol in the rat. *J. Geront.* **14**, 164–73.

SELISKO O., HENTSCHEL G. & ACKERMANN H. (1963) Uber die Abhangigkeit der Mittleren Todlichen Dosis (LD$_{50}$) von exogenen Factoren. *Arch. int. Pharmacodyn.* **145**, 51–69.

SETNIKAR I. & MAGISTRETTI M.J. (1964) The toxicity of central nervous system stimulants in rats of different ages. *Proc. Eur. Soc. for the Study of Drug Toxicity,* **4**, 132–8 (International Congress Series No. 81). Excerpta Medica Foundation, Amsterdam.

SIEGERT M., ALSLEBEN B., LIEBENSCHÜTZ W. & REMMER H. (1964) Unterschiede in der mikrosomalen oxydation und acetylierung von Arzneimitteln bei verschiedenen Arten und Rassen. *Naunyn-Schmiedebergs Arch exp. Path. Pharmak.* **247**, 509–21.

SILVER S.D. (1946) Constant flow gassing chambers: Principles influencing design and operation. *J. Lab. clin. Med.* **31**, 1153–61.

SMYTH D.H. (1964) Alimentary absorption of drugs: Physiological considerations, in *Absorption and Distribution of Drugs,* ed. BINNS T.B., pp. 1–15. Baltimore, Williams & Wilkens Co.

SPIEGL C.J., LEACH L.J., LAUTERBACK K.E., WILSON R. & LASKIN S. (1953) Small chamber for studying test atmospheres. *A.M.A. Arch ind. Hyg.* **8**, 286–8.

STERNE J. & HIRSCH C. (1964) Seasonal variations in the toxicity of a synthetic hypoglycaemic drug. *Proc. Eur. Soc. for the Study of Drug Toxicity* **4**, 83–5 (International Congress Series No. 81). Excerpta Medica Foundation, Amsterdam.

STOUGHTON R.B. (1965) Physiology of normal skin: Factors influencing percutaneous absorption, in *The Evaluation of Therapeutic Agents and Cosmetics*, eds. STERNBERG T.H. & NEWCOMER V.D., pp. 25–32. New York, McGraw-Hill Book Company.

SURTHIN A. & YAGI K. (1958) Distribution in renal cell fractions of sulfhydryl groups in rats on normal and sucrose diets and its relation to renal mercury distribution after mercuric chloride injection. *Am. J. Physiol.* **192**, 405–9.

SWINYARD E.A., CLARK L.D., MILYAHARA J.T. & WOLF H.H. (1961) Studies on the mechanism of amphetamine toxicity in aggregated mice *J. Pharmac. exp. Ther.* **132**, 97–102.

SWOAP O.F. (1955) A collaborative study on the use of mice in acute toxicity testing. *J. Pharm. Sci.* **44**, 11–16.

TAINTER M.L. (1934) Low oxygen tensions and temperatures on the actions and toxicity of dinitrophenol. *J. Pharmac. exp. Ther.* **51**, 45–58.

TONELLI G. (1966) Acute toxicity of corticosteroids in the rat. *Toxic. appl. Pharmac.* **8**, 250–8.

WEBSTER S.H., RICE M.E., HIGHMAM G. & VON OETTINGEN W.F. (1957) The toxicology of potassium and sodium iodates: Acute toxicity in mice. *J. Pharmac. exp. Ther.* **120**, 171–8.

WESTON R.E. & KAREL L. (1946) An application of the dosimetric method for biologically assaying inhaled particles. *J. Pharmac. exp. Ther.* **88**, 195–207.

WEIL C.S. (1952) Tables for convenient calculation of median effective dose (LD_{50} or ED_{50}) and instructions in their use. *Biometrics* **8**, 249–63.

WERNER G. (1965) Fermentdefekte als Ursache unterschiedlicher mydriatischer Wirksamkeit von Atropin und Cocain bei Kaninchen. *Naunyn-Schmiedebergs Arch. exp. Path. Pharmak.* **251**, 320–334.

WHITE L.P. & CLAFLIN E.F. (1963) Nitrogen mustard: Diminution of toxicity in axenic mice. *Science* **140**, 1400–1.

WILCOXON F. (1945) Individual comparisons by ranking methods. *Biometrics* **1**, 80–83.

WINTER C.A. & FLATAKER L. (1962) Cage design as a factor influencing acute toxicity of respiratory depressant drugs in rats. *Toxic. appl. Pharmac.* **4**, 650–5.

WOODARD G. (1965) Principles in drug administration, in *Methods of Animal Experimentation*, ed. GAY W.I., pp. 343–59. New York, Academic Press.

WORDEN A.N. & HARPER K.H. (1964). Oral toxicity as influenced by method of administration. *Proc. Eur. Soc. for the Study of Drug Toxicity* **4**, 107–9 (International Congress Series No. 81). Excerpta Medica Foundation, Amsterdam.

ZBINDEN G. (1963) Experimental and clinical aspects of drug toxicity, in *Advances in Pharmacology*, eds. GARATTINI S. & SHORE P.A., pp. 1–112. New York, Academic Press.

CHAPTER 4

Measurement of Chronic Toxicity

K.-F. BENITZ*

INTRODUCTION

The results of chronic toxicity experiments together with other information derived from acute toxicity studies, pharmacokinetics, teratogenesis, local irritation, perinatal toxicity, etc. form the basis for the evaluation of the possible hazardous properties of a new drug as well as its safety. There are still many discussions and questions with respect to the validity of long-term animal studies and their predictive value for the clinic. An outline primarily concerned with practical approaches for the determination of toxic effects cannot provide an analysis of these problems. The results from laboratory efficacy studies indicative of desirable and therapeutically useful effects have always been accepted, and, therefore, I postulate that similar procedures be accepted for the detection of the undesirable effects that any given chemical may cause in laboratory animals during and after prolonged administration.

One of the main objectives of long-term toxicity studies is to find toxicity: in other words, to determine the undesirable, harmful effects of a given substance. If such effects are absent, the entire study has failed. Therefore, high enough dose levels must be employed to produce toxicity in a reasonable time. The only exceptions to this general principle are carcinogens that, since they must be given for a long period of time to produce their characteristic effect, cannot be given in doses that damage the health of the animal in shorter periods.

* The author is grateful for the editorial assistance rendered by Mrs Doris H. Lennon.

The determination of a safe dose level is another important objective and is needed to determine the margin of safety of a given compound. In addition, subtoxic dose levels may be necessary for successful teratology experiments since toxic dose levels may have a deleterious influence on reproduction and such a study can only be regarded as a fertility experiment. To study malformations, one has to obtain embryos and newborn animals. Also for other experiments, such as enzyme induction studies and multiple dose pharmacokinetic studies, non-toxic dose levels should be used.

The results of toxicity studies provide indications of the undesirable drug effects one should look for in man during the various phases of the clinical trials and also later when a marketed drug is used (and occasionally abused) by the medical profession. These data can serve as guidelines for the clinician as to what signs or changes indicative of toxic drug effects should be sought by laboratory procedures. Furthermore, they allow an estimation of the safety margin on the basis of the ratio of the maximum tolerated dose to the therapeutic dose determined during the pharmacological evaluation. All this information will help the clinical investigator to conduct meaningful clinical trials in man with a minimum of risk. However differences in species, strains, sex, and environmental conditions are some of the factors responsible for the limitations of interpreting toxic manifestations especially with respect to the transfer from animals to man (Rümke, 1964).

In the light of the results obtained with modern refined research methods, the old concept of a 'no-effect' dose is no longer tenable. When anti-infectious agents are studied, the drug-induced effects can be classified in the manner proposed by Dessau and Sullivan (1961). These authors used three categories to classify chlortetracycline-induced morphological changes; namely, toxic, indifferent, and beneficial. The classification proposed by Abrams *et al.* (1965), who advocated distinction between specific and nonspecific toxic manifestations, may also have its limitations. Generally speaking, the mammalian body has a limited number of biological responses, and it is unlikely that a new chemical substance will elicit a completely new type of response (Hoff, 1956). It may be helpful to distinguish between exaggerated therapeutic effects and toxic manifestations that are unrelated to the desirable actions of a drug candidate. Finally, a careful differentiation of all direct or indirect drug effects should be made and put in proper perspective taking other factors into account such as those listed by Abrams *et al.* (1965): the nature of the toxic effect, the dose at which such an effect was encountered, the mechanism of toxogenesis, species differences, and the therapeutic potential of the new compound. Biochemical, physiological, or morphological phenomena related to detoxification or adaptation mechanism should not be classified as 'toxic effects', but their presence indicates that the dose employed was not a 'no-effect' dose level.

It may be presumptuous to present an outline on how to carry out chronic toxicity studies at this time. Also, it may be inappropriate in view of the rapid advances made in recent years. However, as a result of my own activities in this field and my evaluation of toxicity studies from other commercial laboratories and academic institutions, the need to observe certain ground rules to ensure the effectiveness and significance of a safety evaluation programme became obvious. Many of the rules have been violated in the past, and it may be appropriate at this time to summarize some general principles and approaches in safety evaluation without giving undue consideration to details in methodology. Such a practical outline may be of value for the design, execution, and evaluation of toxicity studies and help to fill the rather substantial gap between the postulates that have been made and the actual work that has been carried out in this field.

EXPERIMENTAL DESIGN

General

The safety evaluation of drugs cannot be standardized. Since the experiments are time-consuming, costly, and not easily repeated, careful planning is required. The design, execution, and interpretation of results of a safety evaluation programme should be left to experienced investigators as a joint function of various disciplines in laboratory research. The personnel requirements necessary to conduct these toxicity experiments have been outlined by Beyer (1966) and Peck (1966). The experimental designs are governed by various factors: chemical properties of the compound, its pharmacological activity, and the intended therapeutic use in man. Also, government regulations may exert some influence, and realistic compromises with respect to regulatory demands and commercial interest are necessary to satisfy theoretical, practical, ethical, and legal aspects pertinent to this phase of drug development.

All toxicity studies should be designed to meet the requirements of the initial pharmacological and therapeutic evaluation in the clinic, support more extensive clinical trials, and ultimately permit the commercialization of the new drug candidate.

Experiments with drug combinations are sometimes complicated by drug interactions as shown by Schrogie (1968) and changes in the experimental design are necessary to obtain meaningful information with respect to these interactions and their proper interpretations. All drug combinations should be considered as new therapeutic entities and unless sufficient background data and experience are available on the individual components, each should be studied in comparison with the combination.

On occasion, I have been asked why safety evaluation studies are carried out in normal, so-called healthy animals and not in laboratory species carrying appropriate model diseases. At the present time, I feel that the introduction of such a variable is not warranted. Mayer (1963) has shown the relationship between stimulus, response, and reactivity for pharmacology, toxicology, and pathology. The reactivity of the test animal is defined by the potentially toxic stimulus and the ensuing response. The introduction of a third variable, a second stimulus, either by chemical, surgical, nutritional, genetic, or microbiological factors would definitely disturb the stimulus-reactivity-response triad and may unnecessarily complicate the final interpretation of the toxicity study. These pathological states may modify not only the efficacy but also the toxicity of drugs. Therefore the use of animals with induced model diseases of any kind cannot be generally recommended for toxicity studies. Although the methodology for producing and standardizing model diseases in laboratory animals has made remarkable advances, studies using such animals have to be limited to the area of mechanism of toxicity, usually the next step after the conventional experiments have been concluded.

Choice of Species

Woodard (1965) has summarized some of the factors that govern the selection of animal species to be used for chronic toxicity studies. The most important in this respect are: (i) standardization of species and strain; (ii) experience in terms of past years in other laboratories and by other investigators; (iii) the biochemical or anatomical characteristics of a given animal species in relation to the objectives of the study; and (iv) the presence or absence of physiological response systems similar to those in man.

Certainly the ease of handling, housing, and maintaining laboratory animals under standardized environmental conditions are important factors in the selection of species. However, the most practical considerations when selecting strains are that the stock is healthy and the information on the incidence of spontaneously occurring diseases including tumours is available. As discussed by Barnes and Denz (1954) the use of inbred strains does not offer any advantage with respect to uniformity of response. Wild animals, captured and used for toxicity experiments, pose a special problem in this respect since their genetic background and environmental conditions prior to capture are unknown.

The use of germ-free animals for toxicity studies has been rejected by most laboratories on the basis that in safety evaluation experiments these animals represent a considerable departure from the conditions encountered in the intended use of a drug and their maintenance is too laborious for long-term studies. Specific pathogen free (SPF) and gnotobiotic animals are more useful for toxicity studies as demonstrated by Paget & Lemon (1965). These authors have shown that it is possible to improve the health of a given strain of rodents by SPF breeding practices thus reducing morbidity and mortality without changing the incidence of neoplasias.

These observations indicate that a rigidly controlled environment, which includes not only the obvious factors of caging, temperature, humidity, light, and nutritional requirements, but also a controlled microbial flora, is necessary to breed and maintain a good, uniform, and healthy stock of laboratory animals.

Rats and dogs are used most frequently because all investigators in the field are familiar with these species. One hundred and thirty-four studies of 1 month's duration or longer were published in *Toxicology and Applied Pharmacology* between 1959 and 1966. Of these, 43·3% were carried out in rats, 38·1% in dogs, and 6·7% in monkeys. Mice (3·7%), rabbits (3·0%), chickens and guinea pigs (1·5%), and gerbils (0·7%) played only a minor role.

A study group from the European Society for the Study of Drug Toxicity headed by Bushby (1966) has shown that 71·7% of all laboratories concerned with toxicity testing of drugs used rats and dogs; 16% used monkeys, rats, and cats.

Sufficient biological data have been accumulated on the miniature pig to render this animal useful for toxicity studies (Earl *et al.*, 1964; Pekas & Bustad, 1965; Bustad and McClellan, 1966). However, their large size requires substantial quantities of compounds, and it may not always be feasible to supply these quantities of an experimental drug at an early stage of development.

The physiological and anatomical similarities between subhuman primates and man as well as their phylogenetic relationship seem to make these animals attractive for toxicological research. However, differences in absorption, excretion and drug metabolism patterns, in comparison with man, may render these species of limited value for long-term studies. For example, Owens (1962) claimed that in the area of antineoplastic agents, experiments in monkeys did not yield any information different from that obtained in rats and dogs. Unfortunately the necessary biological background data are widely scattered in the world literature, and it is presently difficult to assemble comprehensive information on this subject. However, unless one raises these animals under standardized conditions which are now certainly an expensive proposition, one is forced to import captured animals. This is an unsatisfactory procedure because a large number of them are true storehouses of diseases such as parasitic infestations, virus infections, dysentery, etc. that are infective to man. Some of these spontaneous disease patterns are bound to be influenced by drug administration, and it may sometimes be difficult to decide whether a biological phenomenon is caused by treatment and has to be regarded as a manifestation of toxicity or constitutes a peculiar, naturally occurring event altered in its intensity or quality by treatment. The formation of primate research and breeding centres might help to raise sufficient numbers of monkeys under standardized conditions.

By extending the range of animal species in preliminary experiments, the chances of finding a species with high sensitivity to a particular drug will be increased. Although the use of such a species should not be disregarded, the results from these experiments would not necessarily have predictive value for man. Therefore, it is questionable that one should always select the most sensitive species for chronic toxicity studies. One species may absorb a given compound at a high rate and form one or more extremely toxic metabolites whereas another species may absorb the same drug at a slower rate and form one or more completely harmless detoxification products that are readily excreted. The conditions prevailing in the first species may have no resemblance to the pharmacokinetic mechanisms in man who may react in a similar manner as the second species.

Brodie (1964) has stated that for toxicity studies, animal species could be selected which inactivate a drug with extreme rapidity. This selection could result in a rather uneventful safety evaluation programme that would have no value for the prediction of toxic effects in man, a species that may handle the drug in a completely different manner. Examples have been collected by Brodie (1966) and these data indicate that some subhuman primates metabolize certain drugs much faster than man.

The decision to use either genetically uniform animals or mixed strains may be of some importance especially in the choice of rodents. Uniform hereditary (for a critique see also Barnes & Denz, 1954) and environmental conditions may occasionally facilitate uniform responses. Inbred strains bred for a particular quality should be avoided since such a selection may enhance or diminish a reaction which is characteristic of the species. Animals obtained from crossbreeding of strains and/or with a limited control of environment may increase the variability of responses and therefore require a larger number of animals.

Golberg (1965) has stated that the objective of animal work is to arrive at reproducible facts. This is certainly a worthwhile requirement; however, I would like to add a second objective. One should also attempt to arrive at meaningful facts since reproducibility *per se* without meaning is of limited or of no value. The thyroid gland hyperplasia in rats induced by sulphonamides may serve as an example. This phenomenon is highly reproducible and has been observed in many laboratories, yet its toxicological significance is nil because morphological activation of the thyroid gland in this species is readily produced by a variety of compounds and the carry-over of this phenomenon to man is extremely poor.

A prime consideration in the selection of a suitable animal for chronic toxicity is that its pattern of absorption, metabolism, detoxification, storage, and excretion should resemble that of man. Boyd (1968) postulates that one should include one species which vomits and another one which does not. This latter species should be the one in which the drug is metabolized as in man and in which toxicity is similar to that in man. This can only be achieved after tolerance studies in man and pharmacokinetics, including identification of metabolites in laboratory animals and man, have been concluded. The principle that toxicity studies should be carried out in species that show signs of the desirable pharmacological effects to be used therapeutically in man should also be considered, especially when similarities with respect to drug metabolism cannot be established or such data are not as yet available or are impossible to obtain.

Number of Animals

The number of animals per experiment depends upon the species used and the length of time required to reach the desired objective. For a long-term chronic toxicity study, the number of animals depends largely upon the results obtained from a range-finding experiment which is usually of rather short duration. Without the benefit of this information no long-term study can be designed with any degree of accuracy. The incidence of toxicological manifestations, the incorporation of a time-sequence study into the long-term experiment, and recovery studies in which animals are sacrificed at various time intervals after the discontinuation of drugs are factors that may change the number of animals considerably. Barnes and Denz (1954) have outlined the statistical problems with respect to the size of treatment groups. If, for instance, a toxic effect occurs in 5% (1 of 20) of the animals, it would take 90 animals to discover this with a probability of $P=0.01$. This statistical uncertainty has led many investigators to use large numbers of animals to enhance the chances of detecting an infrequent toxic effect. Thus individual experiments are enlarged to such a scale that the workload alone may diminish the thoroughness and the care that are necessary for the successful completion of a study. The use of 20 to 30 rodents per dose level and sex together with a control group of 40 to 60 per sex should be sufficient for practical purposes and allows the necessary freedom for interim sacrifices. Groups of four to eight non-rodents per dose level and sex permit intensive investigations using pertinent measurements and parameters indicative of toxicity. The basic concept that more useful information can be obtained in thorough studies carried out in a relatively small number of animals should not be sacrificed in favour of incomplete experiments using an excessive number of animals.

Methods of Administration and Dose Levels

The compound to be tested should be administered 7 days per week. A 5 day per week treatment schedule as advocated by Ther (1965) will result in a 28·6% decrease of exposure and provide a 48-hour weekly recovery period. The introduction of a correction factor as suggested by Boyd (1968) may be acceptable under the premise that the response to a drug given on Monday, after 2 days of recovery, is similar to that observed during Tuesday through Friday. This author determines the total weekly dose, divides the number by 5 (number of working days per week) and then administers that amount of drug on a 5-day per week basis. This purely mathematical correction cannot be recommended as a standard procedure. The difference between the effects of a 5 day per week and a 7 day per week dosing schedule has been shown by Baker and Alcock (1965) who observed cataractogenicity with continued drug administration but no effects using the 5 day schedule. However, if the therapeutic application of a drug calls for an intermittent dosage schedule, the 7 day per week dosing may not be necessary and schedules simulating the administration to man should be used (Paget & Barnes, 1964).

Routes of administration should be identical with the ones to be used therapeutically in man. Paget & Barnes (1964) state that most drugs are given to patients more than once a day and therefore it may be desirable to use equally divided doses. In rodents oral administration can be achieved rather conveniently by using drug diets but the stability of the compound in the feed must be checked. It is good practice to mix no more than a week's supply of diet in advance. The daily drug intake can easily be calculated from the food consumption of the individual animals. Some investigators adjust the drug-diet concentrations on a periodic basis to reflect the body weight changes with the objective in mind to maintain relatively constant dosages. Other investigators prefer giving compounds by stomach tubing or in gelatin capsules. The administration of one dose by gavage results in peak blood levels whereas the continuous ingestion of drug diet leads to a lower and more prolonged drug concentration with less fluctuation. The capability of each method to affect absorption, concentration in blood and tissues, and the subsequent elimination of the foreign substance can account for marked differences in results obtained with the same compound. When the compound is administered by gavage, the determination of food consumption is not obviated since this determination is necessary to evaluate measurements indicative of growth and feed efficiency ratios.

For parenteral administrations (subcutaneous, intramuscular, or intravenous), rotation of injection sites is necessary. An additional groups of animals should receive the vehicle without the drug. Woodard (1965) has summarized principles of dosing for topical preparations to be applied to certain regions of the body (skin, eyes, ears) or internal surfaces (oral cavity, vagina). The inhalation of medicated aerosols can be achieved by the procedures outlined by Jemski & Phillips (1965), Gage (Chapter 9), and Balazs (Chapter 3). Daily intracisternal or intraspinal injections cannot be repeated for prolonged time periods.

Generally pair-feeding experiments, either on an individual basis or on a group basis, are not necessary. However, when marked decreases of food consumption are noticed in one or more treatment groups, it may be advantageous to include pair-fed groups at these diet levels to differentiate between the effects of the compound and semistarvation. Dixon *et al.* (1960) for instance have shown that starvation depresses hepatic microsomal enzymes that are necessary for the metabolic transformation of drugs.

Sometimes escalating doses for a comparison can be useful. An example of this approach has been published by Benitz *et al.* (1965) comparing three different substances using increasing dose levels for various periods of time. Such a dosage schedule may also be of interest when studying tolerance phenomena.

The selection of dose levels for long-term studies can best be achieved by a preliminary toxicity experiment of short duration (up to 4 weeks). The procedure of selecting doses on the basis of the LD_{50} determinations alone should be discouraged since in most instances the LD_{50} values have no relation to the inherent toxic properties of a compound that is administered in multiple doses for an extended time period. The only benefit one can obtain from an LD_{50} determination is that this parameter, together with the ED_{50} values from various pharmacological tests, provides a range for the selection of dose levels. The approach of Janků (1966) utilized the mean lethal time (LT_{50}) in relation to fractions of the LD_{50} administered repeatedly to estimate a safe dose for chronic toxicity studies. Whether this approach is practical remains to be seen but it gives an insight into some mechanisms of toxicity as a function of dose and frequency of administration.

Three or more dose levels, in geometric progression, should be used. There is general agreement that the highest should produce definite, harmful effects that serve as an indication of toxicity to be looked for and avoided in man. If there are no overt signs of toxicity, it is proper to conclude that the dose levels selected were too low, and no matter what other data are obtained they are of no value since the main purpose, that of obtaining toxic effects, has not been achieved. One dose level, hopefully an intermediate or at least the lowest, should not produce any adverse physiological, biochemical, or morphological effects and therefore can be used for the approximation of the margin of safety.

Sometimes one encounters a situation where preclinical (short-term) toxicity experiments in animals have been completed and subsequent clinical trials in man have indicated a therapeutic dose range which, in turn, should be used to select the dose levels for chronic toxicity studies.

Duration of Drug Administration

The rate of cell turnover and cellular metabolism of a given mammalian species is usually inversely related to body weight. The greater rate of metabolic processes per unit of body weight in smaller animals may be reflected by a greater food consumption, greater oxygen usage, greater carbon dioxide production, and greater turnover of body water. The higher rate of metabolism can be accompanied by a higher rate of metabolizing and excreting foreign substances as evidenced by the ability of smaller species to tolerate larger doses of most exogenous chemicals per unit of body weight.

The signs of ageing are rather similar in various species, including man, and begin to appear during the second half of the average life span. For example, in man the entire life cycle occupies almost seven decades but in the rat this is telescoped to 2–4 years. Since all the phases of a normal life cycle are telescoped into a much shorter time span for a small mammal, it is probable that most harmful

Table 4.1 Time relationships between drug exposure, life span, and time equivalents in man.

Duration of study in months	Rat		Rabbit		Dog		Pig		Monkey	
	Percentage life span	Human equivalent in months	Percentage life span	Human equivalent in months	Percentage life span	Human equivalent in months	Percentage life span	Human equivalent in months	Percentage life span	Human equivalent in months
1	4·1	34	1·5	12	0·82	6·5	0·82	6·5	0·55	4·5
2	8·2	67	3·0	24	1·6	14	1·6	14	1·1	9
3	12	101	4·5	36	2·5	20	2·5	20	1·6	13
6	25	202	9·0	72	4·9	40	4·9	40	3·3	27
12	49	404	18	145	9·8	81	9·8	81	6·6	53
24	99	808	36	289	20	162	20	162	13	107

reactions to the chronic administration of foreign substances are also telescoped in a similar manner. The data in Table 4.1 relate the months of drug administration for man to the per cent of the life span of laboratory animals and the duration of the study. It becomes apparent from this tabulation that the month for month equivalence of toxicity studies versus the time period of human exposure is not rational and that some other factors must be considered to account for the species differences.

The duration of dosing has been a subject of controversy for a long time. All vague terms such as subacute, subchronic, or chronic studies should be avoided. As indicated in Table 4.2, various investigators have attached different definitions to these terms.

Table 4.2   Definitions of terms with respect to duration of drug administration.

Fitzhugh (1959)	Abrams *et al.* (1965)	Ther (1965)	WHO (1966)
	13 weeks (subacute)	4 weeks (?)	< 3 months short term (subacute)
3 months (sub-acute)		3 months (?)	3–6 months long term (chronic)
6–18 months (chronic)	6–18 months (chronic)	6–12 months (chronic)	Life span studies

In 1965 Boyd felt that long-term toxicity tests in laboratory animals called for repeated drug administration through the life-span or a major portion of it. This postulate seems somewhat unrealistic since the life-span of larger animals such as dogs, rabbits, pigs and monkeys ranges from 5 to 20 years. Later, in 1968, the same author restricted the time of drug exposure to 100 days. Paget and Barnes (1964) feel that a duration of twice the maximum exposure intended to be used in man is a convenient guide. Generally speaking, it seems adequate to limit drug administration to periods from 3 to 6 months which is also the recommendation of the World Health Organization issued by the Scientific Group on Rationale of Drug Testing (1966). There seems to be general agreement (Barnes & Denz, 1954; Bein, 1963) that little additional information is gained from longer periods of testing. However, Goldenthal (1968) mentions some toxicological manifestations such as changes in the eye and endocrine system after the administration of certain psycho-tropic and anticonvulsant agents that were only seen after the sixth month of drug administration. These observations point to the necessity for employing longer testing periods in special cases. In cases of suspected carcinogenicity, experiments of even longer duration are warranted. Finally there might be a few agents that are used therapeutically for a prolonged time period in the therapy of extremely chronic diseases that also require experiments of longer duration.

Use of Standards for Comparison

The use of standards is a widely accepted procedure for screening and testing new compounds but it is not common practice to use standards in chronic toxicity experiments to evaluate the safety of a new compound. Table 4.3 shows a semiquantitative comparison of two phenothiazine derivatives (unknown and standard) and illustrates how simple observations during life can be used for the safety evaluation of a new drug. Hallesy and Benitz (1963) published the results of a study comparing two diuretic drugs (unknown and standard). Both compounds caused renal concretions, and no safe dose level for either one was obtained. If the standard had not been used, one would have been forced to conclude that the high incidence of renal concretions in the treated animals receiving the new drug (unknown) constituted a serious toxic effect. However, since the standard caused quantitatively and qualitatively the same changes, these findings were disregarded in the final evaluation of the safety, especially in view of the fact that the standard had not shown this phenomenon in man during several years of wide therapeutic use.

Time Sequence Studies

After the conclusion of a certain phase of safety evaluation, it may be of considerable practical and academic interest to study the course of development of the toxic phenomena. Special time sequence experiments can be designed with this goal in mind, and the investigators can focus their attention on a limited number of functional and structural abnormalities. This limitation permits the use of refined pharmacological, biochemical, and morphological techniques that may be impractical during the course of some of

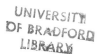

Table 4.3 Toxicological comparison of two phenothiazine derivatives.

Concentration of drug in diet	UNKNOWN						STANDARD					
	High dose		Medium dose		Low dose		High dose		Medium dose		Low dose	
	Drug effect	Score	Drug effect	Score	Drug effect	Score	Drug effect	Score	Drug effect	Score	Drug effect	Score
Mortality	Marked	3	Absent	0	Absent	0	Marked	3	Absent	0	Absent	0
Decrease of food intake	Marked	3	Slight	1	Absent	0	Marked	3	Moderate	2	Absent	0
Decrease of body weight gain	Marked	3	Slight	1	Absent	0	Marked	3	Slight	1	Absent	0
Sedation	Marked	3	Moderate	2	Absent	0	Marked	3	Moderate	2	Absent	0
Ptosis	Marked	3	Slight	1	Absent	0	Marked	3	Slight	1	Absent	0
Perioral irritation	Moderate	2	Slight	1	Absent	0	Moderate	2	Slight	1	Absent	0
Urinary incontinence	Marked	3	Slight	1	Absent	0	Moderate	2	Slight	1	Absent	0
Score per dose level		20		7		0		19		8		0
Total score per compound			27						27			

Mortality figures were converted into the following scores: 0 = Absent (0%); 3 = Marked (100%).

the main experiments. Fitzhugh (1955) has recommended that during the course of a chronic toxicity study one or two animals of each sex should be sacrificed at various intervals before the study is terminated. This approach seems to be impractical since it only allows conclusions with respect to toxic effects that occur in 100% of the animals within a certain dose level and does not allow a statistical comparison. In most instances, information with respect to toxicity is available from short-term toxicity studies and there is really no need to decrease the number of animals during the course of a long-term study. Finally, one should keep in mind that an equal number of control animals have to be sacrificed at the same time which is undesirable since the necessary additional control animals are sometimes not available. It is sometimes practical to combine two phases of a long-term toxicity programme. For example a sufficient number of animals from all dose levels, including controls, can be sacrificed after 90 days of drug exposure while the remaining animals are kept for a longer term.

Occasionally one is forced to design a special experiment focusing one's attention on a phenomenon of special interest. Table 4.4 presents an example of such a time sequence study that was designed after a long-term toxicity study in rats had been completed. Since 10 animals and 8 criteria were used, the maximum lesion score is 80. As one can see from this table, the score almost doubled after each week thus reflecting a time-effect relationship.

Table 4.4 Incidence of antibiotic-induced morphological kidney changes observed at various time intervals.

Morphological findings	Weeks of treatment		
	2	3	4
Mottled surface	0/10	0/10	4/10
Anaemia on surface and cut surface	2/10	5/10	5/10
Loss of zonation	2/10	5/10	5/10
Interstitial fibrosis	2/10	2/10	6/10
Leukocytic infiltration	0/10	2/10	4/10
Tubular dilatation	2/10	3/10	4/10
Casts in tubuli	1/10	2/10	5/10
Necrotic tubular epithelium	0/10	0/10	3/10
Total score/group	9/80	19/80	36/80

Recovery Experiments

It is sometimes important for the safety evaluation of a compound to determine whether certain toxicological phenomena are reversible. Therefore, recovery studies indicating the rate and the extent of reversibility of toxic manifestations seem to be indicated in almost every instance. Benitz *et al.* (1965) have studied a recovery pattern 2, 4, and 16 weeks after the termination of drug administration in rats. Body weight gain and four to seven sets of gross and microscopic criteria were used for changes found in liver, femur, and three endocrine glands. All criteria showed changes in the direction of complete recovery but not all became normal at the same time. It is obvious that a critical synthesis must be achieved using the various criteria indicating reversibility.

The value of recovery studies can also be illustrated by the following example. Rats that received an antithyroid compound in the diet for a year were divided into two groups. One group was sacrificed immediately after termination of treatment, whereas the other group was allowed to recover receiving normal diet. The thyroid glands of the animals that were examined immediately after termination of treatment showed some histological signs such as papillary pattern, vascular invasion, and destructive infiltration indicative of neoplastic changes in 7 of 15 animals. After a 4 month recovery period when the thyroid glands of the 16 rats were examined, none of these signs were found. According to Willis (1953) a malignant neoplasm is defined as an abnormal mass of tissue, the growth of which exceeds and is uncoordinated with that of the normal tissues, and persists in the same excessive manner after cessation of the stimuli which evoked the change. Therefore, as soon as one could demonstrate that a morphological structure with histological signs of malignancy was able to regress, the tentative diagnosis of a malignant neoplasm was no longer tenable. Such a reversibility of a toxic effect plays, of course, a definite role in the final evaluation of toxicity.

OBSERVATIONS DURING LIFE

Mortality

The death of a laboratory animal is the most significant sign of toxicity and the mortality pattern obtained during the course of an experiment can have a significant influence on the continuation or the termination of the study. The morphological examination using animals found dead is usually hampered by various degrees of post-mortem autolysis due to the 8 hour workday and the 5 day workweek in most commercial laboratories. However, all efforts should be made to determine the cause of death especially in view of the fact that the pathological findings in the more susceptible animals of a given dose group may indicate toxicological problems. Thus a separation of drug-induced deaths from spontaneously occurring fatalities can be attempted especially during the first 6 to 10 weeks of drug-diet experiments. As shown by Fitzhugh *et al.* (1944) young rats receive relatively more toxic material (on the basis of mg/kg body weight) than older animals and such high doses may lead to an increased number of early deaths. Generally speaking, material from animals found dead is sometimes of limited value for finer histological analyses. Animals that died prior to the termination of the experiment or are obviously moribund should not be excluded from the morphological examination. The recommendation by Mihich (1966) to eliminate material from animals found dead and cold should be rejected because in a group of animals that died prematurely, one may find clues with respect to the drug-induced morphological changes and this information may be of considerable value in determining the timing of interim sacrifices and the modification of the morphological procedures to be employed for a study. It may be advantageous in rodent experiments to let 50–60% of the animals die spontaneously and obtain a true mortality pattern. Then the remaining animals of that particular dose group, and the controls can be sacrificed to obtain adequate material for morphological studies. Non-rodents should be sacrificed when moribund.

Clinical Observations

The investigators should be thoroughly familiar with their animals, especially those of the larger species. This can be done with relative ease during the 3 to 6 weeks' predose holding period when base line information with respect to hematology, chemical and function tests is obtained.

The general clinical condition of animals can be determined by physical examinations and general observations. Only a few of these methods lend themselves to instrumentation, therefore, all deviations from the norm must be recorded adequately and accurately. Qualitative toxic signs observed in groups of animals can be counted and, according to Boyd (1968), may be tabulated as incidences or intensities or treated as regressions with time and dose.

Food and water consumption should be determined not only in rodents but in the large animals as well. Since body weight gain and food intake are intimately related, any data on one without the other are meaningless. The procedures for obtaining body weight gain and food intake data for large numbers of rodents can be automated. Modern data acquisition equipment can be used effectively from the initial weighing of individual animals and feed containers to the final computer print-out that provides a finished tabulation including statistical analyses.

The statistical analysis of body weight data has been reviewed by Jackson (1962) who emphasized that not only body weight curves should be considered for the evaluation of growth, but also weight gain data should be included in such an analysis. Furthermore this author advocates the use of non-parametric analogues of conventional parametric statistical procedures. Generally speaking, the evaluation of body-weight gain data has been somewhat overemphasized, and there are certainly other criteria of a physiological, biochemical or morphological nature equally or even more important than the results of lengthy statistical evaluation of body weight data.

Body weight gain is not the only measurement that can be made during the life of a laboratory animal. The skeletal growth is sometimes also informative and can be measured *in vivo* by determining the distance between two prominent landmarks of one bone. In rodents, the tail length (distance between anus and tip) provides a convenient measure for skeletal growth during life.

Observations to detect toxic signs should be made daily especially during the first weeks of a study. Changes in general behaviour and locomotor activity as well as the character and frequency of respiration can be noticed easily. The occurrence of emesis, diarrhoea, discolouration of faeces and urine should be noted. The appearance of eyes, ears, nose, mouth, mucous membranes, skin, and external genitalia can be examined and recorded.

Physical examinations should be carried out at regular intervals or as the condition of the animals indicates. The diagnostic procedures used in veterinary clinical medicine can provide suitable guidelines for the methodology for these examinations for nonrodent species. The list of observations compiled by Balazs (Chapter 3) intended to be used for the examination of rodents can be used as an example of how to detect toxic effects during a chronic toxicity study.

Electrocardiograms complete the cardiological examination of large animals. The basic studies published by Detweiler *et al.* (1960) and Detweiler and Patterson (1965) provide suitable guidelines for the electrocardiographic analyses, especially for dogs. At the present time, the three standard limb leads I, II, and III, together with three augmented limb leads and three precordial leads, have been useful for the electrocardiographic analysis of drug-induced cardiac malfunctions. A standardized position of the animal is essential since the loose connective tissue of the mediastinum permits considerable shifts in the position of the heart.

Recent observations with respect to eye toxicity have put more emphasis on ophthalmologic examinations. Ophthalmoscopic and slit-lamp examinations are now established routine procedures not only for larger animals as outlined by Krawitz (1965) and Magrane (1965) but also for rats.

Routine X-ray examinations are usually not necessary. However, one should consider such diagnostic measures when postural changes without neurological signs are observed or when clinical chemical data indicate a disturbance of bone metabolism.

Clinical Chemistry

Cornelius and Kaneko (1963) have collected methods in clinical pathology for veterinary use. Street (Chapter 12) has compiled function tests and clinical chemical determinations that are especially useful for toxicity studies. New methods will always be added and to prove their biological significance they should be used with the old ones for some time. It does not necessarily follow that if a large battery of function tests has been applied to a chronic toxicity experiment that such a study is superior to one in which a smaller number was used. It is more judicious to select the most meaningful tests for the problems that manifest themselves during the preliminary toxicity studies or in the early phase of a long term study. Results from the pharmacological efficacy studies may also give some hints or even definite indications as to what problems can be expected.

Function tests and clinical chemical determinations are usually carried out at various stages of the experiments. These procedures are necessary to detect and characterize toxic effects as expressed by abnormal biochemical and physiological functions. They provide some guidance for post-mortem studies and help the pathologist who is participating in these experiments to concentrate his efforts on certain organs or systems that require special attention.

Sampling techniques to obtain body fluids (blood, lymph, urine, or cerebrospinal fluid) have been outlined by Moreland (1965). One of the most important prerequisites for any test is that sampling procedures do not impair the health of the animal. The amount of blood that can be obtained at frequent intervals is extremely limited in smaller animals and therefore only meaningful determinations should be carried out. Larger animals like rabbits, dogs, monkeys, and pigs allow more freedom in this respect. Regardless of the species used, micro methods play an important role for analytical procedures using blood, serum, or plasma. Twenty-four hour urine collections provide sufficient quantities for analysis in all species. Usually there is no shortage of faeces. Predose determinations should be repeated two or three times in large animals so that each animal can serve as its own control.

When rodents are used and especially when they receive treatment immediately after weaning, it is more desirable to use untreated animals as controls rather than do predose function tests since a valuable period of body weight gain would be wasted by carrying out these determinations. At this stage the animals are still small and the corresponding circulating blood volume does not allow extensive sampling. In addition, a considerable variability is sometimes noticeable making the final interpretation of data difficult or almost impossible. Since rodents can easily be obtained in large numbers, it is more economical to determine specific organ functions at suitable intervals during the drug administration period or prior to sacrifice. A chronic toxicity study in rodents consists of a rather large number of animals per dose level and sex and it may not be possible to subject all animals to a set of function tests. A random selection of 8–10 males and females per dose level will usually give sufficient information.

Another guideline for the selection of clinical chemical determinations is that these tests should be applicable to man. Identical, or at least similar, procedures should be used in the clinic to look for toxic effects when a drug candidate goes into the early phases of clinical trial. Street (Chapter 12) however has stated that there are some procedures that are regarded as quite useful in clinical medicine but have little or no value for studies in animals.

Some of the function tests currently in use have been mentioned by Abrams *et al.* (1965) and Peck (1966). It is impossible to give an exhaustive list of all function tests or to make specific recommendations for certain classes of chemicals. As shown in Table 4.5 a group of clinical chemical determinations are listed that were used for a study of a psychotropic agent in dogs which presented few toxicological problems. Such a selection must vary with the pharmacological nature of a given compound, e.g. a diuretic agent requires special emphasis on kidney function tests such as glomerular filtration rate, effective renal blood flow, tubular maximal excretory capacity for para-aminohippurate, osmolar clearance, free water clearance and filtration fraction as studied by Ewald (1967) and urinary transaminase determinations as suggested by Balazs (1963). Some of the commoner tests, such as the determination of calcium, chloride, magnesium, inorganic phosphorus, carbon dioxide, urea nitrogen, uric acid, creatinine, total protein, albumin, bilirubin, glucose, cholesterol alkaline phosphatase, glutamic oxalacetic transaminase, and glutamic pyruvic transaminase have been conveniently automated and substantial additions to this list can be expected. In accordance with Street (Chapter 12) one should not rely on normal values obtained elsewhere but one should establish the normal ranges for normal animals in each individual laboratory. Constant monitoring with respect to accuracy and precision is necessary especially in view of the fact that small variations in the environment may cause changes that could distort the interpretation of results.

Haematology

Most haematological methods used in man have been adapted to animals and have been standardized. Sampling procedures should be kept constant. Blood samples from the various vascular provinces differ in cell counts as pointed out by Hulse (1965). Table 4.6 lists a number of haematological procedures that are useful for

Table 4.5 List of clinical chemistry determinations.

Measurement	Method	Reference
	Blood	
pH	Beckman micro blood pH assembly and expanded scale pH meter	Hoffman, 1937
Fasting glucose	Technicon[a] methodology adaptation	
	Plasma	
Urea nitrogen	Technicon[a] methodology adaptation	Skeggs, 1957; Marsh et al., 1957
Glutamic pyruvic trans-aminase	Sigma methodology[b]	Sigma Technical Bulletin No. 505
Glutamic oxalacetic transaminase	Sigma methodology[b]	Sigma Technical Bulletin No. 505
Tyrosine transaminase	Sigma methodology[b]	Waalkes & Udenfriend, 1957
Creatine phosphokinase	Phosphatabs ®-alkaline, quantitative[c]	Sigma Technical Bulletin No. 660
Alkaline phosphatase		
Creatinine		Hawk et al., 1947
	Serum	
Total solids and protein	Goldberg refractometer (Model B)[d]	Smith, 1960
Proteins	Zone electrophoresis with densitometer quantification	
Electrolytes		
Sodium	Technicon[a] methodology adaptation	Israeli et al., 1960
Potassium	,,	Israeli et al., 1960
Chloride	,,	Zall et al., 1956
Calcium	,,	Kesseer & Wolfman, 1964
Inorganic phosphate	,,	Fiske & Subbarow, 1925

Triglycerides	Extraction	Nicolaysen & Nygaard, 1963
	Determination	Van Handel, 1961
Phospholipids	Extraction	Nicolaysen & Nygaard, 1963
	Determination	Bartlett, 1959
Cholesterol	Determination	Trinder, 1952
	Saponification	Zlatkis et al., 1958
BSP retention	Determination	Seligson et al., 1957

Urine

pH, protein, glucose, occult blood, acetone bodies	Labstix ®[e]	
Electrolytes (Na, K, Cl, P)	Technicon[a] methodology adaptation	
Calcium	Technicon[a] methodology fluorometric determination	
Urobilinogen	Wallace & Diamond	
24 hour nitrogen	Kjeldahl digestion and a modification of the method of Folin & Wu	Bloom, 1960; Hawk et al., 1947
Sediment	Microscopy	
Dilution–concentration test	One hour after the removal of drinking water the animals were catheterized (U_0). One hour later 20 ml of water per kg body weight was given. Subsequent catheterizations were carried out 2(U_1) and 20 hours (U_2) after the water load. Osmolality was determined by a freezing point depression method	

[a] Technicon Instrument Corporation, Chauncey, New York.
[b] Sigma Chemical Co., St Louis, Missouri.
[c] Warner–Chilcott Laboratories, Morris Plains, New Jersey.
[d] American Optical Co., Keene, New Hampshire.
[e] Ames Company, Elkhart, Indiana.

Table 4.6   List of haematological measurements.

Measurement	Method	Reference
	Erythropoietic System	
Haemoglobin concentration	Measured as cyanmethaemoglobin using a Klett–Summerson photoelectric colorimeter[a]	Wintrobe, 1961
Haematocrit (packed cell volume)	Drummond microhaematocrit apparatus[b]	
Erythrocyte counts	Coulter counter[c]	Grant, Britton & Kurtz, 1960
Erythrocyte glucose-6-phosphate dehydrogenase	Spot test[d]	Fairbanks & Beutler, 1962
Reticulocyte counts	Number per 1,000 erythrocytes	
Sedimentation rate	Citrated blood in Wintrobe haematocrit tubes for 1 hour	
	Leukopoietic System	
Leukocyte counts	Coulter counter[c]	Richar & Breakell, 1959
Differential counts	Conventional counts	
	Coagulation System	
Clotting time		Lee & White, 1913
Platelet counts	Levy–Hausser counting chamber	Björkman, 1959
Fibrinogen		Goodwin, 1961
Prothrombin time	Quick's test using Simplastin ® reagent[e] with an Oxford Prothrometer[f]	Cartwright, 1963

[a] Klett Manufacturing Co., New York.
[b] The Drummond Scientific Co., Philadelphia.
[c] Coulter Electronics, Inc., Hialeah, Florida.
[d] Calbiochem, Box 54282, Los Angeles, California.
[e] Warner–Chilcott Laboratories, Morris Plains, New Jersey.
[f] Oxford Laboratories, San Mateo, California.

long-term toxicity studies. Not all methods have the same degree of reliability as shown by Wintrobe (1961). For instance, the number of red cells shows considerable variability whereas haemoglobin determinations and haematocrit values do not. Therefore, red cell counts could be eliminated as a routine measure since anaemias and polycythemias readily manifest themselves by changes in haemoglobin and haematocrit values. However, if a haematological problem arises, the number of red cells should be available for calculating corpuscular constants, such as corpuscular haemoglobin, corpuscular volume, etc. Besides numerical values, qualitative morphological changes should be taken into account for the assessment of haematological damage. The appearance of abnormal cells, changes in stainability and the formation of pathological cellular components under the influence of drugs indicate the value of such information.

Total bone marrow nucleated cell counts, a technique developed by Gerarde (1956) and subsequently used by Vogel (1961) for the assessment of bone marrow damage, can only be regarded as a screening technique since individual components of the haemato-poietic system are neglected. Paraffin sections (4 μ) of bone marrow sampled from long bones or imprints seem to give a better oppor-tunity for the qualitative assessment of bone marrow changes. Mayer & Ruzicka (1956) devised a method for the topographical assessment of bone marrow components that can be used in small rodents, but it should not be regarded as a routine procedure since it is too laborious and time-consuming. For routine work the bone marrow can be removed from the femur shaft either at autopsy or after fixation. Due to topographical variability, the sampling sites in larger animals such as dogs, swine, monkeys, etc., should be standardized. Femur marrow sampled at a given distance from the joint surface or segments of sternum should give reproducible results. Sections, imprints and smears of bone marrow have been used to study morphological alterations. Each technique has its advantages and disadvantages. For instance, smears will not yield enough information with respect to the histotopographical com-position of the bone marrow as outlined by Mayer (1963).

Pliess & Fassbender (1961) have used the mitotic index (number of mitoses/1,000 cells of each system) in the bone marrow for the erythropoietic and leukopoietic system to study hypoplastic and hyperplastic bone marrow changes under the influence of cyclophos-phamide. The same authors have used histochemical techniques for acid and alkaline phosphatases, peroxidase reaction, haemoglobin, fat, and glycogen to study qualitative aspects of bone marrow dam-age. Generally speaking, bone marrow counts are time-consuming and laborious and can be replaced by ranking individual compon-ents using a system as outlined in the section on Quantification of Morphological Structures, p. 120, and as shown in Table 4.7. Unless one has to deal with a complex haematological problem that defi-nitely requires bone marrow counts, such a grading procedure for individual details serves the purpose of documenting bone marrow changes.

Table 4.7 Quantification of bone marrow changes by ranking individual components.

Treatment	Control	Low dose	High dose
Cellularity	Normal 8/9 Slight decrease 1/9	None 6/8 Slight decrease 1/8 Moderate decrease 1/8	Slight decrease 1/6 Moderate decrease 3/6 Marked decrease 2/6
Fat	Normal 8/9 Moderate increase 1/9	Normal 6/8 Slight increase 1/8 Moderate increase 1/8	Slight decrease 2/6 Moderate increase 3/6 Marked increase 1/6
Erythoid elements	Normal 8/9 Moderate decrease 1/9	Normal 4/8 Slight decrease 3/8 Moderate decrease 1/8	Moderate decrease 3/6 Marked decrease 3/6
Myeloid elements	Normal 8/9 Slight decrease 1/9	Normal 5/8 Slight increase 1/8 Slight decrease 1/8 Moderate decrease 1/8	Slight decrease 2/6 Moderate decrease 2/6 Marked decrease 2/6
Mega-karyocytes	Normal 9/9	Normal 8/8	None 1/6 Slight decrease 2/6 Moderate decrease 2/6 Marked decrease 1/6

As soon as one encounters severe changes either in the peripheral blood or in the composition of the bone marrow, extramedullary haematopoesis should be studied morphologically using sections from lymph nodes, spleen, and liver.

Drug Concentration in Serum

Methods for the determination of drug concentration in serum are being developed in increasing numbers. In addition, the qualitative and quantitative determination of metabolites has gained more and more importance. When the more recent sulphonamides and anti-biotics were introduced, results of laboratory efficacy studies were not only expressed on a mg/kg basis (drug diet basis or oral dosage basis) but also on the basis of serum concentrations. This approach can also be used for toxicity problems providing sensitive enough methods with acceptable specificity are available.

The opportunity should not be missed to obtain sufficient quanti-ties of serum at the end of an experiment when the animals are to be sacrificed. The sampling time with relation to the last dose should be chosen carefully on the basis of the pharmacokinetics for a given compound. Intermediary sampling during the drug administration period may sometimes also be of value especially with compounds that accumulate in the body. This offers an opportunity to corre-late the increasing signs of toxicity with rising blood levels. The relation of drug concentration in serum to biochemical or morpho-logical changes allows toxicity data to be expressed in terms of blood levels. These data are also useful since in the early phases of clinical trials multiple dose studies are usually carried out in man to assess not only its efficacy but also the inherent toxic properties of a potential drug candidate. Drug serum concentration data may be obtained sometimes with relative ease from these studies thereby permitting a comparison with animal toxicity data on a blood level basis. An example is given in Table 4.8. An anti-

Table 4.8 Relation of antibiotic-induced toxicity to antibiotic serum concen-trations in various species after 1 month of drug administration. Values in ( )=ranges.

Species	Dose (mg/kg/day)	Route of administration	Mean serum concentrations (μg/ml)	Drug-induced toxicity
Rat	8	Oral	0·86 (0·34–1·10)	Present in 3/20
Dog	5	Intravenous	2·09 (0·32–3·82)	Present in 2/2
Monkey	30	Oral	21·1 (20·8–21·5)	Present in 3/6
Man	10	Oral	12 h=5·16 (2·22–12·91)	Absent in 9/9

biotic was given to the following species: rats, monkeys, dogs, and man. The doses as tabulated in the second column of this table resulted in blood levels shown in the fourth column and the inci-dence of toxic effects in the fifth. This comparison indicated that toxic effects could be found in three laboratory species whereas man did not show any effect. The serum concentrations in the monkeys showed the highest value yet toxicological effects were only found in half of the animals. The antibiotic serum concentrations in man were higher than serum concentrations shown to produce toxicological effects in rats and dogs. These data, therefore, indicate that the latter two species showed a different reactivity both qualitatively and quantitatively with respect to drug-induced harmful effects.

It should be emphasized at this point that not only anti-infectious agents should be evaluated on the basis of drug concentration in serum but this approach lends itself to almost all types of drugs provided a sufficient quantity is absorbed from the site of application and remains unchanged for a reasonable period of time in the bloodstream.

Frequency of Observations

The long standing controversy, how often clinical observations should be carried out, can be resolved easily. These observations, including clinical chemistry and haematology, should be made when necessary. Any preconceived, rigid schedule is impracticable and only valid if no significant toxicological changes occur in the animals. As a rule, significantly abnormal results of function tests are accompanied by subtle or even pronounced clinical signs of illness that can be detected by careful observation. To repeat a battery of function tests every month or every three months for a study of one year's duration is neither scientifically nor economically warranted. The truly toxic dose level selected on the basis of the results of preliminary toxicity experiments for the high dose group of animals should lead, in almost all instances, to physical signs of illness. These sick animals are then subjected to a sequence of diagnostic procedures to pinpoint the nature and the degree of functional abnormalities. The results from the predose period together with the data from the control animals should enable the investigator to arrive at some interpretation of the drug-induced changes. It depends on the nature of the toxicity whether these abnormal results of the various function test procedures should be correlated with morphological changes at this time. Biopsy procedures for bone marrow, liver and kidney devised by Reutner & Kaump (1967) can be used for such a purpose. Immediately after drug induced changes have been found in the high dose animals, a suitable set of function tests can be selected and applied to the animals of the lower dose groups. These tests should be repeated at reasonable intervals to determine the onset of functional disturbances which is usually later (if they occur at all) in the animals of the lower dose groups.

Special attention should be devoted to the entire set of experimental animals (including controls) during the first 6 weeks of drug administration. All toxicologists have experienced transient changes during the course of the long term safety experiments and Table 4.9 can serve as an example of how toxic effects disappear during the course of an experiment.

Table 4.9 Clinical signs of toxicity observed in a group of dogs receiving toxic doses of a psychotropic active agent for 12 weeks.

Clinical signs	Weeks of dosing				
	1	2	4	8	12
Decreased food intake	+ +	+	−	−	−
Increased water intake	+	−	−	−	−
Increased urine volume	+	−	−	−	−
Melena	+ +	+	−	−	−
Elevated body temperature	+	−	−	−	−
Emesis	+	−	−	−	−
Salivation	+	−	−	−	−
Increased motor activity	+ +	+ +	+ +	+ +	+ +
Aimless, athetoid movements	+ +	+ +	+ +	+	−
Ulcerations in oral cavity	+	+	−	−	−
Congestion of mucous membranes and interdigital skin	+	−	−	−	−
Swelling and cracking of foot pads	+ +	+	−	−	−

− = absent   + = slight   + + = marked

Any lackadaisical attitude with respect to clinical observations is usually linked with an unwarranted expectation that the postmortem examination of the animals at the end of the treatment period will reveal morphological changes indicative of toxicity. Such a reliance is fallacious since the correlation between function and morphology is by no means complete. The observations during life should be made in such a manner that their results alone give a clear indication of the toxicity pattern at hand.

POST-MORTEM STUDIES

General

The practice of eviscerating animals and preserving the contents of the three body cavities in acid formaldehyde for later sampling of tissues for histopathological examination is an unacceptable procedure. The mistakes made at autopsy can never be corrected and the successful completion of a toxicity experiment depends on proper dissection and fixation techniques.

Following the lead of human pathology, one should advocate the performance of complete autopsies with uniform procedures. The thoracic, abdominal, and cranial cavities in each animal should be autopsied according to a definite schedule. The most careful microscopic investigation cannot substitute for a thorough gross autopsy. For instance, in a severely anaemic animal the gross dissection of the gastrointestinal tract may reveal bleeding ulcers. If this point has been missed during the gross examination, the most elaborate microscopy of haematopoietic tissues will be of little value. Other examples of this kind are the condition of the common bile duct, the portal vein, and the ureters. It is also easier to estimate the quantity of lymphatic tissue in an animal during the autopsy rather than in histological sections. In spite of the fact that standardization of these morphological procedures is desirable, certain variability of emphasis is inevitable.

The practice of examining only organs found to be abnormal at autopsy is unjustifiable since considerable harmful effects may be found histologically. This is especially true in small rodents where the macroscopic evaluation of tissue damage has limitations.

Abrams *et al.* (1965), have listed 18 tissues that should be routinely sampled for histopathological examination. Rather than adhering to such standardization one should preserve as many tissues as possible in suitable fixatives. After all, a long-term toxicity study cannot be repeated easily and it is always good practice to sample as completely as possible for the full evaluation of toxic effects.

This is in contrast to a recommendation made by Frazer (1958) who claimed that this procedure is wasteful and does not yield any valuable information. His suggestion, to limit the morphological examination to liver and kidney, is not justified since the morpho-

112

logical effects of new and unknown chemicals are unpredictable and require an extensive histological investigation. To limit the microscopic examination to grossly abnormal organs and structures supplemented by the material of two or three representative animals as suggested by Boyd (1968) may not yield the optimum amount of morphological data.

The recommendation that only 'major organs' should be examined is also questionable. Major organs (in contrast to minor organs) cannot be defined and therefore such recommendations are of little meaning.

A gross and microscopic comparison between controls and the animals receiving the highest dose should, in almost all cases, single out one or more targets (organs or systems). These morphological sites of drug toxicity can then be studied using material from animals of the lower dose groups to establish a dose-response relationship and a safe dose level.

The extent of the morphological examination is also governed by previous experience with a particular agent or its chemical relatives, the observations during life, and the pharmacological nature of the drug. The incidence of drug-induced pathological lesions encountered in our laboratories during the last 10 years as shown in Table 4.10 indicates that all organ systems are sites of toxic effects. Such an incidence profile must of course vary according to the selection of compounds studied. As expected, the liver and the kidney, the two organs of prime importance for detoxification and excretion, showed the highest incidence of pathological lesions. A rather high number of chemically induced morphological changes was also found in the endocrine system.

Generally speaking, one should perform complete autopsies on a sufficient number of rodents (8–12) and on all non-rodents. Well-trained autopsy teams can perform these procedures in a short time with reasonable reliability.

When results of a special type are wanted quickly, usually it is not possible or even necessary to perform complete autopsies. These incomplete autopsies should be used in special studies that supplement the main experiments. There are different ways of abbreviating an autopsy. The opening of the cranial cavity may be omitted or the thoracic and abdominal organs may be inspected from their surfaces only, without being dissected systematically. It is evident that less weight should be attached to such incomplete autopsies than to the complete ones.

The morphological changes that were encountered in the various organ systems listed in Table 4.10 could be divided into the follow-

Table 4.10 Incidence (in per cent) of drug-induced pathological changes encountered over a 10 year period in approximately 14,000 animals.

Systems and organs	Incidence	
	By organ	By system
Cardiovascular system		4·3
Respiratory system		5·3
Alimentary system		20·6
Liver	15·8	
Gastrointestinal tract	3·8	
Pancreas	1·0	
Urinary system		13·0
Kidney	12·0	
Ureter and urinary bladder	1·0	
Reproductive system		7·7
Males	4·8	
Females	2·9	
Ductless glands		22·1
Thyroid	11·5	
Adrenal	4·8	
Pituitary	5·3	
Islets of Langerhans	0·5	
Hematopoietic system		3·3
Lymphoid and reticuloendothelial system		7·2
Central nervous system		3·3
Sensory system		1·9
Eye	1·4	
Ear	0·5	
Locomotor system		10·5
Skin		1·0

ing categories: in 76·5%, dystrophic (degenerative) changes were found, inflammatory lesions were encountered in 14%, circulatory disorders in 7·%, and neoplastic changes including precancerous lesions in 1·8%. These figures show that dystrophic changes play the most important role in the safety evaluation of drugs. Therefore, optimal sampling and fixation procedures should be selected to detect these types of lesions. It may be relatively easy to recognize pronounced dystrophic changes, but sometimes it may be difficult to detect, grade, and document less obvious alterations of this kind.

Organ Weights and Skeletal Measurements

The determination and recording of organ weights are an integral part of the macroscopic diagnostic procedures. They provide the first morphological signs of dystrophic or dysplastic changes.

Barron (1965) and Peck (1966) have stated that organ weights are of limited or no value. The latter author claims that these data are only of value if the drug has a specific effect on a target organ. This is certainly true but not always known at the time of autopsy. Therefore, if these weight determinations were eliminated, valuable information may be lost. The removal of the surrounding connective tissue and the weighing require some additional effort at autopsy but the results may pinpoint problems of toxicological importance.

As an example, the oral administration of an antiparasitic agent caused enlargement of the adrenal glands in rats. Since it was known that hypocholesteremic agents can cause this weight increase, the serum of these animals was analysed for total sterols which were found to be decreased. The cross sections of the adrenal glands from the treated animals showed an enlarged cortex indicating the portion of the gland responsible for the increase in weight. After the drug concentrations in serum were determined, the correlations, as shown in Table 4.11, were found using the simple rank correlation method of Litchfield & Wilcoxon (1955).

Organ weight decreases usually indicate hypoplastic or atrophic changes; increased weights are more difficult to interpret. Hyperaemia, hyperplasia, hypertrophy, enzyme induction phenomena and neoplastic changes play a role in this respect. Golberg (1966) has given an example of how increased relative liver weights can be classified with respect to their significance in toxicity.

Some investigators have limited themselves to the presentation of relative organ weights. These data can be misleading since relative weights by themselves do not indicate whether an increase is due to reduced body weight gain that left the organ growth comparatively unaffected or whether the organ showed a genuine increase. There-

Table 4.11 Correlation coefficients for absolute and relative weights of adrenal glands and total sterol and drug concentrations in serum obtained from male rats receiving various dose levels of an antiparasitic agent for 30 days.

Correlations	Correlation coefficients	P values
Absolute weight vs drug concentration	$+0\cdot64$	$\leq 0\cdot05$
Relative weight vs drug concentration	$+0\cdot81$	$\leq 0\cdot01$
Absolute weight vs total sterol concentration	$-0\cdot70$	$\leq 0\cdot01$
Relative weight vs total sterol concentration	$-0\cdot80$	$\leq 0\cdot01$
Drug concentration vs total sterol concentration	$-0\cdot70$	$\leq 0\cdot01$

fore, relative organ weights should always be accompanied by body weights and absolute organ weights so that a decision can be made in respect to the factors that led to the weight changes. My experience suggests that one should limit the interpretation of relative organ weights to groups of animals with comparable body weights. This procedure is only applicable to organs that are related to body weight during the entire growth period of an animal. The weights of thymus, testes, seminal vesicles, ovaries, and uteri can present special problems in this respect.

In most instances pathological organ weights are associated with histological abnormalities. Jackson & Cappiello (1964) concluded in their study using organ weights of beagles that in nearly 80% of the organs examined, the histopathological diagnoses agreed with the weight changes.

Water content of organs may be determined by subtracting the weight after drying (72 hours at 110°C) from the wet weight. These data can be used to differentiate hypertrophy from oedema or establish the presence of both as shown by Benitz *et al.* (1961) and Benitz & Diermeier (1964) for kidneys. Since the water content shows considerable fluctuation related to the age of the animals as show by Peters (1967) an adequate number of control animals of the same age should be available for comparison.

Paired organs such as kidneys or adrenal glands pose no problems since one of them can be used for histological examination while the other is used for wet weight/dry weight determinations. Single organs like the heart or the pancreas have to be divided using distinct topographical landmarks in order to obtain comparable samples. This may be relatively easy in larger laboratory animals. but almost impossible when small rodents are used. If the number of rodents per sex and treatment group is large enough to allow additional sacrifices, animals of such a group can be used for these weight determinations. The same principles apply to all other chemical analyses of organs such as lipids, glycogen, protein, etc.

Skeletal measurements can be used to supplement body weight and organ weight data indicative of growth. In rats the femur length can be easily measured at autopsy with a Vernier caliper. Disproportionate growth of the skull can also be easily detected. A few simple weight determinations and skeletal measurements are shown in Table 4.12. This example was taken from a publication

Table 4.12 Summary of measurements indicative of growth in three groups of male rats[a]

Group	Controls	Underfed controls	Toxic dose of an antithyroid agent
No. of animals/group	12	12	6
Avg food intake/rat (g)	20·4	13·2	13·3
	(14–22)	(11–17)	(11–17)
Body weight (g)	407	251[b]	217[b,c]
	(351–501)	(224–278)	(166–257)
Dry carcass weight (g)	114	68[b]	47[b,d]
	(98–134)	(59–73)	(35–59)
Water content of carcass (%)	61·6	62·7	67·4[b,d]
	(59·9–63·8)	(60·5–65·2)	(64–69·7)
Head length (mm)	53	50[b]	49[b]
	(51–58)	(48–51)	(45–51)
Head width (mm)	28	25[b]	25[b]
	(26–29)	(24–26)	(23–26)
Cephalic index, $W:L$	0·52	0·50	0·51
	(0·47–0·54)	(0·48–0·52)	(0·48–0·52)
Femur length (mm)	38	35[b]	35[b]
	(36–41)	(33–37)	(32–37)

[a] From Benitz *et al.*, 1965.
[b] Significantly different from controls at $P \le 0.01$.
[c] Significantly different from underfed controls at $P \le 0.05$.
[d] Significantly different from underfed controls at $P \le 0.01$.

Values in parenthesis = ranges.

by Benitz *et al.* (1965) reporting the effects of anti-thyroid compounds using a group pair-feeding experiment. Wet weight minus dry weight data were used to document generalized oedema (water content of carcass) that occurred in the treated animals. The decreases in skeletal measurements were caused by starvation and did not result in a disproportionate growth of the skull as expected with a potent antithyroid drug as shown by Goddard (1948).

Histological Techniques

The fate and the ultimate value of tissue samples for microscopical examination are decided at the autopsy table. Although formaldehyde fixation and haematoxylin-eosin stain are widely used, there are better ways to bring out special histological details. Multiple fixations allow the use of special stains and histochemical procedures.

It would be presumptuous to make specific recommendations for the use of fixatives and stains since most pathologists have developed their own tastes and preferences. Neutral buffered formaldehyde in conjunction with Bouin's, Zenker's, Helly's, Carnoy's, and SUSA solutions offer sufficient choices for multiple or special fixation. Numerous special stains for various normal and pathological tissue components are available and can be used with advantage for tissue samples (4–5 mm thick) fixed immediately after death.

Specific histochemical methods for substances such as metals, minerals, lipids, carbohydrates, and endogenous and exogenous pigments are available as outlined by Thompson & Hunt (1966).

So far enzyme histochemistry has played a minor role in the routine morphological examination of tissues obtained from animals used for chronic toxicity experiments. Usually biochemical *in vitro* techniques are used first to study chemically induced enzymatic changes using material from animals that received a small number of doses. If the results from these short term experiments indicate the need to investigate histotopographical changes in enzyme content, tissue samples of the organ under study can be frozen quickly for cryostat sectioning. Such autopsy material can be obtained at the termination of a long term study. The large number of histochemical enzyme techniques available makes a reasonable selection necessary. The results obtained from *in vitro* or short term experiments should be available to aid in the selection. The conclusions derived from enzyme histochemistry plus observations from conventional microscopy may lead to a better understanding of the pathogenesis and the biological significance of drug induced pathology.

Electron microscopy has established its value in three areas of application: (a) the earlier detection of morphological changes, (b) the more definitive interpretation of pronounced morphological lesions that are already visible with ordinary light microscopy, (c) the detection of ultrastructural changes that do not manifest themselves in stained preparations regardless of dose or duration of exposure.

The early detection of lesions is more of an academic problem. It is of little interest in detecting drug induced morphological changes 6–24 hours after exposure to a chemical stimulus if the experimental design for the safety evaluation of such a substance calls for an experiment of 3–12 months' duration. However, if one is interested in the development of such changes, the combination of electron microscopy with conventional light microscopy in a time sequence study is certainly worth while.

Electron microscopy can provide diagnostic assistance to morphological problems already recognizable by conventional light microscopy. Usually pronounced, chemically-induced lesions that can be seen readily with an ordinary light microscope do not need supplementation by electron microscopy. But many exceptions are possible and examples for such a supplementation have been presented by Benitz *et al.* (1967) and Koss (1967).

The use of electron microscopy is limited by the number of samples that can be processed and examined, and by the sampling procedures themselves, especially in organs with distinct morphological zonations (e.g. kidney, adrenal cortex) or microtopographical biochemical differences (hepatic lobule). Continuous transitions in magnification (dissecting microscope, phase microscopy of unstained thick sections, low power electron micrographs, ×5,000–12,000) may help to define the origin of the samples by proper microtopographical orientation.

Since electron microscopy has its limitations, one should carefully formulate the problems to be studied by ultrastructural analysis. Pease (1964) has stated that it would take more than 7 years of continuous photography to record the structures within 1 cm², an area which can be surveyed by a pathologist in 5 min or less. The practice of fixing every liver from a toxicity study in buffered glutaraldehyde has no justification and points to the improper use of electron microscopy. Peculiar morphological findings from previous experiments or from animals that died prior to the scheduled termination of the study, abnormal results of function tests and clinical chemistry determinations, and special storage and metabolism phenomena help to pinpoint morphological problems worthy of ultrastructural investigation.

Quantification of Morphological Structures

The quantification of drug-induced morphological changes should not be limited to qualitative descriptions that are occasionally accompanied by illustrations. The pathologist participating in toxicity studies usually works in close cooperation with scientists from other disciplines such as pharmacology, toxicology, biochemistry, and biophysics. These branches of biological science have used the quantitative approach to problems whereas morphology remained largely qualitative. Mere descriptions of morphological changes in qualitative terms are no longer acceptable and attempts should always be made to quantify drug-induced morphological changes.

The most widely used method is the assignment of grades to pathological changes or normally-existing structures as outlined in Table 4.13. These semiquantitative procedures provide fairly

Table 4.13   Rank estimates or grades

For pathological changes, absent = normal in control population			For changes of normally occurring structures and their components			
Degrees	Numbers	Symbols for Degrees or Numbers		Increases	Symbols	Decreases Symbols
Absent	Absent	0	0	Normal	N	Normal N
Doubtful	Doubtful	$+/-$	?	Question-able	$N+$	Question- $N-$ able
Slight	Few	$+$	1	Slight	I1	Slight D1
Moderate	Several	$++$	2	Moderate	I2	Moderate D2
Marked	Many	$+++$	3	Marked	I3	Marked D3

accurate estimates of morphological changes. Generally, these grades are obtained from some unsystematical ranking procedure and the number of useful ones is limited. According to Mayer (1963), plus signs, grades in excess of 4, or intermediary grades such as 2 to 3 plus make the final tabulation of data complicated and thus defeat the purpose.

Rank methods such as developed by Wilcoxon (1945, 1947) and Litchfield & Wilcoxon (1955) avoid these difficulties and there is no problem of intermediary steps since the number of rank places is unlimited. The ranking of morphological changes shows good correlation with biochemical analyses. Mayer (1963) has demonstrated a good comparison of histochemical and chemical estimates of glycogen in rat livers and Sparano (1965) has used the same procedure to establish a positive correlation between Sudan-positive material and chemical estimates of fat.

Hennig (1958), Weibel (1963) and Weibel *et al.* (1966) have reviewed point and line sampling techniques and better methods than the one published by Chalkley (1943) are now available. Some practical examples using various combinations of morphological quantification techniques have been published by Benitz and Dambach (1964).

The determination of nuclear volume in target organs can be helpful in assessing the functional state on the basis of swelling or contracting of nuclei as introduced by Benninghoff (1950). These measurements can be carried out relatively easily by determining the largest and smallest diameter of a sufficient number of nuclei. These values are then put into the formula for the rotation ellipsoid and the nuclear volume can be determined by calculators or computers. Some authors have limited their morphological investigation to these measurements alone. In some cases this may not be sufficient and the addition of other quantitative procedures may be helpful. In our control population of rats, we found two animals with thyroid glands of different size. One was grossly and microscopically normal. The amount of epithelium was 66·2% and the respective amount of the colloid was 20·7% of the glandular volume. The nuclear volume in this particular gland was 94·6 μ^3. The other gland was slightly enlarged; microscopically, marked hyperplasia and hypertrophy were noted. The amount of epithelium was increased to 87·5%, and the amount of colloid was decreased to 3·8%. However, the nuclear volume in this particular gland was 92·5 μ^3, which

Table 4.14 Summary of histological quantification methods and their applications for chemically induced lesions.

Procedures	Histological substrates	Comments
Counts	Bile plugs, giant cells, mast cells, calcification sites, mitoses, etc.	Expressed as average number/field; total number/ section, etc.
Linear measurements	Thinning of femoral epiphyseal disc; hyperplasia of zona glomerulosa in adrenal cortex; reduction in height of spermatogenic epithelium; decrease of tubular diameter of testes	Calibrated micrometer, results in micrometer units or μ
Area measurements	Muscles: necrosis Uterus: atrophy of mucosa and myometrium Brain: hydrocephalus	Components expressed in planimeter values obtained from tracings or projections
Nuclear volume	Hyperplasia of thyroid gland; dystrophy of adrenal cortex; atrophy of liver due to starvation	Two perpendicular measurements using computerized formula of rotation ellipsoid for calculating μ^3
Composition of organs	Hyperplasia of thyroid gland: epithelium colloid, open capillaries, etc. Atrophy of ovaries: ratio of primary follicles to corpora lutea Cirrhosis of liver: density of reticulum fibres Composition of submaxillary glands: ratio of mucous to serous terminal portions	Point sampling[a] Components expressed in percentage of organ volumes
Nuclear density	Dystrophy in zona fasciculata of adrenal cortex	
Internal surface measurements	Alveolar surface in lungs altered by inflammation, fibrosis, or emphysema. Trabecular surface in femoral epiphysis altered by osteodystrophy	Line sampling[a] Results expressed in mm^2/mm^3 of organ volume

[a] For methodology and examples see Hennig (1958) and Benitz & Dambach (1964).

was within the normal range of the population examined. In this instance the use of the nuclear volume alone would have been misleading.

Table 4.14 gives a summary of histological quantification methods that can be used for the assessment of drug-induced morphological changes. Many of these procedures can be combined so that the investigator does not have to rely on one method alone.

According to Pease (1964), electron microscopy should not accept problems that are primarily statistical. This statement could be interpreted in such a manner that the quantification of ultrastructural changes would be almost impossible. This is mainly due to the small number of samples that can be examined and photographed. However, attempts have been made recently to quantify ultrastructural components by simple counts (Fletcher & Yusa, 1967) and by point and line sampling procedures (Loud *et al.*, 1964; Weibel *et al.*, 1966; Sitte, 1967).

PRESENTATION OF RESULTS

It may be pertinent in a chapter concerned with practical procedures that are used in chronic toxicity experiments to devote some lines to the presentation of results of these studies. A computerized operation for the evaluation of chronic toxicity data as outlined by Small (1967) may be helpful in retrieving and assembling information but such a system cannot replace a well organized, logical final presentation of the data that originate from these studies.

Nelson (1965) and Mayer (1963) have published some ground rules with examples of how pathology data should be recorded and reported. Similar principles should be applied to the results obtained by other disciplines, such as toxicology and biochemistry, which are also involved in a safety evaluation programme. Clarity should have priority over elegance; toxic effects should be presented clearly; all material should be organized logically; tables and figures should be self-contained requiring no reference to the text. One should always keep in mind that toxicity studies have to be reviewed by many persons in industrial or academic laboratories, government agencies, and by clinicians who need this information in order to conduct meaningful clinical trials. Kilogram quantities of raw data are incomprehensible. Very often the most essential information is found only after a long search through pages and pages of documentation. This must be avoided but does not necessarily mean that detailed and individual data should be omitted from the presentation of results. Such material can be attached as appendices for handy reference if the need arises.

After having read numerous reports, manuscripts and publications, I feel that an outline as shown in Table 4.15 may be helpful for the organization and presentation of toxicity data.

Table 4.15 Outline for organization and presentation of toxicity data.

I. Origin and Purpose of Study
II. Materials and Methods
    A. Experimental design
    B. Chronological sequence
    C. Identification of drug or foreign chemical including purity and stability data
    D. Species and strain of animal used
    E. Animal maintenance and environmental conditions
    F. Methods for clinical observations
    G. Methods for function tests, clinical chemistry, and haematology
    H. Methods for the determination of concentration of drugs in serum or tissues
    I. Autopsy techniques and histological procedures
    J. Morphological quantification techniques
    K. Statistical evaluation of numerical data
III. Results
    A. Observations during life
        1. Mortality
        2. Body weight gain
        3. Clinical observations
        4. Function tests, clinical chemistry, and haematology
        5. Concentration of drug in serum
    B. Post-mortem studies
        1. Body weights, organ weights, and skeletal measurements
        2. Treatment-induced morphological changes in various organ systems
        3. Influence of treatment on incidence and severity of spontaneous diseases
        4. Concentration of drug in tissues
IV. Discussion and Interpretation
V. Summary and Conclusions
VI. List of References

In most chronic toxicity experiments the results should be discussed in terms of previous knowledge with the class of compound under study. A critical evaluation should be made of the chemically induced physiological, biochemical, and morphological findings with respect to the intended use of the compound. Species differing with respect to reactivity and the interpretation of the findings in terms of what is known in the literature with respect to certain biological phenomena may help to put the results in proper perspective.

There should be a definite statement as to which dose levels appear safe and which produce toxic effects. This can be easily achieved by a summary table limiting its contents to the pertinent facts that resulted from any given experiment. If the results do not lend themselves to drawing definite conclusions, one should not hesitate to say so. Mayer (1963) has stated that clear cut conclusions, hypothetical interpretations, and recommendations for future work add to the value of a report, yet many investigators are reluctant to commit themselves presumably under the assumption that the results of future experiments may show that they were wrong. According to Hoff (1956) a fear of correlating individual observations and data inhibits the formulation of hypotheses and results in the mere presentation of unconnected fragments and in the stifling of new scientific concepts. This fear is not justified since honest mistakes are unavoidable in any developing science. It is especially true in toxicology which is a young science that has to absorb the approaches and methodology from various disciplines of biological research.

REFERENCES

ABRAMS W.B., ZBINDEN G. & BAGDON R. (1965) Investigative methods in clinical toxicology. *J. new Drugs* **5,** 199–207.

BAKER S.B. DE C. & ALCOCK S.J. (1965) An apparent change in toxicity of a compound when dosed for seven days a week instead of five. *Experimental studies and clinical experience—the assessment of risk, Proc. Eur. Soc. for the Study of Drug Toxicity* **6,** 213–18 (International Congress Series No. 97). Amsterdam, Excerpta Medica Foundation.

BALAZS T. (1970) Measurement of acute toxicity, in *Methods of Toxicology,* ed. PAGET G.E. Oxford, Blackwell Scientific Publications.

BALAZS T. (1970) Measurement of acute toxicity, in *Methods of Toxicology,* toxicity studies on rats. *Toxic. appl. Pharmac.* **5,** 661–74.

BARNES J.M. & DENZ I.A. (1954) Experimental methods used in determining chronic toxicity. *Pharmac. Rev.* **6**, 191–242.

BARRON C. (1965) Discussion of organ weights following: The recording and reporting of pathology data by A.A. NELSON, in *The Pathology of Laboratory Animals*, eds. RIBELIN W.E. & McCOY J.R. Springfield, Illinois, Charles C. Thomas.

BARTLETT G.R. (1959) Phosphorus assay in column chromatography. *J. Biol. Chem.* **234**, 466–8.

BEIN H.J. (1963) Rational and irrational numbers in toxicology. *Viewpoints on the study of Drug Toxicity, Proc. Eur. Soc. for the Study of Drug Toxicity* **2**, 15–26 (International Congress Series No. 73). Amsterdam, Excerpta Medica Foundation.

BENITZ K.-F. & DAMBACH G. (1964) Quantification of drug-induced morphologic changes with Hennig's point- and line-sampling methods using Zeiss integrating eyepieces I and II. *Arzneimittel-Forsch.* **14**, 929–35.

BENITZ K.-F. & DIERMEIER H.F. (1964) Renal toxicity of tetracycline degradation products. *Proc. Soc. exp. Biol. Med.* **115**, 930–5.

BENITZ K.-F., KRAMER A.W. & DAMBACH G. (1965) Comparative studies on the morphologic effects of calcium carbimide, propylthiouracil, and disulfiram in male rats. *Toxic. appl. Pharmac.* **7**, 128–62.

BENITZ K.-F., MORASKI R.M. & CUMMINGS J.R. (1961) Relation of heart weight, ventricular ratio, and kidney weight to body weight and arterial blood pressure in normal and hypertensive rats. *Lab. Invest.* **10**, 934–46.

BENITZ K.-F., ROBERTS G.K.S. & YUSA A. (1967) Morphologic effects of minocycline in laboratory animals. *Toxic. appl. Pharmac.* **11**, 150–70.

BENNINGHOFF A. (1950) Funktionelle Kernschwellung und Kernschrumpfung. *Anat. Nachr.* **1**, 50–2.

BEYER KARL H. Jr. (1966) Perspectives in toxicology. *Toxic. appl. Pharmac.* **8**, 1–5.

BJÖRKMAN J.E. (1959) A new method for enumeration of platelets. *Acta Haemat.* **22**, 377–9.

BLOOM F. (1960) *The urine of dog and cat.* New York, Gamma Publishing Co.

BOYD E.M. (1965) Part I: Preclinical testing, (2) Toxicological studies, in *Clinical Testing of New Drugs*, eds. HERRICK A.D. & CATTEL M. New York, Revere Publishing Co.

BOYD E.M. (1968) Predictive drug toxicity: Assessment of drug safety before human use. *Can. Med. Ass. J.* **98**, 278–93.

BRODIE B.B. (1964) Kinetics of absorption, distribution, excretion, and metabolism of drugs, in *Animal and Clinical Pharmacologic Techniques in Drug Evaluation*, eds. NODINE J.H. & SIEGLER P.E. Chicago, Year Book Medical Publishers, Inc.

BRODIE B.B. (1966) The mechanisms of adverse reactions, in *Mechanisms of Drug Toxicity, Proc. of the Third International Pharmaceutical Meeting*, ed. RASKOVA H., Vol. 4, pp. 23–47. Oxford, Pergamon Press.

BUSHBY S.R.M., LECHAT J. & SANTARATO R. (1966) Hematological investigations in the toxicity testing of drugs. *Experimental Study of the Effects of Drugs on the Liver, Proc. Eur. Soc. for the Study of Drug Toxicity.* **7,** 208–15 (International Congress Series No. 115). Amsterdam, Excerpta Medica Foundation.

BUSTAD LEO K. & MCCLELLAN ROGER O. (1966). Swine in biomedical research. (Proc. of a symposium at the Pacific Northwest Laboratory, Richland, Washington). Battelle Memorial Institute, Pacific Northwest Laboratory, Richland, Washington.

CARTWRIGHT G.E. (1963) *Diagnostic Laboratory Hematology*, 3rd Edition. New York, Grune & Stratton.

CHALKLEY H.W. (1943) Method for the quantitative morphologic analysis of tissues. *J. Nat. Cancer Inst.* **4,** 47–53.

CORNELIUS C.E. & KANEKO J.J. (1963) Clinical biochemistry of domestic animals. New York, Academic Press.

DESSAU F.I. & SULLIVAN W.J. (1961) A two-year study of the toxicity of chlortetracycline hydrochloride in rats. *Toxic. appl. Pharmac.* **3,** 654–77.

DETWEILER D.K., HUBBEN K. & PATTERSON D.F. (1960) Survey of cardiovascular disease in dogs—preliminary report on the first 1,000 dogs screened. *Am. J. Vet. Res.* **21,** 329–59.

DETWEILER D.K. & PATTERSON D.F. (1965) The prevalence and types of cardiovascular disease in dogs. *Ann. N.Y. Acad. Sci.* **127,** 481–516.

DIXON R.L., SHULTICE R.W. & FOUTS J.R. (1960) Factors affecting drug metabolism by liver microsomes. IV. Starvation. *Proc. Soc. exp. Biol. Med.* **103,** 333–5.

EARL F.L., TEGARIS A.S., WHITMORE G.E., MORISON R. & FITZHUGH O.G. (1964) The use of swine in drug toxicity studies. *Ann. N.Y. Acad. Sci.* **3,** 671–88.

EWALD B.H. (1967) Renal function tests in normal beagle dogs. *Am. J. Vet. Res.* **28,** 741–9.

FAIRBANKS V.F. & BEUTLER E. (1962) A simple method for detection of erythrocyte glucose-6-phosphate dehydrogenase deficiency (G-6-PD Spot Test). *Blood* **20,** 591–601.

FISKE C.H. & SUBBAROW Y. (1925) The colorimetric determination of phosphorus. *J. Biol. Chem.* **66,** 375–400.

FITZHUGH O.G. (1955) Procedures for the appraisal of the toxicity of chemical in foods, drugs and cosmetics. Part VI. Chronic oral toxicity. *Fd. Drug and Cosmetics Law J.* **16,** 712–19.

FITZHUGH O.G., NELSON A.A. & BLISS C.I. (1944) Chronic oral toxicity of selenium. *J. Pharmac. exp. Ther.* **80,** 289–99.

FLETCHER R.D. & YUSA A. (1967) Electron microscopic study of the effect of 2-diethylaminoethyl 4-methylpiperazine-1-carboxylate on influenza virus. *Virology* **31,** 382–5.

FRAZER A.C. (1958) Discussion following chapter on morphological evaluation of toxic action (chapter by PAGET G.E.), in *The Evaluation of Drug Toxicity*, eds. WALPOLE A.L. & SPINKS A. London, J. & A. Churchill.

GERARDE H.W. (1956) Toxicological studies on hydrocarbons. *A.M.A. Arch. ind. Hlth* **13,** 331–5.

GODDARD R.F. (1948) Anatomical and physiological studies in young rats with propylthiouracil-induced dwarfism. *Anat. Rec.* **101,** 539–76.

GOLBERG L. (1965) Part I: Preclinical testing, (3) The predictive value of animal toxicity studies carried out on new drugs in *Clinical Testing of New Drugs, eds.* HERRICK A.D. & CATTELL M. New York, Revere Publishing Co., Inc.

GOLBERG L. (1966) Liver enlargement produced by drugs: its significance. *Experimental Study of the Effects of Drugs on the Liver, Proc. Eur. Soc. for the Study of Drug Toxicity* **7,** 171–84 (International Congress Series No. 115). Amsterdam, Excerpta Medica Foundation.

GOLDENTHAL E.I. (1968) *Current Views on Safety Evaluation of Drugs.* Washington, DC., FDA Papers. U.S. Government Printing Office. Division of Public Documents, May 1968.

GOODWIN J.F. (1961) Estimation of plasma fibrinogen, using sodium sulphite refractionation. *Am. J. clin. Path.* **35,** 227–32.

GRANT J.L., BRITTON M.C. & KURTZ T.E. (1960) Measurement of red blood cell volume with the electronic cell counter. *Am. J. clin. Path.* **33,** 138–43.

HALLESY D.W. & BENITZ K.-F. (1963) Toxicity studies on quinethazone. *Arzneimittel-Forsch.* **13,** 665–73.

HAWK P.B., OSER B.L. & SUMMERSON W.H. (1947) *Practical Physiological Chemistry,* 12th edition. Philadelphia, Blakiston Co.

HENNIG A. (1959) A critical survey of volume and surface measurements in miscroscopy. *Zeiss-Werkz.* **6,** 3–12.

HOFF F. (1956) Kritische Betrachtungen zu Grundproblemen der Krankheitslehre. *Von Ärztlichem Denken und Handeln,* pp. 5–36. Stuttgart, Georg Thieme Verlag.

HOFFMAN W.S. (1937) A rapid photoelectric method for the determination of glucose in blood and urine. *J. Biol. Chem.* **120,** 51–5.

HULSE E.V. (1965) Laboratory animals in experimental haematology. *Fd. Cosmetics Toxic.* **3,** 735–48.

ISRAELI J., PELAVIN M. & KESSLER G. (1960) Continuous automatic integrated flame photometry. *Ann. N.Y. Acad. Sci.* **87,** 636–49.

JACKSON B. (1962) Statistical analysis of body weight data. *Toxic. appl. Pharmac.* **4,** 432–43.

JACKSON B. & CAPPIELLO V.P. (1964). Ranges of normal organ weights of dogs. *Toxic. appl. Pharmac.* **6,** 664–8.

JANKŮ I. (1966) Quantitative aspects of chronic toxicity. *Mechanisms of Drug Toxicity, Proc. of the Third International Pharmacological Meeting,* ed. RASKOVA H., **4,** 65–73. Oxford. Pergamon Press.

JEMSKI J.V. & PHILLIPS G.B. (1965) Aerosol challenge of animals, in *Methods of Animal Experimentation,* ed. GAY W.I. New York, Academic Press.

KESSLER G. & WOLFMAN M. (1964) An automated procedure for the simultaneous determination of calcium and phosphorus. *Clin. Chem.* **10,** 686–703.

Koss L.G. (1967) A light and electron microscopic study of the effects of a single dose of cyclophosphamide on various organs in the rat. I. The urinary bladder. *Lab. Invest.* **16,** 44–65.

Krawitz L. (1965) Clinical examination of the canine and feline eye. *J. Am. vet. med. Ass.* **147,** 33–7.

Lee R.I. & White P.D. (1913) A clinical study of the coagulation time of blood. *Am. J. med. Sci.* **145,** 495–503.

Litchfield J.T. Jr. & Wilcoxon F. (1955) The rank correlation method. *Anal. Chem.* **27,** 299–300.

Loud A.V., Barany W.C. & Pack B.A. (1964) Quantitative evaluation of cytoplasmic structures in electron micrographs, in *Quantitative Electron Microcopy,* eds. Bahr G.F. & Zeitler E.H., pp. 258–70. Baltimore, The Williams & Wilkins Co.

Magrane William G. (1965). *Canine Ophthalmology.* Philadelphia, Lea & Febiger.

March W.H., Fingerhut B. & Kirsch E. (1957) Determination of urea nitrogen with the diacetyl method and an automatic dialyzing apparatus. *Am. J. clin. Path.* **28,** 681–8.

Mayer Edmund (1963) Introduction to Dynamic Morphology. New York, Academic Press.

Mayer E. & Ruzicka A.Q. (1945) A method for studying numerical and topographic problems in the whole femoral marrow of rats and guinea pigs, with the use of undecalcified sections. *Anat. Rec.* **93,** 213–28.

Minich E. (1966) Prediction of the potential toxicity of anticancer agents from studies in animals. *Methods of Drug Evaluation, Proc. of the International Symposium,* eds. Mantegazza P. & Piccinini F., pp. 393–410. Amsterdam, North Holland Publishing Co.

Moreland A.F. (1965) Collection and withdrawal of body fluids and infusion techniques, in *Methods of Animal Experimentation,* ed. Gay W.I. New York, Academic Press.

Nelson A.A. (1965) The recording and reporting of pathology data in *The Pathology of Laboratory Animals,* eds. Ribelin W.E. & McCoy J.R. Springfield, Illinois, Charles C. Thomas.

Nicolaysen R. & Nygaard A.P. (1963) The determination of triglycerides and phospholipids. *Scand. J. clin. lab. Invest.* **15,** 79–82.

Owens A.H. Jr. (1962) Predicting effects of anticancer drugs in man from laboratory animal studies. *Cancer Chemother. Rep.* **16,** 557–60.

Paget G.E. & Barnes J.M. (1964) Toxicity tests, in *Evaluation of Drug Activities: Pharmacometrics,* eds. Laurence D.R. & Bacharach A.L., Vol. 1, pp. 135–66. London & New York, Academic Press.

Paget G.E. & Lemon P.G. (1965) The interpretation of pathology data, in *The Pathology of Laboratory Animals,* eds. Ribelin W.E. & McCoy J.R. Springfield, Illinois, Charles C. Thomas.

Pease Daniel C. (1964) *Histological Techniques for Electron Microscopy,* 2nd edition. New York, Academic Press.

Peck Harold M. (1966) Evaluating the safety of drugs. *BioScience* **16,** 696–701.

PEKAS J.C. & BUSTAD L.K. (1965) A selected list of references (1960–1965) on swine in biomedical research. Atomic Energy Commission Research and Development Report (BNWL-115). Pacific Northwest Laboratory, Richland, Washington.

PETERS J.M. (1967) Organ weights and water contents of fully grown female rats. *Toxic. appl. Pharmac.* **10,** 21–6.

PLIESS G. & FASSBENDER D. (1961) Die Wirkung subletaler Dosen von Endoxan (R) auf die Hämopoese der Ratte. *Arzneimittel-Forsch.* **11,** 179–88.

REUTNER T.F. & KAUMP D.H. (1967) Personal Communication. Parke Davis and Co., Departments of Experimental Therapeutics, Pathology and Toxicology, Ann Arbor, Michigan.

RICHAR W.J. & BREAKELL E.S. (1959) Evaluation of an electronic particle counter for the counting of white blood cells. *Am. J. clin. Path.* **31,** 384–93.

RÜMKE C.L. (1964) Some limitations of animal tests, in *Evaluation of Drug Activities: Pharmacometrics,* eds., LAURENCE D.R. & BACHARACH A.L. Vol. 1, pp. 125–33. London & New York, Academic Press.

SCHROGIE J.J. (1968) Drug Interactions. *FDA Papers,* pp. 11–13. November.

SELIGSON, I., MARINO J. & DODSON E. (1957) Determination of sulforbromophthalein in serum. *Clin. Chem.* **3,** 638–45.

Sigma Technical Bulletins (No. 505 and No. 660). St Louis. Missouri, Sigma Chemical Co.

SITTE H. (1967) Morphometrische Untersuchungen an Zellen. In *Quantitative Methods in Morphology,* eds. WEIBEL E.R. & ELIAS H., pp. 167–98. Berlin & Heidelberg, Springer-Verlag.

SKEGGS L.T. (1957) An automatic method for colorimetric analysis. *Am. J. Clin. Path.* **28,** 311–22.

SMALL R.M. (1967) Use of computers in the evaluation of chronic toxicity studies. *Drug Inf. Bull. of the DIA,* Jan./March, pp. 48–53.

SMITH I. (1960) *Chromatographic and Electrophoretic Techniques,* Vol. 2: *Zone electrophoresis.* New York, Interscience Publishers, Inc.

SPARANO B.M. (1965) Sex difference in chlortetracycline-induced fatty livers in rats. *Lab. Invest.* **14,** 1931–8.

STREET A. (1970) Clinical Biochemistry in Toxicology. A technical discussion. In *Methods in Toxicology, ed.* PAGET G.E. Oxford, Blackwell Scientific Publications.

THER L. (1965) *Grundlagen der experimentellen Arzneimittel-Forschung.* Stuttgart, Wissenschaftliche Verlagsgesellschaft m. b. H.

THOMPSON SAMUEL W. & HUNT RONALD D. (1966) *Selected Histochemical and Histopathological Methods.* Springfield, Illinois, Charles C. Thomas.

TRINDER P. (1952) The determination of cholesterol in serum. *Analyst* **77,** 321–5.

VAN HANDEL E. (1961) Suggested modification of the microdetermination of triglycerides. *Clin. Chem.* **7,** 249–51.

VOGEL A.W. (1961) Tumour-marrow index: A means of laboratory evaluation of antineoplastic compounds. *Cancer Res.* **21,** 1450–4.

WAALKES T.P. & UDENFRIEND S. (1957) A fluorometric method for the estimation of tyrosine in plasma and tissues. *J. Lab. clin. Med.* **50**, 733–6.

WEIBEL E.R. & ELIAS H. [eds.] (1967) *Quantitative Methods in Morphology.* Springer-Verlag.

WEIBEL E.R., KISTLER G.S. & SCHERLE W.F. (1966) Practical stereological methods for morphometric cytology. *J. Cell Biol.* **30**, 23–38.

WORLD HEALTH ORGANIZATION (1966) Principles for pre-clinical testing of drug safety. *Tech. Rep. Ser. Wld Hlth Org.* 341. Geneva.

WILCOXON F. (1945) Individual comparisons by ranking methods. *Biometr. Bull.* **1**, 80–3.

WILCOXON F. (1947) Probability tables for individual comparisons by ranking methods. *Biometrics* **3**, 119–22.

WILLIS, R.A. (1953) *Pathology of Tumors*, 2nd edition. London, Butterworth.

WINTROBE M.M. (1961) *Clinical Hematology*. Philadelphia, Lea and Febiger.

WOODARD G. (1965) Principles in drug administration, in *Methods of Animal Experimentation*, ed. GAY W.I. New York, Academic Press.

ZALL D.M., FISHER D. & GARNER M.Q. (1956) Photometric determination of chlorides in water. *Anal. Chem.* **28**, 1665–8.

ZLATKIS, A., ZAK B. & BOYLE A.J. (1958) A new method for the direct determination of serum cholesterol. *J. Lab. clin. Med.* **41**, 486–92.

CHAPTER 5

Detection of Teratogenic Actions

The late C.S. DELAHUNT

INTRODUCTION

Eight thousand children were estimated as having been born malformed from thalidomide. There is no device or concept of measurement that can describe the parental grief or emotional suffering nor the problems these deformed children will encounter in their lives. However, present and future generations of scientists, or more especially toxicologists, should never forget this utterly sad event encountered because of a hiatus in our scientific knowledge. At that time, none of the animal testing procedures in vogue could have predicted this tragedy.

Landauer (1945) was one of the early workers to show a drug to be teratogenic in experimental animals. He demonstrated that insulin treatment of developing chick embryos produces morphological abnormalities. Chomette (1955) induced several different types of malformations in rabbits from injections of this hormone. Pregnant mice given insulin also produce deformed offspring (Smithberg et al., 1956). Some investigators feel that if an agent is teratogenic in three species of laboratory animals, it will be deleterious to the human embryo. Needless to say, insulin has never been implicated as a teratogen in man; on the contrary, it prevents the malformations that may occur in infants born of untreated diabetic mothers (Hoet, 1960). The majority of teratologists agree that most pharmacologically active agents tested under certain circumstances, can be shown to be teratogenic in experimental animals.

How then can teratogenic testing in animals of a prospective human therapeutic agent provide meaningful predictive results? The most meaningful assessment of animal experimentation comes from comparative, animal-to-man, retrospective analysis. There are eight known human teratogenic agents or groups of agents that will cause morphological abnormalities. They are thalidomide, excessive vitamin D, radiation, androgens, cytotoxic agents, rubella, cytomeglic virus, and toxoplasmosis. There may also be agents which will produce functional alterations. This latter subject is briefly discussed later.

Teratogenic studies, as a phase of animal safety evaluation of drugs, must encompass all the aspects of toxicology applied to the process of reproduction, with emphasis on the investigation of the effect of a drug on the foetus itself. Therefore, it is worthwhile to consider in some detail the usual procedures for a toxicity study, as related to teratology. Each facet of the toxicity testing programme will be discussed separately. Those parameters which appear to be most useful for a meaningful teratogenic system will be combined in an attempt to construct a programme for what might be considered an ideal system for the detection of teratogenic action of a new drug.

This chapter will not be a comprehensive review of teratology. There are numerous excellent articles on this subject: Kalter & Warkany (1959), Cahen (1964), Karnosky (1965), Ciba Symposium (1960), European Society for the Study of Drug Toxicity Symposium (1963), First and Second International Conferences on Congenital Malformations (1961, 1964), Wilson & Warkany (1965), and Teratogenesis (1964).

SELECTION OF SPECIES

As in general toxicity studies, selection of the proper experimental animal will govern the accuracy with which the possible adverse effects of a drug in man may be predicted (Delahunt *et al.*, 1965). Almost all the laboratory species have been examined, at one time or another, in the study of congenital malformations. The advantages and disadvantages of each common laboratory animal will be discussed briefly.

CHICK EMBRYO
Landauer's work with insulin has already been cited. Somers (1963) was not able to induce defects in the chick embryo by treatment with thalidomide. William *et al.* (1963) demonstrated that

thalidomide could cause some anomalies in the chick embryo, but sand and other inert materials could cause similar defects. The solvent, dimethylsulfoxide, was tested in three different types of laboratory animals (Caujolle, 1965); defects were noted only on the chicken embryo; none were reported to have occurred in mice or rabbits. The cytotoxic cancer therapeutic agents appear to be teratogenic in all mammalian species, as well as the fertilized chicken egg.

Some compounds could conceivably be metabolized in the mother from a nonteratogen to a teratogen. Tests conducted in developing chick embryos would fail to reveal this effect, for the compound would not pass through a maternal alimentary canal and other usual physiological pathways followed by a drug administered orally. For this reason, the chick embryo is not considered a prime species in which to detect drug-induced malformations. However, it is useful in antimetabolite investigations. The chicken embryo could be utilized in pesticide work to determine an insecticide's effect on game bird embryos (Marliac, 1964). The various authors cited have described methods in this and other cases that are completely satisfactory for problems oriented to a specific need.

MOUSE
Fraser & Fainstat (1951) and other workers have reported cleft palates in mice treated with cortisone. This discovery was utilized (Pinsky & DiGeorge, 1965) as a technique for evaluating the potency of steroids. The potency of corticosteroids in inducing this remarkable effect in the mouse appears to closely parallel anti-inflammatory activity in man. Fortunately, cleft palates have not been a problem in children whose mothers have been treated with steroids (Bongiovanni & McPadden, 1960).

Courrier (1962) reported that thalidomide produced congenital anomalies but his results have not been confirmed. The defects he reported in mice did not resemble the 'thalidomide syndrome' observed in man.

Many drugs have been tested in this species but the results have little or no predictive value for effects in man. The only exception to this statement appears to be the current cancer chemotherapeutic agents (Karnosky, 1965). For example, aminopterin (Sansone & Zunin, 1964) has induced CNS malformations in this species similar to those noted in man (Thiersh, 1952).

RAT

Kim *et al.* (1960) conducted several very interesting studies in rats that were made 'subdiabetic'. These studies provided a good method for investigating the action of insulin on pregnancy. Insulin administered throughout pregnancy prevented prolongation of gestation and reduced foetal mortality. No hormonal-induced malformations were reported in these studies. Tuchmann-Duplessis (1958) reported that massive amounts of the oral hypoglycaemic agent BZ-55, administered to pregnant rats, produced cataracts in rat pups, as well as other defects.

Cyclizine has been shown to be capable of inducing cleft palates, cataracts and bone growth retardation (Tuchmann-Duplessis, 1963). King (1963) tested a related antihistamine, meclizine, which produced cleft palates, but no cataracts, in the rat. He also utilized the rat to evaluate thalidomide, and found the results in no way similar to the syndrome induced in man by this drug. Lenz (1964) has commented on the teratogenic capabilities of the two latter compounds (meclizine and thalidomide) in man. In contrast to the devastating effects of thalidomide on the human foetus, Lenz has pointed out that meclizine has not been shown to be teratogenic in humans. Thus, the rat has demonstrated some false positive as well as some false negative responses. These data are presented in Table 5.1.

Table 5.1 Teratogenic effects of thalidomide and meclizine in rat and man.

Drug	Reference	Species	Dose (mg/kg)	Teratogenic
Meclizine	King, 1963	Rat	125	Yes
Meclizine	Lenz, 1964	Man	2	No
Thalidomide	King, 1962	Rat	50	No
Thalidomide	Lenz, 1964	Man	4	Yes

RABBIT

Girls born of mothers treated with testosterone during pregnancy show evidence of masculinization (Jacobson, 1962). Courrier & Jost (1942) have demonstrated a similar developmental abnormality in the female progeny of pregnant rabbits that received ethinyl testosterone.

Somers' (1963) work with thalidomide has focused interest in this species. By administering 150 mg/kg of the drug to pregnant rabbits, phocomelia, the external skeletal defect of the thalidomide syndrome, was induced. Some pharmacologic and toxicologic correlations with man have been demonstrated in this species. Pharmacologically, the rabbit or man treated with thalidomide has an EEG pattern compatible with induced sleep (Giurgea & Moeyersoons, 1963). Toxicologically, we have been unable to reproduce in the rabbit, or even the monkey, the peripheral neuritis noted in some older human patients treated with this hypnotic (Florence, 1960; Howe, 1961). In our studies, however, only a few animals were treated, all of them young, and the limited numbers and age range may have been inappropriate for the detection of this type of toxicity. The unique ocular toxicity of chloroquine observed in man has only been manifested in pigmented rabbits (Dale *et al.*, 1965).

There are, however, several cases where tests in rabbits have given false results. Tuchmann-Duplessis (1963) describes malformations due to cyclizine in the rabbit. This compound has not been shown to be a human teratogen. Nevertheless, the rabbit shows more parallelism with man than do most other species. Therefore, it is recommended for inclusion in a primary teratogenic screen for drug safety.

Yeary (1964a), Staemmler *et al.* (1964) and others have pointed out the problem associated with spontaneous abnormalities in this species. There are few reports in the literature on the normal incidence of malformations in the rabbit. Care must be taken to differentiate, as much as possible, between spontaneous and induced malformations. The pharmacological principle of the 'dose-effect relationship' is indeed applicable to all teratogenic investigations.

HAMSTER

Dimethylsulfoxide (DMSO) has produced exencephaly and anencephaly in the golden hamster (Ferm, 1966). Two viruses have been inoculated into hamsters by several workers (Toolan, 1960; Kilham, 1961) and have caused abnormalities. Monif *et al.* (1965) have studied the H-1 and RV viruses in the human population without finding any adverse effects. Fratta *et al.* (1965) had no success producing typical thalidomide defects in the hamster. Somers (1963) gave thalidomide to these animals without producing any defects. Another group of workers (Homburger *et al.*, 1964), using thalidomide, induced a low incidence of congenital anomalies in this species. Chen (1945) published on the pharmacologic response of the hamster to several different drugs. This rodent does not seem to have any attributes which make it superior to the rat.

CAT

A few investigators have utilized cats for teratogenic testing (Yeary, 1964b; Somers, 1963). Thalidomide, administered to cats by these workers, did not result in defects similar to the syndrome induced by thalidomide in the human. The possible teratogenic sequelae of feline diseases has apparently not been investigated. Unless an ideal environment is provided for cats, diseases (especially viral diseases) run rampant. The cat is not recommended as a primary species for testing the teratogenic potential of a drug at this time.

DOG

Weidman *et al.* (1963) administered thalidomide to dogs without significant effects being noted. Delatour (1965) reported phocomelia after he treated dogs with this drug. Friedman (1957) has stated that azaserine causes severe congenital anomalies when pregnant bitches are treated with this drug.

Five or six-month old beagles are commonly used as part of a chronic toxicity study. The bitch usually comes into heat after 6 or 7 months of age. Mating at the first oestrus period is a most practical procedure. This regime would provide two oestrus cycles for a one-year chronic toxicity investigation. Since these animals are so readily available and they are not usually difficult to breed, the low and middle treated groups of dogs should be mated. Determination of drug pharmacokinetics should be attempted. This metabolic information will be of great assistance in interpreting not only the teratogenic but also the toxicity data.

MONKEY

To date, the use of primates in teratogenic testing has been very limited. Yet, in many instances, the monkey has been the only animal which manifested a toxic effect that has been noted in man (Schmidt, 1962; Potts, 1965; and Earl, 1966). The similarity of the reproductive system in the monkey and man renders the primate especially valuable for the testing of a potential teratogen. The reproductive traits of man and monkey are illustrated in Table 5.2.

Table 5.2 Reproductive characteristics of rat, monkey, and human.

	Rat	Monkey	Man
Type of cycle	oestrus	menstrual	menstrual
Length of cycle (days)	5	28	28
Gestation (days)	21	155	270
Uterus	bicornate	pyriform	pyriform
Placenta	haemo-endothelial	haemo-chorial	haemo-chorial
Progeny	12	1	1

The rat is included as an example of a species having an oestrus cycle.

The most useful indication of pharmacologic activity of a hypnotic is the EEG. Lelahunt *et al.* (1965) have reported that the macaque treated with thalidomide had EEG patterns that were characteristic of sleep. This same pharmacologic response was observed in man subsequent to drug treatment. The above-mentioned authors have shown that the thalidomide drug blood levels after one oral treatment were very similar in man and monkey.

Many investigators (Habel, 1942; Cabasso & Stebbins, 1965; Krugman *et al.*, 1953; Sever, 1965; Parkman *et al.*, 1965) have employed the monkey in the study of experimental rubella infection, and consider it an ideal model for this purpose. There is one important exception in that primates do not appear to manifest the rash associated with German measles in the human. The monkey, in general, does contract this disease much like the human. This comparable relationship of rubella in the monkey and man serves as an example of a sound basis for initiating teratogenic investigations of this particular microbiologic agent in the primate. The virus does produce the human rubella syndrome in the offspring from inoculated monkeys (Delahunt & Rieser, 1966). If an experimental animal responds, clinically or biochemically, to a disease or drug similar to man, there would be sufficient rationale to evaluate its teratogenic potential in that species.

One might hope that similarities in toxic responses, biochemistry, and anatomy between the monkey and man might be translated to a comparable teratogenic response. Table 5.3 shows that this has indeed been the case in the small number of experiments reported to date.

Table 5.3   Comparative human to monkey teratogenic data.

Treatment	Man	Monkey	Primate reference
Thalidomide	+	+	Delahunt & Lassen, 1964
Aspirin	0	0	Palotta, 1966
Rubella	+	+	Delahunt, 1966
Rubeola	0	0	Riazantsera, 1959
Testosterone	+	+	Wells & Van Wagenen, 1954
Meclizine	0	0	Little, 1966

Furthermore, latent embryotoxicity which can be very elusive and insidious, can be detected in the infant primate. For example, the monkey infant can manifest metabolic errors much akin to those seen in the human. Two such conditions are kernicterus (Lucey, 1964) and phenylketonuria-induced mental deficiency (Waissman & Harlow, 1965). Windle (1963) also had induced an anoxic condition at birth in the primate which was similar to human beings with cerebral palsy.

ENVIRONMENTAL CONDITIONS

Environmental conditions must be standardized and rigidly controlled in order to eliminate variables other than those on test. Viral infections, such as hog cholera in pigs, will produce congenital malformations in offspring (Jubb & Kennedy, 1963). Feed contaminated with *Veratrum californium* can cause pregnant sheep to produce offspring with congenital cyclopian deformities (Binns, 1959). Starvation of mice can produce congenital anomalies in the offspring. If a drug causes complete anorexia mice could possibly have malformed progeny from secondary nutritional problems rather than primary drug-induced effects. Kalter & Warkany (1959) have reported on malformations associated with certain dietary deficiencies.

ROUTE OF ADMINISTRATION

The pregnant rat treated with Vitamin A intraperitoneally, or subcutaneously, produces normal offspring (Gebauer, 1954). However,

Cohlan (1954) administered Vitamen A by the oral route to rats and induced malformations in the progeny.

Horita's (1961) work with monoamine oxidase (MAO) inhibitors revealed the importance of the route of administration. The subcutaneous administration of pheniprazine and phenelzine cause a greater MAO activity in the brain than in the liver. When these drugs were given orally greater MAO blockade in liver was found.

Dekker & Mehrizi (1964) employed oil as a vehicle for thalidomide treatment of their rabbits. A more striking and complete syndrome resulted: atonia, facial capillary haemangioma, phocomelia, and amelia were recorded. It may be that the vehicle delayed absorption and provided a prolonged blood level.

The route of administration in animals should mimic that used clinically. In man, oral administration is the most common one because it is the most convenient. Medication should not be administered to rabbits, dogs, monkeys, and large experimental laboratory animals in the drinking water, but rather in the dosage form to be used clinically, or in specially prepared capsules. If an animal drinks only a little medicated water at one time, a significant or meaningful drug blood level may never be obtained.

Lucey & Behrman (1963) administered thalidomide to monkeys orally and found no resultant embryopathy. The test dose that they administered was placed in the drinking water. Since thalidomide is very insoluble, at best only an uneven suspension could have been obtained. The studies of Delahunt & Lassen (1964) with thalidomide in monkeys were performed using gavage. It was found that a considerable amount of drug adhered to the tubing, making it almost impossible to wash all of the drug down the tube. We have found that administering compounds in cherry flavoured syrups on bread, in bananas, candy, or ice cream is much more satisfactory. Since the monkey likes these foods, the probability of his consuming all the drug at one time is practically assured. Such a system of administration also avoids unnecessary handling of the animal. Where drugs are prepared in various oral pharmaceutical formulations, the incipients can also be tested at the same time. This type of oral administration is especially favourable, since it works equally well with different forms of the drug and permits comparison between them.

The absorption of any orally administered substance may be altered by the presence of food in the digestive tract. Certain compounds, such as the tetracyclines, should be administered before, rather than after, feeding, since food impairs absorption of most tetracyclines. Thus, to single out for observation the effects of a drug alone, it is desirable that any compound orally administered be given to fasted animals. The common practice of giving a drug first thing in the morning, after a nocturnal fasting, is recommended.

If emesis or signs of marked pharmacological activity occur, or if a drug is to be given in a multiple daily dose to man, the experimental animal could be dosed on a twice-a-day basis. The oral administration of drugs by stomach tube is extremely time-consuming. If all animals undergoing teratogenic evaluation were treated by gavage tubing, once a day, it would take two men at least 5 hours a day. If the treatment schedule called for twice-a-day administration, it would take two shifts to complete the work. Rats usually eat most of their food at night in three or four large meals. This pattern somewhat resembles a four-times-a-day treatment schedule. Therefore, including the drug in the feed has obvious advantages by comparison to the daily stomach tubing procedure in rats. Additional viewpoints regarding the ideal system for drug dosage will be discussed under the next heading, where comparative blood drug levels are considered.

DRUG DOSAGE LEVELS

Obviously, selection of an appropriate dosage level is vitally important. This point cannot be over emphasized. Drug treatment schedules and the species of animal chosen are the two most important factors in any toxicity study. A useful approach for estimating approximate dosage 'equivalence' can be made, in the case of drugs that are measurably localized in serum, by the administration of the drug at various dosage levels, and subsequent measurement of blood levels of the drug. From comparative animal-to-human blood level data of drugs that do locate in the serum compartment, more meaningful dosage regimens may be selected than are often realized by consideration of dose ingested alone. Naturally, it is important to consider the possible distorting influence of other dynamic properties of drugs, which can and do vary from species to species, and between close chemical analogues. Among the most important of these are drug half-life, and drug localization in tissue.

A classical example of this technique is the work of Schmidt *et al.* (1962) with ethambutol. The monkey, but not the rat or dog (Kaiser, 1964), manifested the ocular toxicity observed in man (Carr & Henkind, 1962) as a result of ethambutol therapy. The former group of workers found that if the monkey's daily drug blood level was kept below 15 μg/ml no toxicity would result. Human studies show that blood levels in excess of 15 μg/ml resulted in eye damage. Human toxicity can be predicted with greater precision, if comparative animal-to-man drug blood levels and potency are considered in the interpretation.

Another example of the application of comparative blood levels to pharmacologic and teratogenic action is our own work with

Table 5.4 Pharmacologic vs teratogenic effect of thalidomide.

Species	EEG		Blood level ($1\gamma/cm^3$)		Embryo-pathy
	Onset (min)	Duration (hr)	Onset (min)	Duration (hr)	
Rabbit	8	2	8	2	incomplete
Monkey	15	6	15	5	complete
Man	30	6	30	6	complete

REFERENCES

	EEG	Blood level	Embryopathy
Rabbit	Giurgea & Moeyersoons, 1963	Delahunt *et al.*, 1965	Somers, 1963
Monkey	Delahunt *et al.*, 1965	Ibid.	Delahunt & Lassen, 1964
Man	Wallenhorst, 1957 Lasagna, 1960	Ibid.	McBride, 1961 Lenz, 1964

thalidomide. Table 5.4 presents a comparison of blood level, pharmacologic effect, and teratogenicity in the rabbit, monkey, and human. Analyses of the blood level data in reference to the EEG response to thalidomide, show that CNS activity became observable when roughly 1 μg of thalidomide per millilitre of blood was obtained. The onset and duration of CNS activity corresponded well with drug blood levels. It certainly seems likely that the teratogenic results achieved by Dekker (1964) in rabbits, where this agent was suspended in oil, are a reflection of prolonged drug blood levels, which exposed the developing embryo to higher concentrations of drug, for longer periods of time, than can be achieved after oral administration. This, in turn, would produce a more complete embryopathologic state.

Comparison of the pattern of metabolism of a drug in man and animals is also important to the selection of an appropriate species for toxicological experimentation. Paper chromatographic finger-printing of urine samples from treated human subjects, and various treated animals, can give a rough indication of the species that best parallels man. It is important to remember that the interaction of drug metabolism and toxicology, as described by Williams (1959) applies equally to teratogenic work. The more complete and quantitative the results of comparative metabolic investigations, the more meaningful will be the prediction of human toxicity or teratogenicity from animal data.

Massive overdosage is not desirable in teratogenic studies. Excessively high doses can produce obvious or subtle maternal toxicity either of which may obscure interpretation of the teratology experiment. Meclizine administered at 125 mg/kg to rats causes mild to marked decreases in water consumption, hypotension, and anorexia (Delahunt, 1964). These may alter embryonic nutrition, and hence a nonspecific teratogenic effect which is not really meaningful in the circumstances of normal clinical use of the drug. Moreover, excessive drug dosage may produce different drug metabolic patterns, quantitatively, qualitatively, or both than would therapeutic levels.

The rat, rabbit, monkey, and man produce a common metabolite, norchlorcyclizine, after oral treatment with meclizine (Figdor, 1966). His metabolism studies suggest that at low levels norchlorcyclizine is cleared relatively rapidly, whereas at excessively high treatment levels the presence of this metabolite inhibits its own clearance to an extent that it leads to accumulation. This is another reason why human therapeutic dosage levels and small multiples thereof should be used in teratologic studies unless comparative man-to-animal drug blood level data are available. The use of dosages more nearly in the range of therapeutic levels might be expected to minimize the likelihood of this kind of metabolic artifact. A human therapeutic dose of thalidomide was capable of producing malformations in the monkey (Wilson, 1966).

Excessive doses may also give a biphasic response. An example of this is the depressant action of hydroxyzine on gastric secretion in dogs. Although the drug suppresses secretion at 1 mg/kg, excessive levels of this agent results in anomalous stimulation of gastric secretion (Harrison *et al.*, 1959).

DURATION OF DRUG TREATMENT

To exclude the variables of a drug's effect on ovulation and implantation, one should treat after implantation. Table 5.5 summarizes implantation and gestation times for some of the laboratory animals.

Table 5.5 Implantation and gestation time of some laboratory animals (after Spector, 1957).

Species	Implantation time (days)	Gestation time (days)
Mouse	4–5	19
Rat	5–6	21
Hamster	5+	15–18
Rabbit	7–8	30–35
Dog	13–14	53–71
Monkey	9–11	155–180
Man	8–13	274–280

Obviously, not all potential embryonic defects will be seen if the embryo is not exposed to the drug throughout the whole period of organogenesis. Fraser (1964) has shown that treatment at various stages during embryonic development will result in different malformations.

The possible stimulation of microsomal enzyme systems by the drug must be considered in the protocol. Burns (1963) has published a simple test for drug-induced stimulation of drug metabolism. If possible, this evaluation should be made before a teratogenic test is initiated, as part of the preclinical toxicity study. Where there is no stimulation, drug treatment can commence before mating and throughout the entire reproductive process, including the period of lactation. This procedure would ensure demonstration of the largest possible number of potential defects because the new organism would be exposed to a drug throughout its entire development.

Drug-induced functional impairment to the foetus also can occur late in pregnancy. Schmidt & Hoffmann (1954) injected ACTH into pregnant monkeys during the last third of gestation. There was a typical maternal response to this hormone in the form of a reduction in circulatory eosinophils. More important, there was a significant reduction in the size of the foetal adrenal gland.

It is important to extend the study to include investigation of whether the drug passes, accumulates, or is in any way altered in the milk. Thus, drug administration should be continued through the nursing period. Even though the proportion of women on medication that breast-feed has declined, in many countries breast-feeding is still the predominant method of infant rearing.

Lutwak-Mann (1964) has reported an experiment in which the mating of a male treated with thalidomide and an untreated female resulted in deformed rabbit pups. Although this report has not been confirmed, it stands as an important, although unique, example of a possibly distinct latent type of embryotoxicity. Therefore, one must not overlook treatment of the male. Since spermatogenesis may require several weeks for the complete cycle, a drug would have to be given to a male for a prolonged period before the test mating occurs. Pretesting would be necessary in order to clear the epididymis of stored normal sperm. Alternatively, electro-ejaculation can be employed, as suggested by Mastroianni & Manson (1963). However, with the Mastroianni technique chemical restraint (tranquillization) for monkeys is necessary. This introduces another drug variable which influences the practicality of this procedure.

If drug treatment is limited to the period before (or after) a critical period of development, no foetal defects should occur. The offspring of pregnant rats treated with X-ray for the first 8 days of gestation had no observable defects (Wilson, 1954). When thalidomide was administered to monkeys after limb formation was complete, no anomalies were induced (Drobeck *et al.*, 1965). As would be expected, classical embryopathy results only when thalidomide or rubella affects a human or primate embryo during a particular period of organogenesis.

RECOVERY AND EVALUATION OF OFFSPRING

The only way to be sure of securing all the products of conception is to perform Caesarean sections prior to the estimated time of delivery. All animals should be examined during the course of pregnancy. If at any time abnormal bleeding or vaginal discharge occurs, surgical intervention should be employed. From our experience, the monkey foetus can be recovered by Caesaeran section after the 155th day of gestation. Caged monkeys have weak musculature, and if a dystocia occurs, foetal death may result.

Standard autopsy procedures may be used, or gross macrosectioning via the Wilson method (1965) may be employed in the internal evaluation of the offspring. The Dawson technique (1926) is common procedure for skeletal staining. Histologic preparations can be easily made from the macrosections. It would be advisable to examine the microscopic appearance of any organs which appear abnormal, and perhaps routinely examine the brain, eye, and gonads, especially if no animals are allowed to grow to maturity. When an abnormality is noted, the textbook, *Pathology of the Fetus and the Infant* (Potts, 1962) is a very valuable diagnostic reference.

Paget & Thorp (1965) have demonstrated the value of rearing some of the offspring from teratogenic studies. A drug-induced maloclusion of the incisor teeth would not have been observed if these authors had not allowed some rats to grow to be weanlings. Latent functional drug-induced abnormalities must be guarded against, especially ones which have a CNS locus (i.e. lowered IQ or personality aberrations). If progeny from drug-treated mothers are allowed to grow to maturity, all the tests common to toxicological investigations may be applied to these animals, including conditioned avoidance, to test behaviour and learning when so indicated. If the osseous system need be examined, whole skeletal mounts (Miller, 1949) of mature large animals (i.e., rabbits and dogs) would be preferable to preparation by the Dawson method.

The classic and elegant autoradiographic studies of Andre (1959) showed the distribution of tritium-labelled antibiotics in pregnant animals and their foetuses. Such studies can be utilized to indicate placental passage of a specific compound. For example, Hansson & Schmiterlöw (1961) demonstrated that Promethazine passed through the placental barrier, whereas Aprobit, a quaternary analogue, did not. These autoradiographic methods may even be used for mechanism of teratogenic actions studies. When labelled material is not available, (cold) drug foetal organ distribution investigations can be undertaken if chemical assays are available. Certainly, the electron microscope, histochemistry, microchemistry, etc. techniques can be suitably applied to these offspring where there needs to be additional sophisticated interpretation of a specific problem. With large numbers of offspring and other pertinent data being rapidly accumulated, automation is a worthwhile consideration. Small & Anderson's electronic processing approach (1965) to toxicologic data can be easily utilized for teratogenic programs. Stevenson *et al.* (1966) have published a report on congenital malformations in humans with an appendix that contains WHO reporting procedures for human malformations.

HUMAN DRUG TRIALS

It would be remiss to conclude an evaluation of teratological methodology without considering how pregnant humans may first be exposed to a new drug. If clinical pharmacology of a compound in normal individuals, Phase I, can be evaluated in male prisoner volunteers only, this should be encouraged. In this event, the question of teratogenic potential of a given new drug need not be considered until the desired clinical response has been demonstrated in man. Urine and blood samples should be taken during Phase I for comparative metabolic studies. From the results an assessment of comparative animal and human pharmacology, toxicity, and drug metabolism, some early indication of the preferred animal species for toxicologic and teratologic investigations may emerge. When there is no clear-cut correlation between a certain animal species and man, a rabbit teratogenic (Table 5.6) study should be initiated

Table 5.6   A primary teratogenic evaluation–protocol outline.

Species	Rabbit (mouse or rat)
Dose level	Small multiple of human treatment
Number	Ten pregnant females
Route	Feed or tube
Gestation time	(a) Day 1 to 8
	(b) Day 8 to 16
	(c) Day 16 to parturition
Delivery	Caesarean section prior to parturition

first. Obviously, if there is good animal-to-man metabolic relationship, the species (perhaps mouse or rat) most similar to man should
be included in the teratogenic investigation.

If, when the first teratogenic study has been completed, there are
no abnormalities in the progeny, a few women of childbearing
potential should be included in the therapeutic evaluation (Phase
II) of a drug. When malformations result in a rabbit study, women
of childbearing potential should obviously not be exposed to the
new agent, pending an evaluation of the probable significance of
the animal results. If the compound is very promising therapeutically and comparative metabolic data are not available, a Primate
Teratogenic Investigation (Table 5.7) or a Primate Chronic Toxicity

Table 5.7 A specific example of primate teratogenic–protocol
outline.

Drug	P-4657B
Species	Macaca mulatta
Dose route	Oral
Dose levels	0, 1, and 3 mg/kg/day
Number per level	Three[a]
Dose duration	One year
Time of treatment	Before mating, and throughout gestation
Observation intervals	Weekly
Haematology	Blood drug levels
Urinalysis	Urine drug levels
Determination interval	0, 1, and 3 months
Disposition	Returned to reproductive colony

[a] Four monkeys were used at the 3 mg/kg level of P-4657B.

and Teratogenicity Study (Table 5.8) can be started. As data become
available from the monkey teratogenic study and from metabolic
investigations, a judgment can be made as to whether or not human
therapeutic drug trials should include women of the childbearing
age.

Either of these primate protocols is practicable. As an example,
the findings from the primate teratogenic evaluation of P-4657B
are presented in Table 5.9. Chemically, P-4657B is 2-dimethyl-sul-
famyl-[9-(4-methyl-1-piperazinyl)propylidene]-thioxanthene. In a
pilot study and in the teratogenic one, the monkeys manifested
various degrees, depending on the dose level, of the classical pharmacologic signs for tranquillizers; reduced aggression (tranquilliza-

Table 5.8 A general protocol for a primate chronic toxicity and teratogenic test.

Drug	Drug X
Species	Macaca philippensis
Dose route	Oral, syrup suspension
Dose levels	0, 5, 25, and 50 mg/kg/day
Number per level	Four (two per sex per level) mated at appropriate times
Dose duration	One year
Haematology	Haemoglobin, WBC, and differential
Urinalysis	Including microscopic examination of the sediment
Clinical chemistry	BUN, SGOT, SGPT, and alkaline phosphatase
Blood drug level determinations	1 day, 7 months, and terminal
Determination intervals	0, 3, 6, 9, and 12 months
Disposition	Sacrifice top level at one year; if no abnormalities present, remaining animals returned to breeding colony

Table 5.9 Results from a primate teratogenic evaluation of P-4657B.

Dosage (mg/kg)	Pregnancies	Abortions	Live births	Normal infants[a]
3	4/4[b]	0/4	4/4	4/4
1	3/3	1/3[c]	1/2	1/2[d]
0	3/3	1/3[e]	2/2	2/2
3[f]	3/3	0/3	3/3	3/3

[a] Anatomically and physiologically.
[b] Fractions = number effected/number treated.
[c] Aborted at $3\frac{1}{2}$ months due to strep infection.
[d] Foetal death due to dystocia.
[e] Aborted at $4\frac{1}{2}$ months, foetus decomposed.
[f] Taractan.

tion), tremors, sedation, catatonia, etc. The highest dose level employed was sufficient to produce a maximum degree of sedation without adversely effecting normal breeding activity of either sex. The low dosage was equivalent to the therapeutic level. Wilson (1966) has demonstrated that thalidomide induced defects in the monkey at the human therapeutic dose. Taractan was employed as a positive control since it is in the same chemical and pharmacologic family. Thiothixene or P-4657B was reported by Simpson &

Igbal (1965) to be a potent antipsychotic agent in male schizo-phrenics. On the basis of the above-described primate teratogenic study, thiothixene was considered a safe therapeutic agent for the treatment of schizophrenic women of childbearing potential.

After a decision has been made to conduct a drug investigation (either Phase II or III) in women, certain steps should be taken. As in the initial evaluation of any new compound, exposure should be limited initially to only a few individuals. A few pharmaceutical firms are said to have evaluated early embryo toxicity of drugs in countries where legalized abortions take place. Patients who are scheduled for interruption of pregnancy are given an experimental drug before the surgical procedure. This would make possible the ideal situation of obtaining the maximum possible assurance of a drug's safety before exposing a large number of patients to its effect. It certainly would prevent the highly undesirable possibility of malformed children being born. It should be stressed, however, that such a programme would have profound moral and legal ramifications, and such experiments are not recommended here.

With the new immunological tests, early pregnancy can be rapidly and easily detected. As soon as pregnancy is diagnosed, it would be prudent, if medically practical, to withdraw any medication except the compound being tested, from ingestion by the female patient. Needless to say, the environment, nutrition, state of health, etc. of the patient should be monitored very closely. A mild febrile episode, without a rash, in a pregnant woman could easily pass without being recorded, and such an attack of occult rubella might give rise to malformations. Pretreatment serum samples (2 ml) should be drawn, frozen, and stored from any women of the child-bearing age who are to receive a new drug. In the event that a patient becomes pregnant and a deformed infant is born, a comple-ment fixation test for toxoplasmosis, rubella neutralizing antibody titres, and if possible, cytomegalic inclusion virus should be carried out on the samples. Obviously, this is important in order to rule out possible microbiological causes of subsequently discovered congenital defects. Sever (1965) has reported a complement fixation test for rubella which, when it becomes widely available, will be of additional aid in making a positive diagnosis for rubella.

It is felt that a few women should be included in either or both Phase II or Phase III human drug studies. If this is not done, a large number of pregnant women might subsequently become exposed to the drug without adequate knowledge of its effect on the foetus or adequate control. This is a highly undesirable situation.

As previously mentioned, the male should not be overlooked in regard to adverse drug effects on his reproductive capabilities. Inability to ejaculate not infrequently occurs in men taking anti-hypertensive medications with ganglionic blocking activity (Grollman, 1965). This is not considered a serious problem. It is reversible and only discussed as an example of a drug's effect on the male reproductive physiology.

Preliminary human pharmacologic investigations in the United States are, to a large degree, conducted on male prison volunteers. Routine semen counts could be part of the drug testing protocol when these trials are initiated. The more esoteric problems can be evaluated at later stages (Phase II or III). Such aspects as chromosomal breakage should be evaluated. Ingalls *et al.* (1964) have observed fragmented chromosomes in the bone marrow cells of mice treated with 6-aminonicotinamide. Both maternal and foetal cells were affected. There was one unpublished account of a drug being conjugated in the vagina to a more toxic substance than the parent compound. Bearing this in mind, it would seem advisable that post-coital semen samples might also be examined.

DISCUSSION

This chapter has intentionally avoided the problem of detecting teratogens that induce a low incidence of malformations. It does, however, appear practicable at the present time to improve the state of our knowledge to the point where all high incidence (50–100%) teratogens can be predicted. Known human teratogens, thalidomide (Delahunt & Lassen, 1964) or rubella (Delahunt & Rieser, 1966) can be detected in a few (2–4) monkey foetuses. Large numbers of monkeys are not required to detect a human teratogen of the potency of thalidomide. For this reason, it is practicable to incorporate a teratogenic component in a standard primate chronic toxicity study.

The potentiation of drug toxicity or teratogenicity is not uncommon. Wilson (1964) has demonstrated this phenomenon can occur with six known teratogens. This problem certainly exists in drug toxicity and will have to be critically analysed in the near future.

6—M.T.

One other point that has not been considered is the value of comparative pharmacological actions, when comparative metabolic data are not available. Comparative pharmacology should always be considered, in making judgements about dosage, and in the interpretation of experimental results; it can go far to clarify experimentation in the absence of rigorous metabolic data.

CONCLUSION

There is no simple formula to solve all the problems attached to the detection of the teratogenic action of a drug. Only prudent, intellectually and scientifically sound judgement will accomplish this end, through carefully planned and executed experiments. Comparative pharmacological studies including toxicology and metabolism will make available two major factors necessary for meaningful detection of toxicity or teratogenicity, firstly species of animal that most closely correlates metabolically or pharmacologically, or both, to man, and secondly the appropriate parallel blood level information. A primary rabbit teratogenic test and a secondary primate teratogenic test are suggested if the above-mentioned data are not available. These two investigations are considered by the writer, at the present time, to be the most nearly ideal system for the detection of teratogenic actions of a new drug.

REFERENCES

ANDRE T. (1956) Studies on the distribution of tritium-labelled dihydro-streptomycin and tetracycline in the body. *Acta radiol.*, Suppl. 142.

AREY L.B. (1947) *Development Anatomy*, 5th edition. Philadelphia, W.B. Sanders.

BARNES, J.M. & DENZ F.A. (1954) Experimental methods used in determining chronic toxicity. *Pharmac. Rev.* **6**, 191–242.

BINNS W., THACKER E.J., JAMES L.F. & HOFFMAN W.T. (1959) A congenital cyclopian-type malformation in lambs. *J. Am. vet. med. Ass.* **134**, 180.

BONGIOVANNI A.M. & MCPADDEN A.J. (1960) Steroids during pregnancy and possible fetal consequences. *Fert. Steril.* **11**, 181–6.

BURNS J.J., CONNEY A.H. & KOSTER R. (1963) Stimulatory effect of chronic drug administration on drug-metabolizing enzymes in liver microsomes. *Ann. N. Y. Acad. Sci.* **104**, 881–93.

CABASSO V.J. & STEBBINS M.R. (1965) Study of spread of rubella virus from inoculated to uninoculated contact cercopithecus monkeys. *J. Lab. clin. Med.* **65**, 612–16.

CAHEN R.L. (1964) Evaluation of the teratogenicity of drugs. *Clin. Pharmac. Ther.* **5**, 480–514.

CARR R.E. & HENKIND J. (1962) Ocular manifestations of ethambutol. *Arch. Ophth.* **67**, 566–71.

CAUJOLLE F., CAUJOLLE D., CROS S. *et al.* (1965) Teratogenic power of dimethylsulfoxide and diethylsulfoxide. *C. r. Acad. Sci.* (Paris) **268**, 300–27.

CHEN K.K., POWELL C.E. & MAZE W. (1945) Response of hamsters to drugs. *J. Pharmac. exp. Ther.* **85**, 348–55.

CHOMETTE G. (1955) Entwicklungsstörungen nach insulinshock beim trächtiger kaninchen. *Beitr. path. Anat.* **115**, 439–51.

CIBA FOUND. *Symp. Congenital Malformations* (1960) Boston, Little, Brown & Company.

COHLAN S.Q. (1954) Congenital anomalies in rat produced by excessive intake of Vitamin A during pregnancy. *Pediatrics* **13**, 556–7.

COURRIER R. & JOST A. (1942) Intersexualité foetale provoqueé par le prégnéninolone au cours de la grossesse. *C. r. Soc. Biol.* **136**, 395–6.

COURRIER R. (1962) Teratology embryology-production of congenital malformations in mice after administration of low dose of thalidomide. *C. r. Acad. Sci.* **255**, 1646–8.

DALE A.J.D., PARKHILL E.M. & LAYTON D.D. (1965) Studies on chloroquine retinopathy in rabbits. *J. Am. med. Ass.* **193**, 141–4.

DAWSON A.B. (1926) Note on the staining of the skeleton of cleared specimens with alizarin red S. *Stain Technol.* **1**, 123–5.

DEKKER A. & MEHRIZI A. (1964) The use of thalidomide as a teratogenic agent in rabbits. *Bull. Johns Hopkins Hosp.* **115**, 223–30.

DELAHUNT C.S. & LASSEN L.J. (1964) Thalidomide syndrome in monkeys. *Science* **146**, 1300–5.

DELAHUNT C.S. (1964) Unpublished data.

DELAHUNT C.S., KISS N., FELDMAN E. & OAKES M. (1965) Some comparative pharmacological studies in man and the monkey with thalidomide. *Toxic. appl. Pharmac.* **7**, 481–2.

DELAHUNT C.S. (1965) Teratogenic effects of thalidomide in the rabbit, monkey, and man. Supplement to *Teratology Workshop Manual*, pp. 51–84.

DELAHUNT C.S. (1966) Rubella induced cataracts in monkeys. *Lancet* **i**, 7441, 825.

DELAHUNT C.S. & RIESER N. (1966) In press.

DELATOUR P., ADAMS R. & FAVRE-TISSOT M. (1965) Thalidomide embryopathies chez le chien. *Thérapie* **20**, 573–89.

DROBECK H.P., COULSTON F. & CORNELIUS D. (1965) Effects of thalidomide on fetal development in rabbits and on establishment of pregnancy in monkeys. *Toxic. appl. Pharmac.* **7**, 165–78.

EARL A.E., DIENER R.M. & SHOFFSTALL D.H. (1966) Effects of various potassium salts on the gastrointestinal tract of monkeys. *Toxic. appl. Pharmac.* **8**, 339.

European Society for Study of Drug Toxicity Symposium (1963). Effects of drugs on the foetus. *Int. Congress Series* **64**.

FARRIS E.J. & GRIFFITH J.Q., Jr. (1949) *The Rat in Laboratory Investigation,* 2nd edition. Philadelphia, J.B. Lippincott Co.

FERM V.H. (1966) Teratogenic effect of dimethylsulfoxide. Lancet **i**, 208–9.

First International Conference on Congenital Malformations (1961) Philadelphia, J.B. Lippincott Co.

FLORENCE A.L. (1960) Is thalidomide to blame? *Brit. Med. J.* **2**, 1954.

FRASER F.C. (1964) Experimental teratogenesis in relation to congenital malformations in man. *Proc. 2nd Int. Conf. Cong. Malf.,* pp. 279–80. New York, The International Medical Congress Ltd.

FRASER F.C. & FAINSTAT T.D. (1951) The production of congenital defects in the offspring of pregnant mice treated with cortisone. A progress report. *Pediatrics* **8**, 527–33.

FRATTA I.D., SIGG E.B. & MAIORANA K. (1965) Teratogenic effects of thalidomide in rabbits, rats, hamsters and mice. *Toxic. appl. Pharmac.* **7**, 268–86.

FRIEDMAN M.H. (1957) The effect of o-diazoacetyl-L-serine (Azaserine) on the pregnancy of the dog. *J. Am. vet. med. Ass.* **130**, 159–62.

GEBAUER A. (1954) Zur A-hypervitaminose und schwangerschaft. *Pharmazie* **9**, 684–5.

GIURGEA C. & MOEYERSOONS F. (1963) Action of thalidomide on the EEG of the conscious unrestrained rabbit. *Medna. exp.* **8**, 66–73.

GROLLMAN A. (1965) *Pharmacology and Therapeutics,* 6th edition, p. 539. Philadelphia, Lea & Febiger.

HABEL K. (1942) Transmission of rubella to Macacus mulatta monkeys. *Publs. publ. Hlth Serv.* **47**, 1126–39.

HANSSON E. & SCHMITERLÖW C.G. (1961) A comparison of the distribution, excretion, and metabolism of a tertiary (Promethazine) and a quaternary (Aprobit[R]) phenothiazine compound labelled with S^{35}. *Arch. int. Pharmacodyn.* CXXXI, 309–24.

HARRISSON J.W.E., ROSSI G.V., PACKMAN E.W., ROSENTHAL M., COMER M. & LEVY K. (1957) The effects of several ataractic agents upon gastric secretion in the dog and rat. *Fourth Pan-American Congress of Pharmacy & Biochemistry, Washington, D.C.*

HOET J.P., GOMMERS A. & HOEF J.J. (1960) Causes of congenital malformations. *Ciba Symposium,* p. 226.

HOMBURGER F., NIXON C.W., BOGDONOFF P.D. & CHAUBE S. (1964) Prenatal morbidity and thalidomide effects in certain inbred strains of Syrian hamsters. *Fourth Annual Meeting Teratology Society Abstracts,* p. 6.

HORITA A. (1961) The route of administration of some hydrazine compounds as a determinance of brain and liver monoamine oxidase inhibition. *Toxic. appl. Pharmac.* **3**, 474–80.

HOWE P. (1961) Neuropathy after thalidomide. *Br. med. J.* **2**, 1084.

INGALLS T.H., INGENITO E.F. & CURLEY F.J. (1963) Acquired chromosomal anomalies induced in mice by injection of a teratogen in pregnancy. *Science* **141**, 810–12.

JACOBSON B.D. (1962) Hazards of norethindrone therapy during pregnancy. *Am. J. Obstet. Gynec.* **84**, 962–8.

JUBB K.V.F. & KENNEDY P.C. (1963) *Pathology of Domestic Animals*, Vol. II, p. 586. New York, Academic Press.

KAISER J.A. (1964) Studies on the toxicity of disophenol (2,6-diiodo-4-nitrophenol) to dogs and rodents plus some comparisons with 2,4-dinitrophenol. *Toxic. appl. Pharmac.* **6**, 232–44.

KALTER H. & WARKANY J. (1959) Experimental production of congenital malformations in mammals by metabolic procedure. *Physiol. Rev.* **39**, 69–115.

KARNOSKY D.A. (1965) Drugs as teratogens in animals and man. *Ann. Rev. Pharmac.* **5**, 447–72.

KILHAM L. (1961) Rat virus (RV) infections in hamsters. *Proc. Soc. exp. Biol. Med.* **106**, 825–9.

KIM J.N., RUNGE W., WELLS L.J. & LAZAROW A. (1960) Effects of experimental diabetes in the offspring of the rat. *Diabetes* **9**, 396–404.

KING C.T.G. & KENDRICK F.J. (1962) Teratogenic effects of thalidomide in the Sprague-Dawley rat. *Lancet* **ii**, 1116.

KING C.T.G. (1963) Teratogenic effects of meclizine HC1 on the rat. *Science* **141**, 353–5.

KRUGMAN S., WARD K.G., JACOBS & LAZAR M. (1953) Studies on rubella immunization. I. Demonstration of rubella without rash. *J. Am. med. Ass.* **151**, 285–8.

LANDAUER W. (1945) Rumpleness of chicken embryos produced by the injection of insulin and other chemicals. *J. exp. Zool.* **98**, 65–77.

LASAGNA L. (1960) Thalidomide—A new nonbarbiturate sleep-inducing drug. *J. Chron. Dis.* **11**, 627–31.

LENZ M.W. (1964) *Second International Conference on Congenital Malformations*, pp. 263–76. New York, International Medical Congress, Ltd.

LITTLE W.A. (1966) cited by Wilson J.G., Teratology in Non-Human Primates, *F.D.A. Conference on Non-Human Primate Toxicology.*

LEHMAN A.J. (1959) *Appraisal of the Safety of Chemicals in Foods, Drugs, and Cosmetics.* Austin, Texas, The Association of Food and Drug Officials of the United States.

LUCEY J.F. & BEHRMAN R.E. (1963) Thalidomide. Effect upon pregnancy in the rhesus monkey. *Science* **139**, 1295–6.

LUCEY J.F., HIBBARD E., BEHRMAN R.E., ESQUIVEL DE GALLAIDE F.O. & WINDLE W.F. (1964) Kernicterus in asphyxiated newborn rhesus monkeys. *Expl. Neurol.* **9**, 43–58.

LUTWAK-MANN C. (1964) Observations of progeny of thalidomide treated male rabbits. *Br. med. J.* **i**, 1090–1.

MARLIAC J. (1964) Toxicity and teratogenic effects of 12 pesticides in chick embryo. *Fed. Proc. Fed. Am. Socs. exp. Biol.* **23**, 105.

MASTROIANNI L. & MANSON W.A. (1963) Collection of monkey semen by electroejaculation. *Proc. Soc. exp. Biol. Med.* **112**, 1025–7.

McBRIDE W.G. (1961) Thalidomide and congenital abnormalities. *Lancet* **ii**, 1358.

MILLER M.E. (1949) *Guide to the dissection of the Dog*, 2nd edition, pp. 12–14. Ithaca, New York, Cornell.

MONIF R.G., SEVER J.C. & COCHRAN A.D. (1965) The H-1 and the RV viruses and pregnancy: serological study of certain groups of pregnant women. *Pediatrics* **67**, 253–6.

PAGET G.E. & THORP E. (1965) A Teratogenic Effect of a Sulphonamide in Experimental Animals. *Brit. J. of Pharmac. & Chemo.* **23**, 305–12.

PALOTTA A. (1966) Personal communication.

PARKMAN P.D., PHILLIPS P.E., KIRSCHSTEIN, R.L. & MEYER H.M. (1965) Experimental rubella virus infection in the rhesus monkey. *J. Immun.* **95**, 743–52.

PINSKY L. & DiGEORGE A.M. (1965) Cleft palate in the mouse: A teratogenic index of glucocorticoid potency. *Science* **147**, 402–3.

POTTS A.M. *et al.* (1966) Studies on visual toxicity of methanol; additional observations on methanol poisoning in primate test object. *Am. J. Ophthal.* **40**, 76–83.

POTTS E. L. (1962) *Pathology of the Fetus and the Infant.* Chicago, Year Book Medical Publishers, Inc.

RIAZANTSEVA N.Y. (1959) Influence of the state of maternal immunity to measles on the immunity of the child. *Probl. Virol.* **1**, 59–62.

SANSONE G. & ZUNIN C. (1964) Experimental embryopathy caused by folic acid antagonists. *Acta Vitam. (Milano)* **8**, 73–9.

SCHMIDT I.G. & HOFFMAN R.A. (1954) Effects of ACTH on pregnant monkeys and their offspring. *Endocrinology* **55**, 125–41.

SCHMIDT L.H., LANG J., GOOD R.C. & HOFFMANN R. (1962) Experimental studies on the toxicity and antituberculosis activity of ethambutol. *Trans. 21st Conf. Pulmon. Dis.* 355–66.

Second International Conference on Congenital Malformations (1964) New York, The International Medical Congress, Ltd.

SEVER J.L. (1965) Simplified test developed for rubella. *J. Am. med. Ass.* **192**, 33.

SIMPSON G.M. & IQBAL J. (1965) A preliminary study of thiothixene in chronic schizophrenics. *Curr. ther. Res.* **7**, 697–700.

SMALL R.M. & ANDERSON R.C. (1965) Semi-Automatic recording and electronic processing of chronic rat toxicity data. *Lab. Anim. Care* **15**, 345–53.

SMITHBERG M., SANCHEZ H.W. & RUNNER M.N. (1956) Congenital deformity in the mouse induced by insulin. *Anat. Rev.* **124**, 441–5.

SOMERS G.F. (1963) The foetal toxicity of thalidomide. *Proc. Eur. Soc. Study Drug Toxicity* **1**, 49–58.

STAEMMLER V.M., HELM & KIEL H. (1964) Angeborene mibbildungen des bei kanninchen. *Medna. exp.* **10**, 22–6.

STEVENSON A.C., JOHNSTON H.A., STEWART M.I.P. & GOLDING D.R. Congenital malformations. *Bull. Wld Hlth Org.* Supplement to Vol. 34.

Teratogenesis (1964) Basle, Switzerland, Schwabe & Co.

THIERSCH J.B. (1952) Therapeutic abortions with a folic acid antagonist, 4-aminopteroylglutamic acid (4-amino P.G.A.) administered by the oral route. *Am. J. Obstet. Gynec.* **63**, 1298–1304.

TOOLAN H.W. (1960) Experimental production of mongoloid hamsters. *Science* **131**, 1446–8.

TUCHMANN-DUPLESSIS H. & MERCIER-PAROT L. (1958) Influence d'un sulfamide hypoglycémiant l'amino phénnurobutane (BZ 55) sur la gestation de la rate. *C. r. Acad. Sci. (Paris)* **246**, 156–8.

TUCHMANN-DUPLESSIS H. & MERCIER-PAROT L. (1963) Action du chlorhydrate de cyclizine sur la gestation et le developpement embryonnarie du rat, de la souris et du lapin. *C. r. Acad. Sci. (Paris)*, **256**, 3359–62.

VAN WAGENEN G. (1950) The Monkey. *The Care and Breeding of Laboratory Animals*, pp. 1–42. New York, John Wiley & Sons, Inc.

WAISSMAN H.A. & HARLOW H.F. (1965) Experimental phenylketonuria in infant monkeys. *Science* **147**, 685–95.

WALLENHORST A. (1957) Das hypnotisch und sedativ wirkende N-phthalyl-Glutaminsäure-imid als geeignetes provokationsmittel bei hirnelektrischen untersuchungen. *Wien. Klin. Wchnschr.* **69**, 334–9.

WEIDMAN W.H., YOUNG H.H. & ZOLLMAN P.E. (1963) The effect of thalidomide on the unborn puppy. *Proc. Staff Meet. Mayo Clin.* **38**, 518–22.

WELLS C.J. & VAN WAGENEN G. (1954) Androgen induced female pseudohermaphroditism in the monkey (Macaca mulatta): Anatomy of the reproductive organs. *Carnegie Contr. Embryology* **35**, 93–106.

WILLIAMS R.T. (1959) *Detoxification Mechanisms.* New York, John Wiley & Sons.

WILLIAMSON A.P., BLATTNER R.J. & LUTZ H.R. (1963) Abnormalities in chick embryos following thalidomide and other insoluble compounds in the amniotic cavity. *Proc. Soc. exp. Biol. Med.* **112**, 1022–5.

WILSON J.G. (1954) Differentiation and reaction of rat embryos to radiation. *J. cell. comp. Physiol.* **43**, 11–37.

WILSON J.G. (1964) Teratogenic interaction of chemical agents in the rat. *J. Pharmac. exp. Ther.* **144**, 429–36.

WILSON J.G. & WARKANY J. (1965) *Teratology: Principles and Techniques.* Chicago, Illinois, The University of Chicago Press.

WILSON J.G. (1966) Dosage and developmental stage in teratogenesis. *Supplement to Teratology Workshop Manual*, pp. 243–6.

WINDLE W.F. (1963) Neuropathology of certain forms of mental retardation. *Science* **140**, 1186–9.

YEARY R.A. (1964a) Teratogenic agents in man and animals. *Lancet* **i**, 831.

YEARY R.A. (1964b) Personal communication.

CHAPTER 6

Tests for Carcinogenic Potential

P.N. MAGEE*

There is an extensive literature on methods for determination of the carcinogenic potential of chemicals. Although the interpretation of the results will vary depending on the nature of the compound tested, the procedures used are essentially the same. Methods for carcinogenicity testing of food additives, pesticides, industrial, and other environmental chemicals are therefore applicable to drugs. Aspects of the problem have been covered in a number of review articles and in several monographs (Berenblum 1964; Boyland 1957, 1958, 1962; Clayson, 1962; Della Porta, 1964, 1967; Druckrey, 1959; Eckardt, 1959; Hackmann, 1959; Hueper, 1963; Hueper & Conway, 1964; Kotin, 1958; Mantel & Brian, 1961; Orris, 1965; Roe, 1966; Schmähl, 1963; Shubik & Sicé, 1956; Starr, 1961; Truhaut, 1963; Walpole, 1964; Weisburger & Weisburger, 1967; and Willis, 1961). The review by Weisburger & Weisburger (1967) and the two chapters in the book by Clayson (1962) are comprehensive and highly recommended. There are also several reports from various official and semi-official committees who have provided more or less detailed suggestions for carcinogenesis testing. These include: United Kingdom, Committee on Medical and Nutritional Aspects of Food Policy (1960); Association of the British Pharmaceutical Industry, Report of the Expert Committee on Drug Toxicity (1964); United States, Food and Drug Administration (1959); Food Protection Committee (1960); The European Society for the Study of Drug Toxicity (1964, 1965); World Health Organization (1958, 1961, 1964, 1967).

* I am deeply indebted to Drs John and Elizabeth Weisburger for allowing me to see the proofs of their article: Tests for Chemical Carcinogens, *Meth. Cancer Res.* **1**, 307–98 (1967).

Although these articles vary considerably in length and detail certain general conclusions do emerge. There is general agreement that, as with all forms of toxicity testing, it is not possible to lay down firm rules of procedure and that each compound for test must be treated on its own merits. There is also agreement that methods at present available are far from satisfactory and that no shortened test for carcinogenicity can substitute for lifetime studies, particularly in attempts to establish the absence of carcinogenic risk.

In the following brief account some practical aspect of carcinogenesis testing will be discussed.

ANIMALS

Species

The selection of the species used in carcinogenesis studies is largely determined by the necessity to continue the test for all or most of the life span of the animal. Although powerful carcinogens may induce tumours in much shorter periods, weak carcinogenic action can only be revealed by prolonged administration of the compound. Ideally, of course, the species selected should be known to absorb, metabolize, and excrete the drug in the same way as man and much recent work has been directed towards this end (World Health Organization, 1966, pp. 18–19). In carcinogenesis testing this goal may not be achieved because many of the species used for short-term studies are unsuitable for the longer duration. This reservation must always be considered in relating the results of animal studies to man. In practice, most authorities recommend the use of rats and mice because these species are well known, can be housed in large numbers in a small space, and are relatively cheap. The only other species that has been used extensively is the dog, mainly in the United States where pure-bred beagles are favoured. The expense involved in maintaining adequate numbers of dogs for statistical evaluation over long periods to reveal weak carcinogenic action has largely precluded their use elsewhere. Similar considerations apply to primates although recently Kelly *et al.* (1966) have induced malignant liver tumours in several strains of monkey by administration of diethylnitrosamine for only about 2 years. The use of other mammalian species including hamster, guinea pig, rabbit, cat, pig, steppe lemming, and mastomys (African rats), also birds and fish has been discussed by Clayson (1962) and by Weisburger & Weisburger (1967). Some of these may have advantages for special purposes but they have not been widely used. The Syrian hamster may prove a useful addition to the range of species in more general use because increasing evidence is becoming available on its responses to a variety of carcinogens (Shubik *et al.*, 1962a). If only one species is to be used, Della Porta (1967) advances arguments in favour of the mouse rather than the rat because of its relative cheapness based on food consumption, space occupied, and life span. It need hardly be mentioned that, whatever species are selected, animals of both sexes should be used for testing compounds of unknown carcinogenic potential.

Further information on the choice of animal species is given in *Laboratory Animals Centre Collected Papers*, Vol. 9 (1960) which are concerned with provision of animals for cancer research.

Type of Animal

The choice between inbred and outbred strains of animals is difficult (Clayson, 1962). Inbred strains of mouse, rat, guinea pig, hamster, dog, and possibly other species are now available. A general introduction to the use of mice as experimental animals in research is given by Staats (1966a) who describes the origin of several of the major inbred strains, most of which were developed for cancer research. By selective inbreeding susceptibility to various types of tumour in predictable frequencies has been established in several genotypes. Resistance to neoplasia was developed in others. Inbred strains offer the advantage of greater uniformity among the experimental animals so that fewer are needed to attain a given standard of accuracy and repeatability in experiments. Their spontaneous tumour incidence can also be predicted with greater reliability than with outbred animals. First generation (F_1) hybrids from crosses between inbred strains may be preferred. These animals are genetically homogeneous although heterozygous for those gene pairs by which the parent strains differ. Such hybrids are as predictable in their response as the parent strains although not necessarily like either one. The greatest general advantage of F_1 hybrids is their increased vigour (Staats, 1966a).

A guide to the nomenclature of the various inbred strains of mice has been provided by Staats (1963, 1966b) and by various publications of the Committee on Standardized Nomenclature for Inbred Strains of Mice (1952, 1960). The third listing of the committee is given in the references as Staats (1964). These publications include valuable data on the spontaneous tumour incidence in the various inbred strains. It must be remembered, however, that the response of inbred strains of mice to carcinogens may differ and that a given strain may be resistant to the drug under tests. If inbred animals are chosen, several different strains should therefore be used. For this reason Clayson (1962) has recommended the use of outbred stock for testing of compounds of unknown carcinogenic potential in order to obtain a wide range of response, reserving inbred strains for tests of comparative carcinogenic potency.

Whatever the species or strain chosen, the incidence of spontaneous disease, especially that of tumours, must be well known to the investigator. There is now a fairly extensive literature on spontaneous disease of laboratory animals and the following selected reviews and articles, listed by species, should provide a useful introduction.

Tuffery & Innes (1963) give an excellent review of diseases of laboratory mice and rats which is mainly directed to bacterial, viral, and parasitic disease with a short chapter on neoplasia. The most comprehensive account of the pathology of laboratory animal disease is in the book by Cohrs *et al.* (1958), written in German, which includes a full account of spontaneous tumours and an extensive bibliography. A valuable collection of essays on laboratory animal pathology has been edited by Ribelin & McCoy (1965) and, recently, another excellent collection of articles on the pathology of laboratory rats and mice has been edited by Cotchin & Roe (1967). The pathology of spontaneous tumours is described in the books by Guerin (1954), Fischer & Kuhl (1958), and in the review by Tamascke (1955). The recent article by Roe (1965) on spontaneous tumours in rats and mice is particularly helpful, and also discusses external factors which may influence the tumour incidence.

Articles devoted to the mouse include: Dunn (1965), spontaneous lesions; Cloudman (1941), Lippincott *et al.* (1942), Horn & Stewart (1952), Murphy (1966), spontaneous tumours; Shimkin

(1955), Stewart (1959), pulmonary tumours; Dunn (1954), tumours of recticular tissue; Dunn (1959), mammary tumours; Gorer (1940), Burns & Shenken (1940), Andervont (1950), Andervont & Dunn (1952), liver tumours. Information on the rat can be found in: Magee (1959), Snell (1966), spontaneous lesions, including tumours; Bullock & Curtis (1930), Ratcliffe (1940), Saxton *et al.* (1948), Davis *et al.* (1956), Gilbert *et al.* (1958), Crain (1958), spontaneous tumours. An account of tumours in domestic animals, including the dog, is given in the German paper by Tamaschke (1951–2) which includes an extensive bibliography of the earlier literature. Publications in English include the text on veterinary pathology by Smith & Jones (1966), the survey on domesticated mammals by Cotchin (1956), and the book by Mulligan (1949). Relevant papers are by Mulligan (1944), Krook (1954), and Cotchin (1954). Spontaneous neoplasia in the hamster is described by Ashbell (1945), Fortner (1957, 1961), Shubik *et al* (1962), Kirkman (1962), and Handler (1965). The article by Handler (1965) includes a review of the literature. Spontaneous tumours of the guinea pig were reviewed by Warren & Gates (1941) who concluded that this species was resistant to spontaneous and induced tumours, except in the gall-bladder. In particular they state that carcinogenic hydrocarbons are much less potent in guinea pigs than in mice. The resistance of the guinea pig to hepatocarcinogenesis was supported by Breidenbach & Argus (1956) but subsequently it was found highly sensitive to the induction of liver tumours by diethylnitrosamine (Argus & Hoch-Ligeti, 1963; Druckrey & Steinhoff, 1962). Blumenthal & Rogers (1965) have recently discussed spontaneous and induced tumours of the guinea pig. They concluded that spontaneous tumours do not develop in this species under the age of three years and that it is readily susceptible to the induction of experimental neoplasms by methylcholanthrene. All the tumours were mesenchymal, however, and there were no induced carcinomas. A high spontaneous incidence of cancer of the glandular stomach in the African rodent *Rattus* (mastomys) *natalensis* has been reported by Oettlé (1957) who suggested the potential value of this species since this type of cancer has proved remarkably difficult to induce in other rodents.

The main conclusion to be drawn from the accounts of spontaneous neoplasia in rats and mice is that the incidence and type of tumour varies greatly in the different strains. For example, liver tumours are specially frequent in older male mice in strains C3H and CBA but are quite rare in some other inbred strains (Murphy, 1966). In the rats studied by Gilbert *et al.* (1958) phaeochromocytomas were common, but in other strains, such as those described by Snell (1965), they are rare. It follows, therefore, that the investigator must be familiar with the types of tumour and their incidence in the particular species and strain of experimental animal that he is using. Weisburger & Weisburger (1967) have presented a number of tables, compiled from the literature, showing the types and incidence of spontaneous tumours in the laboratory animals commonly used in carcinogenesis studies. Very generally speaking, the commonest types of tumour in inbred strains of mice are mammary tumours (in breeding females), lymphocytic leukaemia, primary lung tumours, hepatoma (in males), and reticulum cell sarcoma (in older animals). Spontaneous tumours of the skin have rarely been reported except in mice kept in wooden cages treated with creosote (Murphy, 1966). As emphasized above, the incidence of neoplasia varies considerably in different strains of rat but the investigator should be on the lookout for fibroadenoma of the breast, lymphosarcoma, pituitary tumours, interstitial cell tumours of the testis, and phaeochromocytoma of the adrenal medulla (Weisburger & Weisburger, 1967; Magee, 1959).

Husbandry

Good animal care is essential for successful carcinogenesis testing. Several detailed publications are available which give guidance on all aspects of laboratory animal breeding, husbandry, and maintenance. Of these, the UFAW Handbooks on the Care and Management of Laboratory Animals (Worden & Lane-Petter, 1957; Lane-Petter *et al.*, 1967), the book, Animals for Research (Lane-Petter, W. ed., 1963), and the publication of the Committee on the Guide for Laboratory Animal Facilities and Care, National Academy of Sciences—National Research Council (1965) are among the most comprehensive. Other useful articles are by Porter & Lane-Petter (1962), and Les (1966). These publications give detailed information on animal-house construction, specification of cages, sanitation, breeding, feeding, watering, etc., and provide an extensive bibliography on all aspects of animal care.

Valuable annotated bibliographies on laboratory animals have been prepared by Cass *et al.* (1960, 1963).

Although the care and maintenance of animals for carcinogenesis testing is essentially the same as that for toxicity tests of shorter duration experience has shown that special attention must be paid to certain points (Roe, 1965). The use of creosote as a preservative on wooden mouse cages has led to misleading results in experiments on skin carcinogenesis since the animals showed abnormally high incidence of skin tumours when treated with croton oil only (Boutwell *et al.*, 1957). Mice from the same source also developed abnormally large numbers of apparently spontaneous skin tumours (Shubik *et al.*, 1957). An unexpectedly high incidence of apparently spontaneous lung tumours was also reported in mice bred in creosote-treated boxes (Roe *et al.*, 1958). Another possible source of error has arisen from exposure of bedding to ethylene oxide which appeared to lead to an increase in the incidence of spontaneous tumours in germ-free mice (Reyniers *et al.*, 1964).

Unsuspected carcinogens may be present in the food of the animals. The unexpected occurrence of liver tumours in rats was thought to be due to the presence of aflatoxin in their diet (Schoental, 1961). Chlorinated hydrocarbon insecticides, such as DDT and chlordane, may be present in the diet or applied to the animals. These compounds are well known to increase the activity of microsomal drug-metabolizing enzymes in the liver (Remmer, 1964; Fouts, 1963) and may thus have profound effects on long-term feeding studies. An example of such an effect is the inhibition by methylcholanthrene of hepatocarcinogenesis by 3'-methyl-dimethyl-aminoazobenzene. Conney *et al.* (1956) showed that this inhibitor effect was due to stimulation by methylcholanthrene of the enzymes in rat liver which convert the azo dye into a less active form.

The number of animals per cage may affect the incidence of spontaneous and induced tumours. Graffi & Hoffmann quoted by Fare (1965) found that mice housed in groups gave higher tumour incidences than did animals kept singly. Fare (1964) reported a non-random distribution of time of skin tumour incidence even among mice given apparently identical treatment with a polycyclic hydrocarbon. These observations underline the extreme importance of treating control animals in exactly the same way as the treated groups in every detail (Fare, 1965).

Food

The diet of the experimental animals is known to have a profound general effect on their response to carcinogens and on their incidence of spontaneous tumours (Tannenbaum & Silverstone, 1953; Tannenbaum, 1959; Saxton *et al.*, 1948; Gilbert *et al.*, 1958). Tannenbaum has shown that the critical factor in this general effect is the level of total calories rather than of any particular major dietary component. When animals are maintained on low-calorie diets the incidence of induced and spontaneous tumours may be considerably lower than that with higher calorie levels. Adequate intake of vitamins is essential and deficiencies may effect the induction of tumours. For example, there is a correlation between the level of hepatic riboflavin and the appearance of liver tumours in rats fed azo dyes (Miller *et al.*, 1948; Griffin & Baumann, 1948).

It is essential, therefore, to provide a good, well-tried diet and to ensure that the animals have adequate readily available amounts. When the test compound is mixed with the diet it must be established that the palatability is such that the animals will eat it. Information on nutritional requirements and feeding methods for rats and mice is provided by Morris (1944), Cuthbertson (1957), Porter (1963), Hoag & Dickie (1966), and Worden & Shillam (1967). Other species, including hamster, guinea-pig, cat, and monkey, as well as rat and mouse are covered in the report of the Committee on Animal Nutrition, National Academy of Sciences —National Research Council (1962) which also includes an extensive bibliography. The cubed diet for rats and mice, M.R.C. diet 41B (Bruce & Parkes, 1949, 1956), has proved satisfactory in many laboratories.

SPF Animals

There can be little doubt that specific pathogen free (SPF) animals offer considerable advantages in toxicity work and particularly in long-term carcinogenesis studies. SPF animals are free from their natural infectious diseases and have been defined by Foster (1963) as those initially delivered by caesarian section and subsequently maintained in some type of barrier system. It is insufficiently realized that animals derived from an SPF nucleus can be maintained under relatively simple conditions of isolation and still remain in much better health than conventionally reared animals. Comprehensive information on the breeding and maintenance of SPF animals can be found in the reviews by Davey (1959), Foster (1963), and Bleby (1967). The advantages of SPF rats have been advocated most persuasively by Paget & Lemon (1965) who compared the morbidity and mortality of two groups of Wistar derived rats, one reared under SPF conditions and the other under conventional "dirty" conditions. The most striking difference between the two groups was the virtually complete absence of early mortality in the SPF animals. Chronic murine pneumonia did not occur and other infections were markedly reduced with complete or almost complete abolition of metazoan parasites. The incidence of neoplasia, however, was not affected by the SPF conditions and there was no difference from the conventional rats in the age at which tumours became an important cause of death or illness. Paget & Lemon (1965) concluded that since a higher proportion of animals survive into the tumour-bearing age, SPF animals are clearly more satisfactory for studies of carcinogenesis than conventionally reared animals. A further conclusion from this work is that experiments of 2 years duration in the rat cannot be regarded as "life-time" studies since 2 years is only life-time when the rats are so debilitated as to die prematurely. This has obvious implications for decisions on the proper length of long-term studies for carcinogenesis testing. The susceptibility of SPF rats to induced carcinogenesis is not yet established but the work of Hadidian et al. (1966) gives no indication that it differs appreciably from conventional animals. These authors also report the loss of only approximately 5% of about 5,000 caesarean-derived Fischer rats due to nonneo-plastic disease in an experiment lasting 18 months.

SPF rats, mice, guinea pigs, and rabbits are now maintained at the Laboratory Animals Centre, Medical Research Council Laboratories, Carshalton, Surrey, England, and at other centres. Advice on all aspects of SPF animals can be obtained from the Carshalton centre.

The production of germ-free animals is technically complicated and expensive (Lev, 1963; Pollard, 1964; Dinsley, 1967) and their general use in carcinogenesis testing seems very unlikely in the foreseeable future. They may, however, be valuable for some special purposes. If germ-free rodents prove to be free from viruses they should be valuable for distinguishing direct carcinogenic action from activation of latent viruses. Germ-free rats were used by

Spatz *et al.* (1967) in their demonstration that methylazoxy-methanol is probably the active carcinogenic component of the naturally occurring glycoside cycasin since the glycoside was only active in rats when the intestinal micro-organisms responsible for its degradation were present.

A very important aspect of the care of laboratory animals used in carcinogenesis testing is the safety of the personnel involved. This topic has been given special attention in the book by Hueper & Conway (1964, pp. 409–12) to which the reader is referred for details. As a guiding principle, carcinogenic chemicals should be handled with the same degree of care as radioactive materials and virulent micro-organisms.

Numbers of Animals

The essential point is not the number of animals at the start of the experiment, but the number that will survive to the tumour-bearing age. Another important factor in deciding the numbers of animals to be used is the expected incidence of tumours in the control groups. When inbred strains are used the control incidence can be predicted with a high degree of reliability. With previously untested compounds the incidence in the treated animals can only be conjectured but indications from preliminary experiments of the expected tumour incidence may be very helpful.

The number of animals in each group should be sufficient to yield statistically reliable results. Boyland (1957) has compiled a table showing the lowest incidence of tumours that can be detected at a level of significance of $P=0.025$ with increasing total numbers of animals when experimental and control animals are present in equal numbers and where no tumours appear in the controls. In most cases, of course, tumours do develop in control groups. Another useful table has been derived from the work of B.J. Vos, and appears in the reports of the Food Protection Committee (1959, p. 26) and of the World Health Organization (1961, p. 10). This table shows the differences which must appear between two equal groups to be significant ($P=0.05$) with groups of 50, 40, 30, 20, and 10 animals. If the less affected group has a certain percentage tumour incidence then the more affected group must have a specified larger percentage incidence for the differences to be significant. An example is quoted showing that at least 50 animals per group would be necessary in order to give reasonable assurance ($P=0.05$) that tumour incidences of 25% in the experimental and 10% in the negative control groups are really different. Positive control groups given known carcinogens are useful to check the susceptibility of the animals. Where possible, the carcinogen used as a positive control should be of similar chemical structure to the material under test.

An arbitrary decision must be made on which animals may be included in the total number for statistical analysis. A common practice is to include only those alive at the time of appearance of the first tumour or those alive at the beginning of the fourth month of treatment (Clayson, 1962; Weisburger & Weisburger, 1967). It is also usual to replace animals dying prematurely during the first months of the test. It is clear that the use of SPF animals will lead to a higher proportion surviving to the effective age and will reduce the numbers necessary at the start.

From the above it is apparent that the choice of the numbers in the experimental and in the negative and positive control groups is no easy matter and that each new compound must be considered individually. The reader is particularly referred to Chapter 4 of the book by Clayson (1962) where a clear account of the statistical principles involved is presented. The number of animals chosen per group will also be influenced by the number of different dose levels used. As a rough guide, the Report of the World Health Organization (1961) recommends that in the case of a negative response, at least 20 animals of each sex should survive for 2 years with rats and 80 weeks with mice in each of the different groups.

CONDITIONS OF THE EXPERIMENT

Age of the Animals and Duration of the Experiment

The age at which the test is started is important. Weanling rats and mice are generally used but there has been much interest in carcinogenesis in rodents treated during the neonatal period. There is no doubt that new-born and baby mice are highly susceptible to the action of some known carcinogens (Pietra *et al.*, 1959; Roe *et al.*, 1961; Kelly & O'Gara, 1961) but further work is needed to establish the role of neonatal animals in the testing of compounds of unknown carcinogenic potential.

As already stated, it has been customary to continue administration of the test compound to mice for 80 weeks and to rats for 2
years and regarding these as life-time studies. As SPF animals
become more widely used, these periods may have to be revised.
With dogs anything approaching a true life-time study can rarely
be justified and the duration of the test becomes more arbitrary.
The Food Protection Committee (1960) state that the period of
2 years often used in chronic toxicity studies in the dog is not, in
general, an adequate test for carcinogenicity and recommend a
duration of at least 4 years.

The period of administration of the test compound must be
considered and this is influenced by its toxicity. It is well established that irreversible changes leading to cancer can be induced
by limited periods of exposure to carcinogens and the concepts of
initiation and promotion of tumours and of co-carcinogenesis are
well known (Berenblum & Shubik, 1947; Berenblum, 1954, 1964;
Shubik & Sice, 1956; Salaman, 1958; Salaman & Roe, 1964). With
some very powerful agents such as the nitroso carcinogens, tumours
may follow a single large dose, even though these compounds do
not persist in the body (Magee & Barnes, 1967; Druckrey *et al.*,
1967). In order to reveal weak carcinogenic activity, however, it
is desirable to continue administration of the test compound until
the animals die or are killed after a predetermined period. If, however, losses are severe from toxic reactions, it may be advisable to
treat some groups of animals for limited periods of 40 weeks to
1 year and then observe them for the remainder of their life span.
If some animals are killed and examined at the end of the period
of treatment it may be possible to detect toxic changes which are
reversible (Weisburger & Weisburger, 1967). Druckrey & Schmähl
(1962), on the basis of very extensive studies of dose-response relationships with various carcinogens, have concluded that the final
number of tumours induced is dependent on the total amount of
the compound received by the animal and that the latent period
depends on the daily dose.

Dosage

Considerable help in deciding on the dosage for carcinogenesis
tests can be derived from the previous studies on the short and
intermediate term toxicity of the drug. It is desirable that a dose

level is included which is as high as can be administered without materially reducing the life span of the animals (British Committee on Medical and Nutritional Aspects of Food Policy, 1960). Tumour induction, however, may be restricted to dosage levels which produce other chronic toxic effects and it is therefore advisable also to give the drug at a level which produced a minimal to moderate amount of short-term toxicity. This may be regarded as the maximum dose for measurement of carcinogenic activity (World Health Organization, 1961). This is consistent with the generally accepted principle of chronic toxicity testing (World Health Organization, 1966) that at least one experimental group should receive a dose that is toxic and kills some of the animals. The inclusion of such a high dose group may provide valuable evidence in support of a conclusion that the test compound is not demonstrably carcinogenic. Practical suggestions for selection of dose levels are found in World Health Organization (1961) and Weisburger & Weisburger (1967). If two dose levels are to be employed $\frac{1}{4}$ to $\frac{1}{3}$ of the maximum may be chosen, if three levels, multiples of 1, $\frac{1}{3}$, and $\frac{1}{9}$ the maximum level are suggested. The higher the dose of carcinogen administered, the greater will be the final incidence of tumours and the shorter the time required to elicit them (Food Protection Committee, 1959). Demonstration of a dose-response relationship may therefore be an important factor in establishing weak carcinogenic action in doubtful cases. It is important to remember that cumulative effects of the drug may require reduction of the dose and that the development of tolerance may allow the dose to be gradually increased. It will be apparent that no fixed rules of dosage can be laid down and each drug will require individual consideration. The discussion by Weisburger & Weisburger (1967) will be found particularly helpful in this regard.

Routes of Administration

Few would disagree that a drug should always be tested by the route or routes that are intended for its clinical use. It is less clear, however, what, if any, other routes should be used. These will be determined by the physical, chemical, and biological properties of the drug and, to some extent, by the personal preferences of the investigator.

ORAL

Since most drugs are administered orally this route will be the one mainly used for carcinogenesis studies. The earlier biochemical and pharmacological investigation of the drug will have provided information on the extent of its absorption from the gastro-intestinal tract. The decision to use the oral route will, of course, depend on adequate absorption. The drug may be given either by repeated intra-gastric injection or by addition to the food or drinking water. The oral intubation method has the advantage that dosage can be accurately controlled but the disadvantages of greater involvement of the time of the animal house staff and the possibility of loss of animals through trauma at the time of intubation. In skilled hands the latter hazard need not be great (Moreland, 1965). There is evidence that the toxic action of a compound may vary when it is given five days a week rather than seven (Baker & Alcock, 1965) but the significance of this for carcinogenesis studies is doubtful. If the compound is given in the diet its stability under the conditions of the test should be established by analysis of the food or drink water as used. Drugs may react chemically with the diet, undergo hydrolysis or photo-decomposition or breakdown in other ways, thus possibly causing misleading experimental results. It must therefore, be established that the drug is present in the diet at or very near to the required level throughout the duration of the test. Uniform mixing in the food can be assured by the use of a suitable mechanical mixer, for example that supplied by The Hobart Manufacturing Co. Ltd., New Southgate, London, N.11, England. The necessity to be on guard against the unsuspected presence of carcinogens, co-carcinogens, and enzyme inducers in the diet has already been emphasized.

CUTANEOUS

The cutaneous route has obvious relevance to drugs which are applied to the skin and to cosmetics. The techniques of testing for skin carcinogenesis have been extremely well worked out and are discussed by Berenblum & Shubik (1947), Stewart (1959), Clayson (1962), Hueper (1963), Hueper & Conway (1964), and Boutwell (1964) among many others. The two-stage mechanism of carcinogenesis and the role of initiation and promotion of tumours are of particular importance in skin carcinogenesis. Topical application to the skin is, of course, the method of choice in testing for co-carcinogenic activity. Quantitative methods for measurement of the irritant, co-carcinogenic, and toxic activity of croton oil are described by Hecker (1963).

The recent work of Fare (1966) on topical application of azo dyes shows the possible danger of reliance only on the mouse for skin carcinogenesis studies. Fare showed that a series of azo dyes, of which 3-methoxy-4-monomethylaminoazobenzene was the most active, are potent carcinogens in rat skin but completely inactive in the mouse. This is an exception to the usual experience that topical skin carcinogens are more effective in the mouse than in the rat and suggests the possibility that the dyes may be metabolized by different pathways in the skins of the two species. There seems to be no inherent difference in the capacity of mouse and rat skin to undergo malignant change, since Graffi *et al.* (1967) have shown that both species and also the hamster are highly susceptible to skin carcinogenesis by topical application of the powerful carcinogen N-nitrosomethylurea.

SUBCUTANEOUS

Apart from its use with drugs intended to be given subcutaneously, this route has been chosen when absorption from the gastro-intestinal tract has been in doubt. The repeated subcutaneous injection of a number of food additives, notably food colours, in rats has led to the local production of sarcomas at the injection site (Stewart, 1953). The subcutaneous tissue in the rat is very sensitive to this form of carcinogenesis but the significance of these sarcomas in relation to human hazard has proved very difficult to assess and will be discussed later.

INTRAVENOUS

This route gives very rapid distribution of the drug in the body which is advantageous with unstable and locally irritant materials. Druckrey *et al.* (1967) have used this method for several nitroso carcinogens, including the relatively unstable N-nitrosomethylurea, which gave tumours at multiple sites, including the brain, in rats after repeated intravenous injection (Druckrey *et al.*, 1965). The method has the disadvantage of requiring more skill for its performance than most other methods and also the number of repeated injections into the tail veins of rodents is limited. Grice (1964) discusses the techniques of intravenous injection in laboratory animals.

INTRAPERITONEAL

This route has not been widely used in carcinogenesis testing because it does not correspond to any commonly occurring exposure to a drug, food additive, or pesticide. Recently, however, Shimkin *et al.* (1966) have used the intraperitoneal route for testing a number of alkylating chemicals in strain A mice. A good pulmonary tumour response was obtained, suggesting that intraperitoneal injection could replace intravenous in this system. It is well established that aqueous and protein containing solutions are rapidly absorbed from the peritoneal cavity (Courtice & Steinbeck, 1951). This route has been of value in demonstration of the local carcinogenic activity of metabolites (proximate carcinogens) of some carcinogens which are only active at sites remote from that of injection (Miller *et al.*, 1961; Miller & Miller, 1966). Although the technique of intraperitoneal injection is simple it is liable to error. It has been reported that in as high a proportion as 20% of rats injected part of the material did not enter the peritoneal cavity (Lewis *et al.*, 1966).

INTRAMUSCULAR

The intramuscular route also has not been widely adopted although for certain drugs it would logically be the one of choice. Rhabdomyosarcomas have been induced by single intramuscular injections of cobalt salts (Heath, 1956, 1960). Mannel & Grice (1964) observed rhabdomyosarcoma at the site of repeated subcutaneous injection of the food colour Blue VRS and therefore tested the dye by repeated intramuscular injection into a large muscle mass, using the posterior thigh muscles of the rat. Rhabdomyosarcomas, which frequently metatasized and were successfully transplanted into rats of the same strain, were induced in 50% of the animals. These observations are of interest since the triphenylmethane dyes as a group are thought to be only weakly tumorigenic (Grice & Mannel, 1966).

INHALATION, INTRANASAL, INTRATRACHEAL, INTRAPULMONARY

Administration by inhalation has not been much used in carcinogenicity testing of drugs but it would be reasonable to test volatile anaesthetic agents in this way. If it is decided that a drug must be tested by inhalation there is a large amount of information available on methods and interpretations from work done on tobacco

smoke and air pollutants. Detailed accounts of methods of chronic inhalation toxicity studies are given by Silver (1946), Fraser *et al.* (1959), and Gage (1959). Experiments on the experimental induction of tumours by inhalation exposure are described by Kotin & Falk (1956), Schoental & Magee (1962), Deichman *et al.* (1963), and Kotin & Wisely (1963). The paper by Dontenwill (1964) is recommended for its description of an apparatus in which hamsters can be exposed to tobacco smoke (and therefore, presumably to other gases, vapours, or particulates) in individual chambers over long periods of time. It also includes a useful table of published papers on the experimental induction of lung tumours in mouse, rat, hamster, guinea pig, duck, rabbit, and dog (see also Chapter 3). Technical difficulties are caused by the anatomical features of small animals since much inhaled particulate matter may fail to reach the lungs. Attempts have been made to circumvent this by using the chicken (Peacock, 1955). Problems of inhalation carcinogenesis are discussed in the papers quoted above and by Hueper (1964) and Roe & Walters (1965).

Some workers have ensured penetration into the lungs by intranasal or intratracheal injection. Howell (1961) administered a polycyclic hydrocarbon to rats intranasally and induced squamous cell bronchial carcinoma in four animals as well as bronchiectasis and other lesions. The Syrian hamster has proved very suitable for intratracheal injection. This method has been used by Della Porta *et al.* (1958) who give a detailed description of the technique. Repeated endotracheal installations of 9,10-dimethyl-1,2-benzanthracene in colloidal suspension gave rise to hyperplasia, squamous metaplasia of the tracheobronchial epithelium and later squamous cell and adenocarcinomas. Blacklock (1961) describes a technique for direct injection into the lungs of rats, guinea pigs, and rabbits after thoracotomy.

RECTAL, VAGINAL AND IMPLANTATION INTO URINARY BLADDER AND OTHER SITES

Rectal administration would, in general, only be considered for drugs to be given as enemas or in suppository form. An interesting example of the use of this route is provided by Schmähl *et al.* (1963) who administered diethylnitrosamine by repeated rectal injection and induced tumours of the liver but none in the intestines. In this case the compound was obviously absorbed and exerted a distant carcinogenic action but had no local effect.

The vaginal route has been used for testing contraceptive preparations by Hoch-Ligeti (1957), Boyland *et al.* (1961), and Boyland & Roe (1964). The experiments of Boyland *et al.* (1961) are interesting because the injection vehicle, a polyethylene glycol (Carbowax 1,000) induced a sufficiently large number of tumours to make it impossible to draw conclusions on the carcinogenic potential of the spermicides tested. In subsequent work, Boyland & Roe (1964) used gum tragacanth as the vehicle, which gave rise to no tumours. The test animals were BALB/c mice and the injections were made twice weekly with a syringe and blunt needle, using an injection volume of 0·1 ml.

Implantation into the bladder and other organs has been used for special purposes. The technique of bladder implantation in mice is now well established and has proved valuable in investigations of bladder carcinogenesis (Jull, 1951; Bonser & Jull, 1956; Bonser *et al.*, 1956, 1963; Allen *et al.*, 1957; Boyland *et al.*, 1964; Roe, 1964; Clayson & Bonser, 1965). The chemical under investigation is compressed into a pellet with a supposedly inert vehicle and implanted surgically into the lumen of the bladder. Problems arise, however, in the choice of the vehicle since a variety of the materials that have been used give rise to a moderate incidence of carcinomas in the absence of added carcinogen (Bryan & Springberg, 1966). This may be due to the presence of unknown carcinogens in the vehicle or the pellet may induce epithelial hyperplasia by acting as a foreign body and thus favour carcinogenesis (Clayson & Pringle, 1966).

Implantation of polycyclic hydrocarbons into the wall of the glandular stomach (Stewart *et al.*, 1953) and into the brain (Stewart, 1953) of rodents has led to the induction of tumours in these organs. The value of these procedures, apart from bladder implantations, in the testing of drugs for carcinogenic action is very doubtful.

The Drug and its Vehicle

From what has already been written it will be obvious that both the drug and its vehicle must be in the same state of purity as that intended for clinical use. The presence of trace amounts of a potent carcinogen in either may lead to erroneous conclusions. Stringent chemical and physical specifications are required by most authorities before a drug is released for clinical trial or marketing. These should go a long way towards eliminating carcinogenic impurities from the material used clinically as well as that for carcinogenesis testing.

Formerly the vehicle for the test compound was chosen in a rather haphazard fashion, but there is now extensive experience of the different agents used (Clayson, 1962; Hueper & Conway, 1964; Weisburger & Weisburger, 1967) and certain recommendations can be made.

When the route of administration is by oral intubation the compound may be given dissolved in water if it is sufficiently soluble and stable in aqueous solution. The addition of alcohol to the water may give the necessary increase in solubility. If the compound is insufficiently soluble in water it may be dissolved in arachis or other food oils. When oils are used the volume administered must be taken into account as it may contribute significantly to the total dietary intake of lipid. Excessive amounts of oil may also cause diarrhoea. Water-insoluble materials may be suspended in aqueous media containing gelatine, gum tragacanth, methyl cellulose, etc. The Steroid Suspending Vehicle used at the National Cancer Institute, Bethesda, Maryland, is described by Weisburger & Weisburger (1967). Its composition is: sodium chloride (9 g), sodium carboxymethyl cellulose 7LP (5 g), polysorbate 80 (4 ml) and benzyl alcohol (9 ml) per litre. The use of pills and capsules is confined to dogs and other large animals.

For parenteral administration the same range of vehicles have been used with some additions. Especially for subcutaneous injection it is essential that the vehicle is free from traces of carcinogenic impurities. This can be achieved with vegetable oils as shown by Dickens (1964) who reported no subcutaneous sarcomas in rats given repeated subcutaneous injections of arachis oil as vehicle. Druckrey *et al.* (1966) have discussed the possible contamination of vegetable oils by organic solvents used in their extraction. Such solvents and liquid paraffin (mineral oil) may contain polycyclic hydrocarbon carcinogens (Druckrey *et al.*, 1959). The synthetic oil tricaprylin (trioctanoin) has been used as a vehicle but some samples may give rise to local tumours at the site of injection (Roe, 1964). Dimethylformamide has been used as a solvent in pharmacology but apparently not to any great extent in carcinogenesis testing. Much interest has been aroused in the use of dimethyl sulphoxide as a solvent for drugs and it has been the subject of a recent symposium (Leake, 1967). This agent clearly has considerable potential value because it is completely miscible with water, is a good solvent with remarkable powers of penetration and, as far as is now known, it is not carcinogenic. However, it is by no means biologically inactive and its possible role in carcinogenesis testing remains to be established.

When test compounds are implanted into tissues or organs (e.g. the bladder, see above) they may be compressed into pellets with a solid vehicle. Various materials have been used for this purpose and the possibility of weak carcinogenic action on the part of the vehicle alone must always be kept in mind, e.g. cholesterol (Hieger, 1958), paraffin waxes (Shubik *et al.*, 1962), and various other solid vehicles (Brian & Springberg, 1966).

In tests for skin carcinogenesis acetone now appears to be the solvent of choice, followed by toluene, benzene, and mineral oils. Application by pipette or dropper is now often preferred to painting with a brush since it allows more accurate quantitation of the dose. Hair should be removed by clipper rather than a chemical depilatory agent, but the clipper should not be lubricated with mineral oils.

Termination of the Experiment and Pathological Examination

The duration of the experiment has been discussed above, concluding that it is better to terminate the experiment after a predetermined period rather than waiting for all the animals to die. While stating that customary periods for rats and mice are 2 years and 80 weeks respectively, it was emphasized that these times may be changed with the more extensive use of SPF animals. The animals can be killed by a variety of methods (Lane-Petter *et al.*, 1967) and the choice is best left to the pathologist in charge.

The importance of good pathological examination cannot be over emphasized since insufficient or incompetent work at this stage can ruin an otherwise well planned and executed study. The first essential is that the pathologist concerned with the examination should be thoroughly familiar with the special problems relating to the species under test and with the natural diseases and pathological conditions, including spontaneous tumours, to which it is liable. The value of frequent examination and weighing of the animal is well recognized. In this way it is often possible to pick out sick animals which can be either isolated in individual cages to avoid cannibalism or, if necessary, killed. The decision whether to kill an ageing and sick rodent can be very difficult and the experience of the observer is the best guide. If too many animals die or are killed too early in the test there may not be an adequate number of survivors from which to draw conclusions at the end. It should be stressed, however, that although very undesirable, it may be possible to make an accurate histological diagnosis on material that has undergone fairly extensive post-mortem decomposition and that an attempt should always be made to do this. Even though cytological detail may be lacking, it may be possible to state with reasonable certainty that a lesion is a tumour on histological grounds, particularly if it is a well known type, and expected in the experiment being carried out.

It is highly desirable that the pathologist who will examine the tissues microscopically should either do or be present at the autopsy. Failing this, the autopsy should be done by an experienced and competent observer who is in close and frequent contact with the microscopist. The animals must be examined externally and all the organs carefully scrutinized macroscopically. A hand lens may be invaluable for this. The skull should be opened in rats, since spontaneous pituitary tumours are not uncommon in some strains and induced tumours of the brain may be less uncommon than was formerly thought. Tumours of the spinal cord have recently been reported in high incidence following administration of some nitroso carcinogens (Druckrey *et al.*, 1967) but exposure of the cord in rats is technically difficult and time-consuming and therefore can hardly be required as a routine procedure unless either the chemical structure of the drug or the clinical signs in the animal suggest the diagnosis of these tumours. The value of organ weight measurement at the end of life-time studies in rodents is doubtful.

Opinions differ on how many tissues or organs should be examined microscopically. Clearly all suspected or obvious tumours and all organs with other macroscopically visible lesions must be taken for histology. The decision with regard to macroscopically normal tissues should be left to the pathologist in charge. Considerations of available technical and scientific staff must obviously effect this decision. The methods of fixation, embedding, sectioning, and staining are widely standardized (Lillie, 1954; Drury & Wallington, 1967) and the details will be decided by the pathologist. Haematoxylin and eosin is the staining method favoured by most pathologists for routine purposes with the use of special stains as and when required. The importance of fixing tissues as soon as possible after the death of the animal is not always appreciated by biochemical and chemical workers who may, from time to time, do autopsies. This should be pointed out by the pathologist. Mice, in particular, undergo very rapid post-mortem changes.

Electron microscopy is playing an increasingly important part in toxicology but its value in carcinogenesis testing is not yet established. It cannot be regarded as essential at present. Although certainly not a routine procedure, transplantation may be valuable occasionally in attempts to establish the malignancy of a tumour.

Careful records of all observations made at autopsy are essential. These should be recorded at the time of the autopsy and filed with the reports of the subsequent histological examinations.

PRESENTATION OF RESULTS

The results should be presented in such a way that the chronological sequence of events in each animal can be readily appreciated. Some form of tabular presentation is best for this, showing the time of death of the animals, the number and site of the tumours and the time at which they were observed in the experimental and in the control groups. When there are multiple tumours in an organ, the number should be recorded. Particularly in skin carcinogenesis tests, any regression of the tumours should be noted. The pathological diagnosis should be as precise as possible, distinguishing, where possible, between benign and malignant neoplasms. It is important to record all non-neoplastic pathological changes observed and all changes thought to be precancerous.

Interpretation

Interpretation of carcinogenesis tests is based on the relative numbers of tumours and their time of appearance in the same organs of the treated and control groups of animals. It cannot be over emphasized that the control animals must have been treated in exactly the same way as those given the test drug. Clearly the time of appearance can be determined more accurately with superficial than with deep tumours.

The detection of carcinogenic potential is relatively simple when the test compound is powerful enough to induce many more tumours in an organ or organs than occur at the same sites in the control animals. This is particularly true when the spontaneous tumour incidence is low. With weak carcinogens, however, the problems of interpretation may be very difficult and require careful statistical analysis. In such cases the advice of a professional statistician can be invaluable. If the experiment is to be repeated it may be advantageous to plan it in consultation with the statistician. Clayson (1962) gives a brief account of some of the statistical principles involved. The useful tables on significant differences between control and treated groups given in the reports of the Food Protection Committee (1960) and the World Health Organization (1961) have been mentioned in the section on numbers of animals. A problem arises from the necessity to decide whether only malignant tumours are considered in the total numbers or whether benign tumours should also be included. The problem is further complicated by lack of general agreement on the pathological classification of some rodent tumours, such as pulmonary adenomas and hepatomas. In situations where there is an increased incidence of histologically benign tumours following exposure to a chemical, the term tumorigenic potential may be used (Davis & Fitzhugh, 1962).

DISCUSSION

Subcutaneous Sarcoma

The significance of induced subcutaneous sarcoma in rodents, particularly the rat, is a subject of continuing debate. The problem has great practical importance for food additives as several food colours have been implicated (World Health Organization, 1965) and for drugs where doubts have been raised regarding the safety of iron-dextran complexes used in the treatment of anaemia because they induced subcutaneous sarcomas in animals (Richmond, 1959; Haddow & Horning, 1960). There is no doubt that certain chemicals, specially after repeated subcutaneous injection at the same site, will induce local sarcomas, although they do not induce tumours elsewhere. In some cases the process of tumour formation is associated with local accumulations of injected material and it has been suggested that in such cases the mechanism of sarcoma induction is similar to that with implanted plastics (Oppenheimer *et al.*, 1952). The implication, of course, is that in such cases the process involved is not one of chemical carcinogenesis but a reaction to the foreign material similar to that with plastic films. The significance of subcutaneous sarcoma has recently been reviewed by Grasso & Golberg (1966) who suggest that probably the majority of test compounds that produce sarcoma after administration of high doses continuously for several months act 'indirectly' by derangement of the normal biological processes of connective tissue repair. They regard statistical analysis as an inappropriate means of determining the significance of subcutaneous sarcoma since the spontaneous incidence of this tumour may be less than 1% in rats and mice reaching the tumour bearing age and thus virtually any increase in incidence cannot be regarded as due to chance. Further support for the relative insignificance of subcutaneous sarcomas is claimed from reports by Japanese workers of sarcoma induction by repeated injections of hypertonic saline and sugar solutions. Against this, however, Hueper (1965) has failed to confirm the carcinogenic action of several different sugars after repeated subcutaneous injection in a large number of rats and mice. Druckrey *et al.* (1966a) discuss the possibility that the positive results obtained by the Japanese may have been due to contamination of the sugar solutions used with carcinogenic polycyclic hydrocarbons. The German workers also report failure to confirm the carcinogenic action of subcutaneous injections of hypertonic salt solutions.

Druckrey *et al.* (1966a) also discuss the significance of subcutaneous sarcoma in the rodent and point out that these tumours are not necessarily always induced by a non-specific indirect mechanism. They quote examples of alkylating agents such as dimethyl sulphate (Druckrey *et al.*, 1966b) and some lactones (Dickens, 1964) which are potent inducers of subcutaneous sarcoma in the rat but which certainly do not accumulate at the injection site. They also refer to some unstable nitrosamides which induce local sarcomas after subcutaneous injection in the rat while the stable nitrosamines induce no sarcomas at the site of repeated injection, but give rise to tumours in the liver, oesophagus, lung, and other distant organs.

It seems probable, therefore, that some subcutaneous sarcomas arise by direct local chemical carcinogenesis, similar in mechanism to that in remote organs while others are the result of indirect non-specific reactions. The significance, therefore, of any subcutaneous sarcoma arising at the site of repeated injections of a drug under test can only be assessed after careful consideration of all the physical, chemical, and biological factors involved. The Committee on Medical and Nutritional Aspects of Food Policy (1960) concluded that 'a sarcoma induced in the subcutaneous tissues of the rat following local administration of a substance is not itself decisive evidence that the substance represents a carcinogenic hazard for other species'. More recently a WHO Scientific Group (World Health Organization, 1967) has recommended '(a) that for the *routine* testing of food additives and contaminants the subcutaneous injection test should be considered inappropriate unless special conditions, such as lack of absorption from the gastro-intestinal tract conditions of routine feeding to experimental animals demand additional studies: (b) that the occurrence of a local sarcoma following subcutaneous injection of food additives or contaminants should not, alone, be considered significant evidence of a carcinogenic hazard; such a finding, however, indicates the desirability of a thorough study for systemic manifestations of carcinogenicity by other parenteral or further specific oral investigations'. Although the WHO recommendations apply to food additives they seem equally appropriate for drugs.

Pulmonary Adenomas in Mice

The induction of primary pulmonary adenomas in mice has been a favoured method for quantitative assay of carcinogenic potential (Andervont & Shimkin, 1940; Shimkin, 1955). It has recently been applied by Shimkin *et al.* (1966) for the testing and bioassay of a number of alkylating chemicals including several drugs used in the chemotherapy of cancer and leukaemia. The significance of positive results in this test and their relation to possible human hazard from the drugs are critically discussed. Objections have been raised that these pulmonary adenomas have no human counterpart and that most strains of mice used have an appreciable spontaneous incidence. These objections have been countered by Roe & Walters (1965) who maintain that a proportion of these tumours, however induced, are undoubtedly malignant and that they know of no substance capable of inducing lung tumours in mice which has not also proved carcinogenic in at least one other system when adequately tested. They also point out that spontaneously-arising examples of practically all inducible tumours are seen from time to time. The significance of induced pulmonary adenomas in mice is of great practical importance in relation to the positive action of the drug isonicotinic acid hydrazide in this test system (see Roe, 1966, for discussion).

Liver Tumours in Rodents

The significance of induced liver tumours, particularly in rats, may be hard to assess. The histological appearance of these tumours is varied (Stewart & Snell, 1957) and distinction between hyperplastic or regenerative nodules, benign hepatoma, and hepatocellular carcinoma may be very difficult (Gann Monograph, 1966). Varying resistance by different species to induction of liver tumours adds to the problems of interpretation.

Hormonally Induced Tumours

It is well known that some hormones can induce tumours and much has been written on mechanisms of hormonal carcinogenesis (Furth, 1957, 1961, 1963; Kirschbaum, 1957; Mühlbock & Boot, 1959; Clayson, 1962). According to Mühlbock & Boot (1959) all hormones which have a carcinogenic effect have the common property of stimulating growth in particular target organs which, with few exceptions, include the primary endocrine organs and the secondary sex organs. Thus experimental tumours of the pituitary have been induced by oestrogens and progesterone; of the thyroid by thyrotrophin, of the adrenals by adrenocorticotrophin and of the ovary and testis by gonadotrophins. In the secondary sex organs tumours of the uterus have been induced by oestrogens and of the mammary gland by mammotrophic hormone. The

7—M.T.

exceptions include tumour induction in kidney, liver, bone, and lymphoid tissue. The carcinogenic effect is related to the amount of hormone acting on the target organ and tumours will only develop under continuous growth stimulation by the hormone. Cancer cannot be induced by a single large dose of hormone and the tumour-inciting action of hormones is not irreversible before tumour formation.

It is clear that induction of cancer by hormones differs in many ways from induction by chemical carcinogens and these differences must be borne in mind when interpreting carcinogenesis tests by drugs with hormonal activity. It may be important to distinguish between tumour induction in the target organs from induction elsewhere. It is also important to remember that drugs without hormonal activity may exert an indirect carcinogenic effect by disturbance of hormonal homeostasis. Thus tumours of the thyroid may follow the administration of thiouracil and other antithyroid drugs as a result of excessive production of thyrotrophic hormone.

CONCLUSION

Most of the content of this chapter is equally applicable to the testing of any chemical for carcinogenic activity. In the case of food additives, which may form part of the human diet for virtually the whole life-time of the consumer, there is general agreement that full carcinogenesis testing is essential. With drugs, however, the indications are less clear and for obvious practical reasons only a very small proportion can be tested. It is widely accepted, however, that special attention should be given to compounds which are structurally related to known or suspected carcinogens and to drugs that affect mitosis or may be taken for a long time or are likely to be retained in the tissues (World Health Organization, 1966). Having decided that a drug must be tested for carcinogenic potential a plan of experiments must be made, based on its chemical, physical, and biological properties and on its intended clinical use. If the drug is found to be carcinogenic its therapeutic use must depend on a very careful assessment of the balance of possible benefit against possible risk.

REFERENCES

ALLEN M.J., BOYLAND E., DUKES C.E., HORNING E.S. & WATSON J.G. (1957) Cancer of the urinary bladder induced in mice with metabolites of aromatic amines and tryptophan. *Br. J. Cancer* **11**, 212–28.

ANDERVONT H.B. (1950) Studies on the occurrence of spontaneous hepatomas in mice of strains C3H and CBA. *J. nat. Cancer Inst.* **11**, 581–92.

ANDERVONT H.B. & DUNN T.B. (1952) Transplantation of spontaneous and induced hepatomas in inbred mice. *J. nat. Cancer Inst.* **13**, 455–503.

ANDERVONT H.B. & SHIMKIN M.B. (1940) Biological testing of carcinogens: pulmonary tumour induction technique. *J. nat. Cancer Inst.* **1**, 225–39.

ARGUS MARY F. & HOCH-LIGETI CORNELIA (1963) Induction of malignant tumours in the guinea pig by oral administration of diethylnitrosamine. *J. nat. Cancer Inst.* **30**, 533–51.

ASHBELL R. (1945) Spontaneous transmissible tumours in the Syrian hamster. *Nature (Lond.)* **155**, 607.

ASSOCIATION OF THE BRITISH PHARMACEUTICAL INDUSTRY (1964) *Report of the Expert Committee on Drug Toxicity,* pp 22–3. London.

BAKER S.B. DE C. & ALCOCK SHIRLEY J. (1965) An apparent change in toxicity of a compound when dosed for seven days a week instead of five. *Excerpta Med. int. Congr. Ser.* **97**, 213–18.

BERENBLUM I. (1954) Carcinogenesis and tumour pathogenesis. *Advd. Cancer Res.* **2**, 129–75.

BERENBLUM I. (1964) The experimental basis for carcinogenicity testing. *Excerpta Med. int. Congr. Ser.* **75**, 7–14.

BERENBLUM I. & SHUBIK P. (1947) A new, quantitative approach to the study of the stages of chemical carcinogenesis in the mouse's skin. *Br. J. Cancer* **1**, 383–91.

BLACKLOCK J.W.S. (1961) An experimental study of the pathological effects of cigarette condensate in the lungs with special reference to carcinogenesis. *Br. J. Cancer* **15**, 745–62.

BLACKLOCK J.W.S. & BURGAN J.G. (1962) The carcinogenic effects of various fractions of cigarette condensate. *Br. J. Cancer* **16**, 453–9.

BLEBY J. (1967) Specific-Pathogen-Free Animals, in *The UFAW Handbook on the Care and Management of Laboratory Animals,* ed. LANE-PETTER *et al.* 3rd edition, pp. 201–15. Edinburgh, Livingstone.

BLUMENTHAL H.T. & ROGERS J.B. (1965) Spontaneous and induced tumours in the guinea pig, in *The Pathology of Laboratory Animals,* eds. RIBELIN W.E. & McCOY J.R., pp. 183–209. Springfield, Illinois. Charles C. Thomas.

BONSER GEORGINA M., BOYLAND E., BUSBY E.R., CLAYSON D.B., GROVER P.L. & JULL J.W. (1963) A further study of bladder implantation in the mouse as a means of detecting carcinogenic activity: use of crushed paraffin wax or stearic acid as the vehicle. *Br. J. Cancer* **17**, 127–36.

BONSER GEORGINA M., BRADSHAW L., CLAYSON D.B. & JULL J.W. (1956) A further study of the carcinogenic properties of orthohydroxy-amines and related compounds by bladder implantation in the mouse. *Br. J. Cancer* **10**, 539–46.

BONSER GEORGINA M. & JULL J.W. (1956) The histological changes in the mouse bladder following surgical implantation of paraffin wax pellets containing various chemicals. *J. Path. Bact.* **72**, 489–503.

BOUTWELL R.K. (1964) Some biological aspects of skin carcinogenesis. *Progr. exp. Tumour Res. (Basle)* **4**, 207–50.

BOUTWELL R.K., BOSCH D. & RUSCH H.P. (1957) On the role of croton oil in tumour formation. *Cancer Res.* **17**, 71–5.

BOYLAND E. (1957) The determination of carcinogenic activity. *Acta Un. int. Cancr.* **13**, 271–9.

BOYLAND E. (1962) The determination of carcinogenic activity of chemical substances. *Sci. Repts 1st Super. Sanita* **2**, 439–44.

BOYLAND E., BUSBY E.R., DUKES C.E., GROVER P.L. & MANSON D. (1964) Further experiments on implantation of materials into the urinary bladder of mice. *Br. J. Cancer* **18**, 575–81.

BOYLAND E., CHARLES R.T. & GOWING N.F.C. (1961) The induction of tumours in mice by intravaginal application of chemical compounds. *Br. J. Cancer* **15**, 252–6.

BOYLAND E. & ROE F.J.C. (1964) Tests for carcinogenic activity on constituents of contraceptive preparations intended for intravaginal use. *Rep. Br. Emp. Cancer Campaign* **42**, 22–3.

BREIDENBACH A.W. & ARGUS MARY F. (1956) Attempted tumour induction in guinea pigs. *Quart. J. Florida Acad. Sci.* **19**, 68–70.

BRUCE H.M. & PARKES A.S. (1949) A complete cubed diet for rats and mice. *J. Hyg. (Lond.)* **47**, 202–8.

BRUCE H.M. & PARKES A.S. (1956) A communiqué to the Editor. *J. Anim. Tech. Ass.* **7**, 54.

BRYAN, G.T. & SPRINGBERG P.D. (1966) Role of the vehicle in the genesis of bladder carcinomas in mice by the pellet implantation technic. *Cancer Res.* **26**, 105–9.

BULLOCK F.D. & CURTIS M.R. (1930) Spontaneous tumours of the rat. *J. Cancer Res.* **14**, 1–115.

BURNS E.L. & SHENKEN J.R. (1940) Spontaneous primary hepatomas in mice of strain C3H: a study of incidence, sex distribution and morbid anatomy. *Amer. J. Cancer* **39**, 25–35.

CASS J.S., CAMPBELL IRENE R. & LANGE LILLI (1963) Laboratory animals. An annotated bibliography. *Fed. Proc.* **19**, Suppl. 6, 1–196.

CASS J.S., CAMPBELL IRENE R. & LANGE LILLI (1963) Laboratory animals. An annotated bibliography. Supplement A. *Fed. Proc.* **22**, Suppl. 13, 1–250.

CLAYSON D.B. (1962) *Chemical Carcinogenesis*, pp. 55–100. London, J. & A. Churchill Ltd.

CLAYSON D.B. & BONSER GEORGIANA M. (1965) The induction of tumours of the mouse bladder epithelium by 4-ethylsulphonylnaphthalene-1-sulphonamide. *Br. J. Cancer* **19**, 311–16.

CLAYSON D.B. & PRINGLE J.A.S. (1966) The influence of a foreign body on the induction of tumours in the bladder epithelium of the mouse. *Br. J. Cancer* **20**, 564–8.

CLOUDMAN A.M. (1941) Spontaneous neoplasms in mice, in *Biology of the Laboratory Mouse*, ed. SNELL G.D., pp. 168–233. Philadelphia, Blakiston.

COHRS P., JAFFÉ R. & MEESEN H. (eds.) (1958) *Pathologie der Laboratoriumstiere* (2 volumes). Berlin, Springer-Verlag.

COMMITTEE ON ANIMAL NUTRITION (1962) Nutrient requirements of laboratory animals. *Publication 990*, pp. 1–95. Academy of Sciences, National Research Council, Washington D.C.

COMMITTEE ON THE GUIDE FOR LABORATORY ANIMAL FACILITIES AND CARE (1965) *Public Health Services Publication No. 1024*, pp. 1–45. National Academy of Sciences, National Research Council, Washington D.C.

COMMITTEE ON MEDICAL AND NUTRITIONAL ASPECTS OF FOOD POLICY (1960) Carcinogenic risks in food additives and pesticides. *Mth. Bull. Minist. Hlth Lab. Serv.* **19**, 108–12.

COMMITTEE ON STANDARDIZED NOMENCLATURE FOR INBRED STRAINS OF MICE (1952) Standardized nomenclature for inbred strains of mice. *Cancer Res.* **12**, 602–33.

COMMITTEE ON STANDARDIZED NOMENCLATURE FOR INBRED STRAINS OF MICE (1960) Standardized nomenclature for inbred strains of mice, second listing. *Cancer Res.* **20**, 145–69.

CONNEY A.H., MILLER ELIZABETH C. & MILLER J.A. (1956) The metabolism of methylated amino azo dyes. Evidence for induction of enzyme synthesis in the rat by 3-methylcholanthrene. *Cancer Res.* **16**, 450–9.

COTCHIN E. (1954) Neoplasia in the dog. *Vet. Rec.* **66**, 879–88.

COTCHIN E. (1956) Neoplasms of the domesticated mammals. *Commonw. Bur. Anim. Hlth, Rev. Ser. No. 4*, Commonwealth Agricultural Bureaux, Farnham Royal, Bucks.

COTCHIN E. & ROE F.J.C. (eds.) (1967) *Pathology of Laboratory Rats and Mice*, pp. 1–848. Oxford, Blackwell.

COURTICE F.C. & STEINBECK A.W. (1951) Absorption of protein from the peritoneal cavity. *J. Physiol.* **114**, 336–55.

CRAIN R.C. (1958) Spontaneous tumours in the Rochester strain of the Wistar Rat. *Amer. J. Path.* **34**, 311–35.

CUTHBERTSON W.F.J. (1957) The nutritional requirements of rats and mice. *Lab. Anim. Centre Coll. Papers* **5**, 27–37.

DAVEY D.G. (1959) Establishing and maintaining a colony of specific pathogen free mice, rats and guinea pigs. *Lab. Anim. Centre Coll. Papers* **8**, 17–34.

DAVIS K.J. & FITZHUGH O.G. (1962) Tumourigenic potential of aldrin and dieldrin for mice. *Toxic. appl. Pharmac.* **4**, 187–189.

DAVIS R.K., STEVENSON G.T. & BUSCH K.A. (1956) Tumour incidence in normal Sprague-Dawley female rats. *Cancer Res.* **16**, 194–7.

188 *Methods in Toxicology*

DEICHMAN W.B., MACDONALD W.E., ANDERSON W.A.D. & BERNAL E. (1963) Adenocarcinoma in the lungs of mice exposed to vapours of 3-nitro-3-hexene. *Toxic. appl. Pharmac.* **5**, 445–56.

DELLA PORTA G. (1964) The study of chemical substances for possible carcinogenic action. *Excerpta Med. int. Congr. Ser.* **75**, 29–40.

DELLA PORTA G. (1967) Some aspects of medical drug testing for carcinogenic activity. *U.I.C.C. Monogr. Ser* **7**, 33–47.

DELLA PORTA G., KOLB L. & SHUBIK P. (1958) Induction of tracheobronchial carcinomas in the Syrian golden hamster. *Cancer Res.* **18**, 592–7.

DICKENS F. (1964) Carcinogenic lactones and related substances. *Br. med. Bull.* **20**, 96–101.

DINSLEY MARJORIE (1967) Germfree Animals, in *The UFAW Handbook on the Care and Management of Laboratory Animals,* eds. LANE-PETTER W. *et al.* 3rd edition, pp. 216–38. Edinburgh, Livingstone.

DONTENWILL W. (1964) Experimentelle Untersuchungen zur Genese des Lungencarcinoms. *Arzneimittel-Forsch.* **14**, 774–80.

DRUCKREY H. (1959) Pharmacological Approach to Carcinogenesis, in *CIBA Foundation Symposium on Carcinogenesis, Mechanisms of Action.* eds. WOLSTENHOLME G.E.W. & O'CONNOR MAEVE. pp. 110–30. London, J. & A. Churchill Ltd.

DRUCKREY H., IVANKOVIC S. & PREUSSMANN R. (1965) Selektive Erzeugung maligner Gumoren in Gehirn und Rückenmark von Ratten durch N-Methyl-N-nitrosoharnstoff. *Z. Krebsforsch.* **66**, 389–408.

DRUCKREY H., PREUSSMANN R., IVANKOVIC S. & SCHMÄHL D. (1967) Organotrope carcinogene Wirkungen bei 65 verschiedenen N-Nitroso-Verbindungen an BD ratten. *Z. Krebsforsch.* **69**, 103–201.

DRUCKREY H., PREUSSMANN R., IVANKOVIC S., SO B.T., SCHMIDT, C.H. & BÜCHELER J. (1966a) Zur Erzeugung subcutaner Sarkome an Ratten. Carcinogene Wirkung von Hydrazodicarbonsäure-bis-(methyl-nitrosamid), N-Nitroso-N-*n*-butyl-harnstoff, N-methyl-N-nitroso-nitroguandin und N-nitroso-imidazolidon. *Z. Krebsforsch,* **68**, 87–102.

DRUCKREY H., PREUSSMANN R., NASHED U. & IVANKOVIC S. (1966b) Carcinogene alkylierende Substanzen. 1. Dimethylsulfat, carcinogene Kirkung an Ratten und warscheinliche Ursache von Berufskrebs. *Z. Krebsforsch.* **68**, 103–11.

DRUCKREY H. & SCHMÄHL D. (1962) Quantitative Analyse der experimentellen Krebserzeugung. *Naturwissenschaften,* **49**, 217–28.

DRUCKREY H., SCHMÄHL D. & PREUSSMANN R. (1959) Fluoerszierende Verunreinigungen bei Parraffinum liquidum und Organischen Lösungsmitteln. *Arzneimittel-Forsch,* **9**, 600–4.

DRUCKREY H. & STEINHOFF D. (1962) Erzeugung von Leberkrebs an Meerschweinchen. *Naturwissenschaften* **49**, 497–8.

DRURY R.A.B. & WALLINGTON E.A. (1967) *Carleton's Histological Technique,* 4th edition, pp. 1–432. New York, Oxford University Press.

DUNN THELMA B. (1959) Morphology of mammary tumours in mice, in *The Physiopathology of Cancer,* ed. HOMBURGER F. 2nd edition, pp. 38–84. New York, Hoeberman-Harper.

DUNN THELMA B. (1965) Spontaneous lesions of mice, in *The Pathology of Laboratory Animals*, eds. RIBELIN W.E. & McCOY J.R., pp. 303–29. Springfield, Illinois, Charles C. Thomas.

DUNN THELMA B. (1954) Normal and pathologic anatomy of the reticular tissue in laboratory mice with a classification and discussion of neoplasms. *J. nat. Cancer Inst.* **14**, 1281–433.

ECKARDT R.E. (1959) *Industrial Carcinogens*, pp. 1–164. New York, Grune & Stratton.

EUROPEAN SOCIETY FOR THE STUDY OF DRUG TOXICITY (1964) Evaluation of the potential carcinogenic action of a drug. *Excerpta Med. int. Congr. Ser.* **75**, 1–112.

EUROPEAN SOCIETY FOR THE STUDY OF DRUG TOXICITY (1965) The study of the toxicity of a potential drug—basic principles. *Excerpta Med. int. Congr. Ser.* **97**, 1–45.

FARE G. (1964) Protein binding during mouse skin carcinogenesis by 9,10-dimethyl-1, 2-benzanthracene. The effect of copper acetate and the nonrandom distribution of induction times among mice given identical treatment. *Br. J. Cancer,* **18**, 768–76.

FARE G. (1965) The influence of number of mice in a box on experimental skin tumour production. *Br. J. Cancer,* **19**, 871–7.

FARE G. (1966) Rat skin carcinogenesis by topical applications of some azo dyes. *Cancer Res.* **26**, 2406–8.

FISCHER W. & KUHL I. (1958) *Geschwülste der Laboratoriumsnagetiere*, pp. 1–260. Dresden, Steinkopf.

FOOD AND DRUG ADMINISTRATION (1959) *Appraisal of the Safety of Chemicals in Foods, Drugs and Cosmetics*, pp. 79–82. Association of Food and Drug Officials of the United States, Austin, Texas.

FOOD PROTECTION COMMITTEE (1960) Problems in the Evaluation of Carcinogenic Hazard from Use of Food Additives. *Publication 749*, pp. 1–44. National Academy of Sciences, National Research Council, Washington, D.C.

FOSTER H.L. (1963) Specific pathogen-free animals, in *Animals for Research,* ed. LANE-PETTER W. pp. 110–38. London, Academic Press.

FORTNER J.G. (1957) Spontaneous tumours, including gastro-intestinal neoplasms and malignant melanomas, in the Syrian hamster. *Cancer,* **10**, 1153–6.

FORTNER J.G. (1961) The influence of castration on spontaneous tumourigenesis in the Syrian (golden) hamster. *Cancer Res.* **21**, 1491–8.

FOUTS J.R. (1963) Factors influencing the metabolism of drugs in liver microsomes. *Ann. N.Y. Acad. Sci.* **104**, 875–80.

FRASER D.A., BALES R.E., LIPPMANN M. & STOKINGER H. (1959) Exposure chambers for research in animal inhalation. *Public Health Monograph No. 57*, U.S. Department of Health. Education and Welfare. *Public Health Service Publication No. 662.* United States Government Printing Office.

FURTH J. (1957) Discussion of problems related to hormonal factors in initiating and maintaining tumour growth. *Cancer Res.* **17**, 454–63.

190   *Methods in Toxicology*

FURTH J. (1961) Vistas in the etiology and pathogenesis of tumours. *Fed. Proc.* **20**, 865–73.

FURTH J. (1963) Influence of host factors on the growth of neoplastic cells. *Cancer Res.* **23**, 21–34.

GAGE J.C. (1959) The toxicity of epichlorhydrin vapour. *Br. J. industr. Med.* **16**, 11–14.

Gann Monograph No. 1 (1966) Biological and biochemical evaluation of malignancy in experimental hepatomas, pp. 1–210. Tokyo, Japanese Cancer Association.

GILBERT C., GILLMAN J., LOUSTALOT P. & LUTZ W. (1958) The modifying influence of diet and the physical environment on spontaneous tumour frequency in rats. *Br. J. Cancer* **12**, 565–93.

GORER P.A. (1940) The incidence of tumours of the liver and other organs in a pure line of mice (Strong's CBA strain). *J. Path. Bact.* **50**, 17–24.

GRAFFI A., HOFFMAN F. & SCHÜTT M. (1967) N-methyl-N-nitrosourea as a strong topical carcinogen when painted on skin of rodents. *Nature (Lond.)* **214**, 611.

GRASSO P. & GOLBERG L. (1966) Subcutaneous sarcomas as an index of carcinogenic potency. *Fd Cosmet. Toxic.* **4**, 297–320.

GRICE H.C. (1964) Methods of obtaining blood and for intravenous injections in laboratory animals. *Lab. Anim. Care* **14**, 483–93.

GRIFFIN A.C. & BAUMANN C.A. (1948) Hepatic riboflavin and tumour formation in rats fed azo dyes in various diets. *Cancer Res.* **8**, 279–84.

GUERIN M. (1954) *Tumeurs Spontanées des Animaux de Laboratoire*, pp. 1–215. Paris, Amédée Legrand.

HACKMANN C. (1959) Problems of Testing Preparations for Carcinogenic Properties in the Chemical Industry, in *CIBA Foundation Symposium on Carcinogenesis, Mechanisms of Action,* eds. WOLSTENHOLME G.E.W. & O'CONNOR MAEVE, pp. 308–322. London, J. & A. Churchill Ltd.

HADDOW A. & HORNING E.S. (1960) On the carcinogenicity of an iron-dextran complex. *J. nat. Cancer Inst.* **24**, 109–47.

HADIDIAN Z., FREDERICKSON T.N., WEISBURGER E.K. & WEISBURGER J.H. (1966) Improved tests for chemical carcinogens, report on aromatic amines, nitrosamines, phenols, nitroalkanes, amides, epoxides, aziridines and purine antimetabolites. *Toxic. appl. Pharmac.* **8**, 343.

HANDLER A.H. (1965) Spontaneous lesions of the hamster, in *The Pathology of Laboratory Animals,* eds. RIBELIN W.E. & McCOY J.R., pp. 210–40. Springfield, Illinois, Charles C. Thomas.

HEATH J.C. (1956) The production of malignant tumours by cobalt in the rat. *Br. J. Cancer,* **10**, 668–73.

HEATH J.C. (1960) The histogenesis of malignant tumours induced by cobalt in the rat. *Br. J. Cancer* **14**, 478–82.

HECKER E. (1963) Über die Wirkstoffe des Crotonols. 1. Biologische Tests zur quantitativen Messung der entzündlichen, cocarcinogenen und toxischen Wirkung. *Z. Krebsforsch.* **65**, 325–33.

HIEGER I. (1958) Cholesterol carcinogenesis. *Brit. med. Bull.* **14**, 159–60.

HOAG W.G. & DICKIE M.M. (1966) Nutrition, in *Biology of the Laboratory Mouse*, ed. GREEN E.L., pp. 39–43. New York, McGraw-Hill.

HOCH-LIGETI, CORNELIA (1957) Effect of prolonged administration of spermicidal contraceptives on rats kept on low-protein or on full diet. *J. nat. Cancer Inst.* **18**, 661–85.

HORN H.A. & STEWART H.L. (1952) A review of some spontaneous tumours in non inbred mice. *J. nat. Cancer Inst.* **13**, 591–603.

HOWELL J.S. (1961) Intranasal administration of 9,10-demethyl-1,2-benzanthracene to rats: the development of breast and lung tumours. *Br. J. Cancer* **15**, 263–9.

HUEPER W.C. (1963) The skin as an assay system for potential carcinogens. *Nat. Cancer Inst. Monogr.* **10**, 577–610.

HUEPER W.C. (1964) Methodologic explorations in experimental respiratory carcinogenesis. *Arzneimittel-Forsch.* **14**, 814–22.

HUEPER W.C. (1965) Are sugars carcinogens? An experimental study. *Cancer Res.* **25**, 440–3.

HUEPER W.C. & CONWAY W.D. (1964) *Chemical Carcinogenesis and Cancers*, pp. 403–604. Springfield, Illinois, Charles C. Thomas.

JULL J.W. (1951) The induction of tumours of the bladder epithelium in mice by the direct application of a carcinogen. *Br. J. Cancer* **5**, 328–30.

KELLY MARGARET G. & O'GARA R.W. (1961) Induction of tumours in newborn mice with dibenz(a,h)anthracene and 3-methylcholanthrene. *J. nat. Cancer Inst.* **26**, 651–79.

KELLY MARGARET G., O'GARA R.W., ADAMSON R.H., GADEKAR K., BOTKIN CONSTANCE C., REESE W.H. & KERBER W.J. (1966) Induction of hepatic cell carcinomas in monkeys with N-nitrosodiethylamine. *J. nat. Cancer Inst.* **36**, 323–51.

KIRKMAN H. (1962) A preliminary report concerning tumours observed in Syrian hamsters. *Stanf. med. Bull.* **20**, 163–66.

KIRSCHBAUM A. (1957) The role of hormones in cancer: laboratory animals. *Cancer Res.* **17**, 432–53.

KOTIN P. (1958) Experimentally weak carcinogens: guest editorial. *Cancer Res.* **18**, 1–3.

KOTIN P. & FALK H.L. (1956) Experimental induction of pulmonary tumours in strain-A mice after their exposure to an atmosphere of ozonised gasoline. *Cancer* **9**, 910–17.

KOTIN P. & WISELY D.V. (1963) Production of lung cancer in mice by inhalation exposure to influenza virus and aerosols of hydrocarbons. *Progr. exp. Tumour Res. (Basle)* **3**, 187–215.

KROOK L. (1954) A statistical investigation of carcinoma in the dog. *Acta path. microbial. scand.* **35**, 407–22.

LABORATORY ANIMALS CENTRE COLLECTED PAPERS (1960) *Provision of Animals for Cancer Research*, Vol. 9. Laboratory Animals Centre, M.R.C. Laboratories, Woodmansterne Road, Carshalton, Surrey, England.

LANE-PETTER W. (ed.) (1963) *Animals for Research*, pp. 1–531. London, Academic Press.

LANE-PETTER W., WORDEN A.N., HILL B.F., PATERSON J.S. & VEVERS H.G. (1967) *The UFAW Handbook on the Care and Management of Laboratory Animals*, 3rd edition, pp. 1–1015. Edinburgh, Livingstone.

LEAKE C.D. (ed.) (1967) Biological actions of dimethyl sulfoxide. *Ann. N.Y. Acad. Sci.* **141**, 1–671.

LES E.P. (1966) Husbandry, in *Biology of the Laboratory Mouse*, ed. GREEN E.L. 2nd edition, pp. 29–37. New York, McGraw-Hill.

LEV M. (1963) Germ-free animals, in *Animals for Research*, ed. LANE-PETTER W. pp. 139–75. London, Academic Press.

LEWIS R.E., KUNZ A.L. & BELL R.E. (1966) Error of intraperitoneal injections in rats. *Lab. Anim. Care* **16**, 505–9.

LILLIE R.D. (1954) *Histopathologic Technic and Practical Histochemistry*, 2nd edition, pp. 1–501. New York, Blakiston.

LIPPINCOTT S.W., EDWARDS J.E., GRADY H.G. & STEWART H.L. (1942) A review of some spontaneous neoplasms in mice. *J. nat. Cancer Inst.* **3**, 199–210.

MAGEE P.N. (1959) Pathological changes in old rats in relation to chronic toxicity tests. *Lab. Anim. Centre Coll. Papers* **8**, 59–68.

MAGEE P.N. & BARNES J.M. (1967) Carcinogenic nitroso compounds. *Advd Cancer Res.* **10**, 164–246.

MANNEL W.A. & GRICE H.C. (1964) Chronic toxicity of brilliant blue FCF, blue VRS and green S in rats. *J. Pharm. Pharmac.* **16**, 56–9.

MANTEL N. & BRIAN W.R. (1961) 'Safety' testing of carcinogenic agents. *J. nat. Cancer Inst.* **27**, 445–70.

MILLER ELIZABETH C. & MILLER J.A. (1966) Mechanisms of chemical carcinogenesis: nature of the proximate carcinogens and interactions with macromolecules. *Pharmacol. Rev.* **18**, 805–38.

MILLER ELIZABETH C., MILLER J.A. & HARTMANN H.A. (1961) N-Hydroxy-2-acetylaminofluorene: a metabolite of 2-acetylaminofluorene with increased carcinogenic activity in the rat. *Cancer Res.* **21**, 815–24.

MILLER ELIZABETH C., MILLER J.A., KLINE B.E. & RUSCH H.P. (1948). Correlation of the level of hepatic riboflavin with the appearance of liver tumours in rats fed amino azo dyes. *J. exp. Med.* **88**, 89–98.

MORELAND A.F. (1965) Collection and withdrawal of body fluids and infusion techniques, in *Methods of Animal Experimentation*, ed. GAY W.I., Vol. 1, pp. 1–42. New York, Academic Press.

MORRIS H.P. (1944) Review of the nutritional requirements of normal mice for growth, maintenance, reproduction and lactation. *J. nat. Cancer Inst.* **5**, 115–42.

MÜHLBOCK O. & BOOT L.M. (1959) The mechanism of hormonal carcinogenesis, in *CIBA Foundation Symposium on Carcinogenesis, Mechanisms of Action*, eds. WOLSTENHOLME G.E.W. & O'CONNOR MAEVE, pp. 83–94. London, J. & A. Churchill.

MULLIGAN R.M. (1944) Some statistical aspects of canine tumours. *Arch. Path.* **38**, 115–20.

MULLIGAN R.M. (1949) *Neoplasms of the Dog*, pp. 1–135. Baltimore, Williams & Wilkins Co.

MURPHY E.D. (1966) Characteristic Tumours, in *Biology of the Laboratory Mouse*, ed. GREEN E.L., 2nd edition, pp. 531–62. New York, McGraw-Hill.

OETTLÉ A.G. (1957) Spontaneous carcinoma of the glandular stomach in Rattus (Mastomys) Natalensis an African rodent. *Br. J. Cancer* 11, 415–33.

OPPENHEIMER B.S. OPPENHEIMER ENID T. & STOUT A.P. (1952) Sarcomas induced in rodents by embedding various plastic films. *Proc. Soc. exp. Biol. (N.Y.)* 79, 366–9.

ORRIS L. (1965) Tests for carcinogenicity. Methods and results. *Proc. Sci. Sect. Toilet Goods Ass.* 44, 23–6.

PAGET G.E. & LEMON PHYLLIS G. (1965) The interpretation of pathology data, in *The Pathology of Laboratory Animals*, eds. RIBELIN W.E. & McCOY J.R., pp. 382–405. Springfield, Illinois, Charles C. Thomas.

PEACOCK P.R. (1955) Experimental cigarette-smoking by domestic fowls. *Br. J. Cancer* 9, 461–63.

PIETRA G., SPENCER KATHRYNE & SHUBIK P. (1959) Response of newly born mice to a chemical carcinogen. *Nature (Lond.)* 183, 1689.

POLLARD M. (1964) Germfree animals in biological research. *Science* 145, 247–51.

PORTER G. (1963) Feeding rats and mice, in *Animals for Research*, ed. LANE-PETTER W., pp. 21–45. London, Academic Press.

PORTER G. & LANE-PETTER W. (ed.) (1962) *Notes for Breeders of Common Laboratory Animals*, pp. 1–205. London, Academic Press.

RATCLIFFE H.L. (1940) Spontaneous tumours in two colonies of rats of the Wistar Institute of Anatomy and Biology. *Am. J. Path.* 16, 237–54.

REMMER H. (1964) Drug-induced formation of smooth endoplasmic reticulum and of drug metabolizing enzymes. *Excerpta Med. int. Congr. Ser.* 81, 57–77.

REYNIERS J.A., SACKSTEDER MIRIAM R. & ASHBURN L.L. (1964) Multiple tumours in female germ-free inbred albino mice exposed to bedding treated with ethylene oxide. *J. nat. Cancer Inst.* 32, 1045–56.

RIBELIN W.E. & McCOY J.R. (eds.) (1965) *The Pathology of Laboratory Animals*, 1–436. Springfield, Illinois, Charles C. Thomas.

RICHMOND H.G. (1959) Induction of sarcoma in the rat by iron-dextran complex. *Br. med. J.* 1, 947–9.

ROE F.J.C. (1964) An illustrated classification of the proliferative and neoplastic changes in mouse bladder epithelium in response to prolonged irritation. *Br. J. Urol.* 34, 238–53.

ROE F.J.C. (1964) Discussion of paper by A.L. WALPOLE. *Proc. Eur. Soc. Study Drug Toxicity*, 3, 26–27.

ROE F.J.C. (1965) Spontaneous tumours in rats and mice. *Fd Cosmet. Toxic.* 3, 707–20.

ROE F.J.C. (1966) The relevance of preclinical assessment of carcinogenesis. *Clin. Pharmac. Ther.* 7, 77–111.

ROE F.J.C., BOSCH D. & BOUTWELL R.K. (1958) The carcinogenicity of creosote oil: the induction of lung tumours in mice. *Cancer Res.* 18, 1176–8.

ROE F.J.C., ROWSON K.E.K. & SALAMAN M.H. (1961) Tumours of many sites induced by injection of chemical carcinogens into newborn mice, a sensitive test for carcinogenesis: the implication for certain immunological theories. *Br. J. Cancer*, **15**, 515–30.

ROE F.J.C. & WALTERS M.A. (1965) Some unsolved problems in lung cancer etiology. *Progr. exp. Tumour Res.* (*Basle*) **6**, 126–227.

SALAMAN M.H. (1958) Cocarcinogenesis. *Br. med. Bull.* **14**, 116–20.

SALAMAN M.H. & ROE F.J.C. (1964) Cocarcinogenesis. *Br. med. Bull.* **20**, 139–44.

SAXTON J.A., SPERLING G., BARNES L.L. & MCCAY C.M. (1948) The influence of nutrition upon the incidence of spontaneous tumours in the albino rat. *Acta Un. int. Cancr.* **6**, 423–31.

SCHMÄHL D. (1963) *Entstehung, Wachstum und Chemotherapie maligner Tumoren*, pp. 13–20, Aulendorf i Württ, Editio Cantor.

SCHMÄHL D., THOMAS C. & KÖNIG K. (1963) Leberkrebserzeugende Wirkung von Diäthylnitrosamin nach rectaler Applikation bei Ratten. *Z. Krebsforsch.* **65**, 529–30.

SCHOENTAL REGINA (1961) Liver changes and primary liver tumours in rats given toxic guinea pig diet (MRC diet 18). *Br. J. Cancer* **15**, 812–15.

SCHOENTAL REGINA & MAGEE P.N. (1962) Induction of squamous carcinoma of the lung and oesophagus by diazomethane and N-methyl-N-nitrosourethane, respectively. *Br. J. Cancer* **16**, 92–100.

SHIMKIN M.B. (1955) Pulmonary tumours in experimental animals. *Adv Cancer Res.* **3**, 233–67.

SHIMKIN M.B., WEISBURGER J.H., WEISBURGER ELIZABETH K., GUBAREFF N. & SUNTZEFF V. (1966) Bioassay of 29 alkylating chemicals by the pulmonary-tumour response in Strain A mice. *J. nat. Cancer Inst.* **36**, 915–35.

SHUBIK P., DELLA PORTA G., PIETRA G., TOMATIS L., RAPPAPORT H., SAFFIOTTI U. & TOTH B. (1962) Factors Determining the Neoplastic Response Induced by Carcinogens, in *Biological Interactions in Normal and Neoplastic Growth*, eds. BRENNAN M.J. & SIMPSON W.L., pp. 285–297. Boston, Little, Brown & Co.

SHUBIK P., SAFFIOTTI U., LIJINSKY W., PIETRA G., RAPPAPORT H., TOTH B., RAHA C.R., TOMATIS L., FELDMAN R. & RAMAHI H. (1962b) Studies on the toxicity of petroleum waxes. *Toxic. appl. Pharmac.* **4**, Suppl., 1–62.

SHUBIK P. & SICÉ J. (1956) Chemical Carcinogenesis as a chronic toxicity test. *Cancer Res.* **16**, 728–42.

SHUBIK P., SPENCER, KATHRYNE & DELLA PORTA G. (1957) The occurrence of skin tumours in untreated albino mice from dealer's stock. *J. nat. Cancer Inst.* **19**, 33–6.

SILVER S.D. (1946) Constant flow gassing chambers: principles influencing design and operation. *J. Lab. clin. Med.* **31**, 1153–61.

SNELL KATHERINE C. (1965) Spontaneous lesions of the rat in *The Pathology of Laboratory Animals*, eds. RIBELIN W.E. & MCCOY J.R., pp. 241–302. Springfield, Illinois, Charles C. Thomas.

SPATZ MARIA, SMITH D.W.E., MCDANIEL E.G. & LAQUEUR G.L. (1967) Role of intestinal micro-organisms in determining cyascin toxicity. *Proc. Soc. exp. Biol. (N.Y.)* **124**, 691–7.

STAATS JOAN (1963) International Rules of Nomenclature for Mice, in *Methodology in Mammalian Genetics*, ed. BURDETTE W.J., pp. 517–21. San Francisco, Holden-Day.

STAATS JOAN (1964) Standardized nomenclature for inbred strains of mice, Third listing (Prepared for the Committee on Standardized Genetic Nomenclature for mice). *Cancer Res.* **24**, 147–68.

STAATS, JOAN (1966a) The Laboratory Mouse, in *Biology of the Laboratory Mouse*, ed. GREEN E.L., 2nd edition, pp. 1–9. New York, McGraw-Hill.

STAATS JOAN (1966b) Nomenclature, in *Biology of the Laboratory Mouse*, ed. GREEN E.L., 2nd edition, pp. 45–50. New York, McGraw-Hill.

STEWART, H.L. (1953) Experimental Brain Tumours, in *Physiopathology of Cancer*, eds. HOMBURGER F. & FISHMAN W.H., pp. 84–92. New York, Hoeber-Harper.

STEWART H.L. (1959) Pulmonary Tumors in Mice, in *Psysiopathology of Cancer*, ed. HOMBURGER F., 2nd edition, pp. 18–37. New York, Hoeber-Harper.

STEWART H.L., HARE W.V. & BENNETT J.G. (1953) Tumours of the glandular stomach induced in mice of six strains by intramural injection of 20-methylcholanthrene. *J. nat. Cancer Inst.* **14**, 105–25.

STEWART H.L. & SNELL K.C. (1957) The histopathology of experimental tumours of the liver of the rat, a critical review of the histopathogenesis. *Acta Un. int. Cancr.* **13**, 770–803.

TAMASCHKE, CHRISTIANE (1951/52) Beiträge zur vergleichenden Onkologie der Haussäugetiere. *Wiss. Z. Humboldt-Univ. Berl.* **1**, 37–77.

TAMASCHKE, CHRISTIANE (1955) Die Spontantumoren der kleinen Laboratoriumssäuger in ihrer Bedeutung für die experimentelle Onkologie. *Strahlentherapie* **96**, 150–68.

TANNENBAUM A. (1959) Nutrition and Cancer, in *Physiopathology of Cancer*, ed. HOMBURGER F., 2nd edition, pp. 517–62. New York, Hoeber-Harper.

TANNENBAUM A. & SILVERSTONE H. (1953) Nutrition in relation to cancer. *Adv Cancer Res.* **1**, 451–501.

TRUHAUT R. (1963) Sur les risques de cancerisation pouvant resulter de l'incorporation, volontaire ou fortuite, da'gents chimiques aux aliments. *Acta Un. int. Cancer.* **19**, 472–6.

TRUHAUT R. (1963) Evaluation of carcinogenic activity of food additives and contaminants. *Arch. environm. Hlth* **7**, 351–8.

TUFFERY A.A. & INNES J.R.M. (1963) Diseases of laboratory mice and rats, in *Animals for Research*, ed. LANE-PETTER W., pp. 48–108. London, Academic Press.

WALPOLE A.L. (1964) The properties in the laboratory of known carcinogens. *Excerpta Med. int. Congr. Ser.* **75**, 15–27.

WARREN S. & GATES O. (1941) Spontaneous and induced tumours of the guinea pig. *Cancer Res.* **1**, 65–8.

WEISBURGER J.H. & WEISBURGER ELIZABETH K. (1967) Tests for chemical carcinogens. *Meth. Cancer Res.* **1**, 307–98.

WILLIS R.A. (1961) The significance of experimental tumours for human tumour causation. *Med. J. Aust.* **1,** 393–8.

WORLD HEALTH ORGANIZATION (1958) Procedures for the testing of intentional food additives to establish their safety for use. *Wld Hlth Org. techn. Rep. Ser.* **144.** (Second Report of the Joint FAO/WHO Expert Committee on Food Additives, Rome 1958.)

WORLD HEALTH ORGANIZATION (1961) Evaluation of the carcinogenic hazards of food additives. *Wld Hlth Org. techn. Rep. Ser.* **220.** (Fifth Report of the Joint FAO/WHO Expert Committee on Food Additives, Geneva 1961.)

WORLD HEALTH ORGANIZATION (1964) Prevention of Cancer. *Wld Hlth Org. techn. Rep. Ser.* **276.** (Report of WHO Expert Committee, Geneva 1964).

WORLD HEALTH ORGANIZATION (1965) Specifications for the identity and purity of food additives and their toxicological evaluation: food colours and some antimicrobials and antioxidants. *Wld Hlth Org. techn. Rep. Ser.* **309.** (Eighth Report of the Joint FAO/WHO Expert Committee on Food Additives, Geneva 1964.)

WORLD HEALTH ORGANIZATION (1966) Principles for pre-clinical testing of drug safety. *Wld Hlth Org. techn. Rep. Ser.* **341.** (Report of a WHO Scientific Group, Geneva 1966.)

WORLD HEALTH ORGANIZATION (1967) Procedures for investigating intentional and unintentional food additives. *Wld Hlth Org. techn. Rep. Ser.* **348.** (Report of WHO Scientific Group, Geneva 1967.)

WORDEN A.H. & LANE-PETTER W. (1957) *The UFAW Handbook on the Care and Management of Laboratory Animals*, 2nd edition, pp. 1–951. London, The Universities Federation for Animal Welfare.

WORDEN A.N. & SHILLAM K.W.G. (1967) *The Nutrition of Laboratory Animals*, in *The UFAW Handbook on the Care and Management of Laboratory Animals*, ed. LANE-PETTER *et al.*, 3rd edition, pp. 134–59. Edinburgh, Livingstone.

CHAPTER 7

Detection of Sensitizing Potential

G.E. DAVIES

Sensitization reactions have been defined as 'those reactions to drugs in which clinical symtoms are conditioned by previous exposure to and sensitization to the drug. They are mediated by an antigen-antibody reaction' (Rosenheim & Moulton, 1958). To this definition I would like to add 'or by antibody-like manifestation of cellular reactivity', to include those sensitization reactions, such as contact sensitivity, which are expressions of delayed type hypersensitivity and have not been shown to be dependent on circulating antibody.

On the whole, the term 'allergy' (a condition of altered reactivity) seems preferable to words such as 'sensitivity' or 'hypersensitivity' in discussion of reactions of the types we are here concerned with. Gell & Coombs (1963) have classified allergic reactions into four types (Table 7·1). All these types are represented by allergic

Table 7.1 Classification of allergic reactions (Gell & Coombs, 1963).

Type I (anaphylactic)	(a) Systemic anaphylaxis
	(b) Local anaphylaxis:
	(i) in the skin (urticaria)
	(ii) in the respiratory tract (asthma)
	(iii) in the gastro-intestinal tract and other organs (food allergy)
Type II (cytolytic or cytotoxic)	Antibody reacting with:
	(a) antigenic component of cell
	(b) an antigen or hapten which has become associated with cells
Type III (Arthus reaction; serum sickness)	
Type IV (delayed or tuberculin type)	

197

reactions to drugs, and this classification forms the basis of the present consideration of the possibility of predicting, by laboratory tests, the likelihood that allergic reactions will develop when the drug comes to be used clinically. A broader classification than that of Gell & Coombs is possible. The first, comprising Gell & Coombs Types I to III, depends on the presence of demonstrable antibody and constitutes the so-called immediate allergies. The second group (Gell & Coombs, Type IV) does not require the presence of antibody and belongs to the so-called delayed allergies. The difference between these two groups is important from the point of view of methodology and can be clarified by a consideration of two examples (Table 7·2).

Table 7.2 Comparison of immediate and delayed allergies.

	Immediate	Delayed
Antibody	Immunoglobulin free in serum or fixed to cells: precipitating or non-precipitating	Antibody-like property of lymphocytes
Passive transfer	With serum	With cells
Time course in sensitized individual	Minutes–hours	1–4 days

Injection of a small quantity of horse serum into a guinea-pig stimulates the production of antibodies and renders the animal anaphylactically sensitized so that a second injection of horse serum, given 2 weeks or so later, causes anaphylactic shock. Serum taken from the sensitized animal can, by appropriate techniques to be described later, be shown to contain antibodies capable of reacting specifically with horse serum. Furthermore, injection of this serum into a normal animal will render the recipient passively sensitized so that it too will respond by anaphylactic shock to an injection of horse serum. The characteristic of this type of allergy, which designates it as 'immediate' is the fact that signs of anaphylaxis become apparent within a few minutes of the provoking injection. It should, however, be pointed out that not all allergies in this group are quite so 'immediate' as anaphylaxis. The Arthus reaction, for example, which is an oedematous and often haemorrhagic local reaction to the injection of antigen into a highly sensitized animal, may take 3 hours or more to reach its peak. The Arthus reaction, like anaphylaxis, depends on the presence of antibody and can be passively transferred with serum.

The second group of reactions is typified by the tuberculin reaction. Injection of a suspension of dead tubercle bacilli into a guinea-pig renders the animal allergic to tuberculin. This state becomes apparent as early as 5 days after the injection and will persist for months. It may be demonstrated following the intradermal injection of a small amount of tuberculin when a slowly-developing erythematous reaction, sometimes indurated or necrotic, appears at the site of the intradermal injection and reaches a peak 24 hours or so later. Unlike anaphylactic-sensitivity, tuberculin allergy is not transferable to normal animals by means of serum but can be transferred by the injection of washed spleen cells or lymph node cells taken from sensitized animals. Antibody-dependent allergies may also be transferable by the same cells but in this case the transfer is due to the secretion of antibody by the cells in the recipient. This is not true for tuberculin allergy: antibodies directed to protein constituents of the tubercle bacillus may, in fact, be secreted but they do not mediate the tuberculin reaction. The slowly developing nature of the tuberculin reaction typifies it as a delayed allergy.

The two examples, described above employed complex antigens (horse serum and the tubercle bacillus, respectively). Our present concern is with drugs which are relatively much simpler molecules of low molecular weight. Such compounds cannot by themselves function as complete antigens but may do so after reaction with protein. Molecules whose chemical reactivity is such that they are able to form a firm conjugate with protein are likely to act as haptens and the conjugate, which may even be formed *in vivo* by reaction with the proteins of the injected animal, will act as an antigen and stimulate the production of antibodies. Most drugs are not of this high degree of chemical reactivity and it is necessary to postulate that the reactive intermediate is formed by metabolic or spontaneous breakdown. This theory has recently received strong support from the brilliant work of de Weck, Levine, and others on the immunochemistry of penicillin (reviewed by de Weck & Blum, 1965). If the potential allergenicity of drugs does indeed depend on their ability to react with protein, then an assessment of this potential should be possible from a consideration of their chemical properties. Table 7·3 (Davies, 1964) shows a list of groupings which may confer suitable reactivity on a compound and also the groups in protein which are available for combination. The absence of these reactive groups from most drugs emphasizes the point made earlier that drugs are not, as a class, reactive chemicals. It is true that many, if not all, drugs are to a certain extent protein-bound in the body, but this type of binding is not sufficient to make them act as haptens.

Table 7.3   Reactive groups on haptens and proteins
(Davies, 1964).

On hapten		On protein
Diazonium	$\overset{+}{-}N{=}N$	—OH (serine)
Thiol	—SH	—NH$_2$ (Lysine)
Sulphonic acid	—SO$_3$H	—NHCNH$_2$ (Arginine)
		NH
Aldehyde	—CHO	
Quinone		—SH (Cysteine) —S—S— (Cystine)
Activated halogen		⬡—OH (Tyrosine)

The ability to recognize the allergenic potential of a drug resolves itself then into attempts to detect immunological changes which might occur when the drug is administered to animals. If the actual sensitizing agent in man is a metabolic product then studies such as we are going to consider will have significance only if the appropriate metabolite is produced in the experimental animal. With new drugs, the metabolic pathway will, as a rule, be unknown and animal tests may prove to be positively misleading, since a reactive metabolite may be produced in the animal but not in man. A further and most important consideration is the use that may be made of any results obtained from animal experiments on allergenicity. It is a well recognized fact that most, if indeed not all drugs have produced allergic reactions in man and that with the exception of penicillin it has not proved possible, even in retrospect, to demonstrate by animal experiments that these drugs have allergenic potential. Further, let us suppose that methods will ultimately be developed which would reveal this potential with absolute certainty, what use would then be made of this knowledge? Would compounds potentially as useful as penicillin or streptomycin or chlorpromazine or aspirin (all 'sensitizing' drugs) be rejected on this basis?

It is therefore in the light of these considerations that a discussion of experimental methods will be undertaken but I would venture to suggest that their value may lie more in the field of pure knowledge rather than any practical use that could arise from the findings.

The two main classes of allergy (immediate and delayed types) demand separate treatment.

METHODS FOR INDUCING DELAYED ALLERGIC REACTIONS WITH SIMPLE CHEMICAL COMPOUNDS

The most readily recognizable delayed reaction is that of contact type hypersensitivity which arises when the chemical is applied to the skin of a sensitized animal. For all delayed type reactions the guinea-pig is the animal of choice being the species most easily sensitized (the rabbit does not show contact sensitivity and rats and mice can be sensitized only with some difficulty). Care must be taken to distinguish true allergic reactions from those which are merely expressions of primary irritancy. This distinction is of less importance during the phase of induction of sensitization than during the actual evocation but, nevertheless, must be taken into account. If the compound is very irritant its effects may so damage the site of future tests for sensitivity as to render interpretation difficult. This trouble can be avoided if the ear is used as the site of application of the sensitizing doses and the skin of the flank for the test doses, as suggested by Turk (1964). It is imperative, however, to use non-irritant concentrations to test for actual sensitivity and it is therefore necessary to titrate the compound by application to the skin of normal animals to determine the maximum concentration that can be used without causing a reaction still visible 24 hours later. The first problem is to find a suitable solvent which will be non-sensitizing in its own right. Olive oil, corn oil, acetone or ethanol may be suitable. For water-soluble compounds intradermal injection of a saline solution may be preferable to skin-application. Levine (1960) sensitized guinea-pigs to penicillin with the aid of a solvent consisting of 95% ethanol, 45 parts, methyl cellosolve, 45 parts and Tween 80, 10 parts by volume and this solvent may be found to have more general applicability. Whatever solvent is eventually chosen, control groups of animals, treated with solvent, must be included in each experiment. The usual practice is to apply the material once daily for three days and then to test for allergy by applying a non-irritant concentration to an area of shaven skin 7–9 days after the last sensitizing application. The animals are examined 24 and again 48 hours later and the degree of reaction noted.

For compounds whose allergenic potential is thought to be low, or for the production of more intense levels of hypersensitivity, injection of the material together with Freund's complete adjuvant is recommended. The following method has been suggested by Salvin (1965): Inject 50 μg of hapten in Freund's complete adjuvant into the foot pad of guinea-pigs. Five or six days later apply to the skin 0.005 ml of a freshly-prepared solution containing 5 mg/ml of hapten in 4:1 acetone-corn oil or acetone-olive oil.

METHODS FOR INDUCING ANTIBODY-DEPENDENT ALLERGIES

Contact sensitivities, although common and troublesome do not, in the main, present a serious hazard. Similarly, urticarial and other skin reactions are usually mild and promptly subside when the drug is withdrawn. Anaphylaxis and allergic blood dyscrasias can, however, be of much more serious consequence and since these reactions are dependent on the presence of antibody, it is necessary to consider methods for producing antibodies to drugs. There is probably little need to attempt to produce experimentally every conceivable type of allergic reaction, if this indeed were possible.

The essential requirement for a drug to become allergenic is, as we have seen, its ability to act as, or be transformed into, a hapten. It then follows that antibodies will be formed with specificity for the hapten. But the presence in a person's serum of antibodies to a drug does not necessarily mean that the individual is allergic to that drug.

The development of allergy is determined by genetic factors which govern the type of antibody produced in response to a given antigenic stimulation. Antibodies belong to the globulin fraction of serum proteins and five main types have so far been recognized in human serum (Table 7·4).

Table 7.4 Immunoglobulins.

Immunoglobulin	Synonyms
γG or IgG	γ, 7Sγ, γ2, γSS
γA or IgA	β2A, γ1A
γM or IgM	γ1M, β2M, 19Sγ, γ-macroglobulin
IgD	
IgE[a]	

[a] Contains reaginic activity.

Until very recently it was believed that the reaginic antibodies involved in hay-fever, asthma, etc., belonged to the IgA class but Ishizaka *et al.* (1966) have described a new immunoglobulin, designated IgE, which carries reaginic activity. Reaginic antibodies are heat-labile and will passively sensitize human skin but not that of animals with the exception of monkeys. Analogous immunoglobulins also appear to be involved in anaphylactic reactions of guinea-pigs (Ovary *et al.*, 1963), mice (Nussenzweig *et al.*, 1964), and rats (Binaghi *et al.*, 1964). No specific function has yet been found for IgD (Rowe & Fahey, 1965).

Very little is known about the pathogenic significance of the other classes of antibody in man. It is however certain that both IgG and IgM antibodies to penicillin can exist in the absence of demonstrable allergic sensitivity. This really is the crux of our present problem. It is apparent that small molecules can be induced to become immunogenic but demonstration is not a sufficient requirement for the induction of allergy. What we need to know is why certain individuals produce qualitatively different antibody and studies such as those discussed here tell us nothing about this.

Allergic blood dyscrasias present certain features which separate them, immunologically, from other drug allergies. In thrombo-cytopenic purpura due to Sedormid, for example, addition of the drug to a mixture of the patient's serum and normal platelets will cause agglutination of the platelets or, in the presence of complement, their lysis (Ackroyd, 1962). The association between drug and platelets is extremely loose, and can be reversed even by a simple wash in saline. Such a loose association is not of the kind that might be expected to lead to antigenicity. An acceptable explanation for these findings has been given by Shulman (1964). He proposed that when the drug is administered a complete antigen is formed by reaction of the drug, not with platelets, but with some non-celluar substance with which, presumably, the drug can form a stable complex. Antibodies formed against this conjugate will react *in vivo* or *in vitro* with hapten (i.e. unchanged drug). The resulting hapten-antibody complex is then absorbed loosely and non-specifically on the platelet surface rendering it liable to agglutinate with other platelets. A similar argument could be applied to other allergic blood dyscrasias.

The ability of a patient to develop drug allergy depends then on a multiplicity of factors, including those responsible for:

1 The ability to form a reactive hapten from the drug.
2 The pre-disposition to produce IgE rather than, or in addition to IgM and/or IgG.
3 The constitutional or disease-induced propensity to react in a particular way following interaction of antigen with antibody.

It is apparent that animal experiments cannot take account of all these variables. The most that can be done is to demonstrate that antibodies are formed when the drug or a suitable conjugate is given to animals.

Fortunately, relatively simple and well-established methods are available for the production and detection of antibodies. There are, however, numerous such methods and for a complete list, standard works on immunology should be consulted. (Campbell *et al.*, 1963; Kabat, 1961; Ackroyd, 1964).

The methods for detection of antibodies, described below, have been chosen for their relative simplicity and should be sufficient for our present purposes. They utilize a visible reaction which takes place when antigen reacts with antibody. Soluble antigens precipitate when mixed with antibody in a test tube but maximal precipitation takes place only with a certain ratio of antigen to antibody, the precipitate may be soluble in an excess of either reagent. As an alternative to mixture in a test tube, antigen and antibody may be allowed to diffuse towards one another in an agar gel, a precipitate being formed when the antigen/antibody ratio becomes optimal.

Certain classes of antibody will, after reaction with antibody, fix serum complement. The principle of their estimation depends on a measurable reduction in the haemolytic titre of added complement. In order to avoid possible complication due to the presence of complement in the antiserum itself it is customary to inactivate the antiserum by heating at 56° for 20 min but it must be understood that this heating may also destroy heat-labile antibodies. An alternative method for removing complement from antiserum, without heating, is by the addition of an unrelated antigen-antibody complex. The methods for estimation of complement-fixing antibody are very complex and tedious and should not be necessary in the study of drug allergies. Details of technique are not, therefore, included here but the methods are fully described by Kabat (1961).

Red blood cells and other suitable particles, such as latex, collodion, bentonite, when coated with antigen become agglutinable in the presence of specific antibody and this forms the basis of a very sensitive test for the estimation of antibodies. Finally, the ability of an antibody to induce passive anaphylactic reactions in animals or tissues may be used. The relative sensitivities of these methods are shown in Table 7·5 (Humphrey & White, 1964).

In general we will be dealing with conjugated antigens in which a small molecule (the hapten) has been reacted with a carrier protein to form a complete antigen. Unless the protein carrier has been derived from the actual animal used for the tests, injection of conjugated antigen will lead to the production of three groups of antibodies, directed respectively against (a) the hapten itself, (b) the conjugated protein, (c) any unreacted protein. Since, with drug allergies, we are interested primarily in anti-hapten antibodies some means of distinguishing these must be adopted. Two general methods may be used to make this distinction.

Table 7.5 Sensitivity of various methods of detecting or determining antibodies (Humphrey & White, 1964).

Method	μg of antibody (N/ml)
Specific precipitation:	
(a) Qualitative	
'Ring' test	3–5
Gel diffusion	5–10
(b) Quantitative	
Micro-Kjeldahl nitrogen	10
Colorimetry (Folin & Ciocalteu)	4
Haemagglutination (adsorbed antigen)	0·003–0·006
Haemolysis (lytic antibody + complement)	0·001–0·03
Complement fixation	0·1
Passive anaphylaxis	Total antibody required (μg N)
Whole guinea-pig	30
Guinea-pig uterine muscle	0·01
Guinea-pig skin (passive cutaneous anaphylaxis)	0·03

1 Animals are immunized with the hapten coupled to one protein and antibody tests done with the same hapten coupled to another protein. In principle, it is better to use 'pure' proteins rather than serum for conjugation. Commercially available crystallized egg albumin or bovine plasma proteins are suitable.

2 Hapten itself may be used to inhibit the reaction of antibody injected with the hapten conjugated protein. Thus an animal injected with a hapten 'X' conjugated to a protein A, will form anti-X, and anti-A antibodies. When hapten 'X' is added to this antiserum it will react with its specific antibody and will thus reduce the titre of antibodies directed against other components of the antigen used for immunization.

Production of Antibodies

PREPARATION OF ANTIGEN
Since most of the types of molecules we are considering at present are unlikely to act directly as antigens the first requirement is to prepare suitable conjugates with protein. The actual method chosen for conjugation will of course depend upon the nature of the reactive group in the hapten and the assistance of an organic

chemist should be sought. As a general method, a solution of the hapten in dioxane may be added gradually to a stirred, cooled solution of protein but more specific methods such as diazotization may be required. Whatever method is chosen two conjugates, each with a widely different protein (such as egg albumin, and bovine γ globulin) should be prepared. One of these will be used for immunization and the other as an antigen to test for antibodies directed against the hapten. Care should be taken to remove free hapten from the antigens (e.g. by dialysis).

IMMUNIZATION OF ANIMALS

At least six guinea-pigs and three rabbits are used. The best chance of producing antibodies will be with the use of Freund's complete adjuvant. This may be purchased (Difco) or made according to the following recipe:

Thoroughly mix 8·5 ml of light liquid paraffin, 1·5 ml Arlacel A (Honeywell & Stein Ltd.) and 50 mg of ground dried, heat-killed mycobacteria. Autoclave the mixture for 15 min at 15 lb in^2.

A solution of the conjugate in saline (5–10 mg/ml) is then added gradually to an equal volume of the adjuvant, so as to form an emulsion. This is done conveniently by placing the adjuvant in a dry sterile mortar and the solution of conjugate in a syringe with attached needle. Stirring is continued, as the conjugate is added gradually. The degree of emulsification can be tested by placing a drop on the surface of ice-cold water. If the drop remains intact, the emulsion is suitable but if it spreads more emulsification is required.

Injections are made in one or more foot pads (0·1 ml per site in guinea-pigs and 0·5 ml per site in rabbits). Trial bleedings may be made 3 or 4 weeks later and if necessary booster injections may be given at this time by injecting saline solutions of conjugate (without adjuvant) intradermally. Further blood samples are taken 7–10 days after the boosting injection.

Blood samples are taken from the veins of rabbits or from the hearts of guinea-pigs. After the blood has clotted, the serum is harvested by centrifugation and either tested immediately or stored at −20°C.

Detection of Antibodies

The most readily detectable activity of antibodies directed against soluble antigens is the precipitation which occurs when antigen and antibody are mixed in a test tube. Optimal precipitation takes place only with a certain ratio of antigen to antibody since the precipitate may be soluble in an excess of either antigen or antibody.

(a) *Ring test*

This is a simple, qualitative test. A solution of the antigen is carefully placed on top of the antiserum in such a manner that a sharp liquid interface is formed. As a result of diffusion of the two components a ratio of antigen to antibody is formed which is optimal for precipitation. Care must be taken that both solutions are as clear as possible.

Method. With a Pasteur pipette carefully place the antiserum into two test tubes (6×50 mm) to a height of 4 to 5 mm. As a control, similarly pipette an equal amount of normal serum into two other tubes. With a clean pipette overlay one sample of antiserum and one of normal serum with a solution of antigen (about 0·05%) and the other two tubes with saline. Avoid mixing at the interface during pipetting by slanting the tube and allowing the solution to run slowly down the wall. A positive reaction is indicated by a zone of turbidity which should be visible within a few minutes.

(b) *Double diffusion in agar*

If antigen and antibody are allowed to diffuse towards one another in an agar gel, a zone is formed where antigen/antibody ratio is optimal for precipitation. There are numerous modifications of this technique (Ouchterlony, 1962). The following has been found suitable for most purposes:

1. Agar Solution:

> Agar (Special Agar-Noble 'Difco')   1 part
> Sodium Chloride   1 part
> Distilled water   98 parts
> Dissolve by immersing the container in a boiling water bath.

2. Impregnation agar solution: 0·1% and 0·05% glycerin in distilled water.
3. Sodium Chloride Solution: 1% NaCl in distilled water.
4. Rinsing solution:

Methyl alcohol	45 parts
Acetic Acid	10 parts
Water	45 parts

STAINING SOLUTION

Dissolve 4·5 g of Amido Black in 750 ml of rinsing solution. Filter.

Method. Clean microscope slides with chromic acid solution and store in acetone or ethanol until required for use. Before use allow the solvent to evaporate and apply a film of hot impregnation agar solution with a brush and let the agar dry for at least 15 min. Place the slide on a level surface and pipette 2·5 ml of agar solution at about 80°C on to the slide. Cover the slide and after about 15 min, when the agar has set, place the slide in a humid chamber for at least 30 min. With a small metal punch, punch holes about 3 mm diameter in the agar and remove the agar by suction. The arrangement and distance between the holes will depend on the nature of the experiment.

Leave the slide in a humid chamber for at least 24 hours. Weaker reactions may take much longer to develop. Wash the slide by immersion first in sodium chloride solution for 6 hours, then in fresh sodium chloride solution for 16 hours and finally in distilled water for 1 hour. Before drying the slides, fill the wells with distilled water and cover the slide with a layer of filter paper. Allow the slide to dry overnight, remove the filter paper (if it adheres it may be wetted with water). Immerse in staining solution for 5 min and then in four separate lots of rinsing solution for 10 min each time. Allow the slide to dry. (A complete kit for the study of immuno-diffusion can be obtained from LKB-Produkter, Sweden.)

Haemagglutination Tests

The agglutination of antigen-coated erythrocytes by specific antisera was first described by Boyden (1951). This test is now one of the most widely used of all methods for the estimation of antibody and has been studied in detail, particularly by Stavitsky & Arquilla (1958).

PRINCIPLE OF METHOD

Washed red blood cells are treated with tannic acid, washed and then treated with a solution of antigen which coats ('sensitizes') the tanned cells. The washed, sensitized tanned cells are then added to dilutions of antibody, which causes them to agglutinate. Unagglutinated cells settle in the form of a discrete button whilst various degrees of agglutination are indicated by a pattern of settling which extends from a narrow ring of red around the edge of a smooth mat to a compact granular agglutinate.

MATERIALS

(i) *Antiserum* is heated at 56°C for 30 min (to destroy complement which might otherwise cause lysis) and absorbed with an equal volume of washed sheep red blood cells for 10 min at room temperature. The inactivated antiserum may be stored at 5°C but should be discarded if bacterial contamination becomes evident.

(ii) *Red blood cells:* Sheep blood in Alsever's solution serves as a satisfactory source of red blood cells. It may be stored for 3–6 weeks if collected aseptically and kept at 5°C. It should not be used if lysis has taken place. The blood is centrifuged and the cells washed three times with saline (discard the cells if the supernatant is not clear and colourless at this stage).

(iii) *Antigen solution:* This is a solution of antigen in saline. The proper concentration should be determined by experiment and will probably fall in the range 0·01 to 0·05%, most frequently 0·025%.

(iv) *Diluent:* A 1 : 100 dilution in saline of normal rabbit serum, inactivated by heat and absorbed with red cells as described for antiserum.

(v) *Tannic Acid:* A stock 1% solution of tannic acid in saline may be stored in a refrigerator and diluted in saline to 0.005% before use.

Buffers pH 7·2 and pH 6·4. Equals parts of 0·15 M phosphate buffer and saline.

METHOD

1   Add 10 ml of saline to 3 ml of sheep blood in Alsever's solution. Mix thoroughly and centrifuge at 500g (approximately 2,500 rev/min if rotating radius is 7 cm) for 5 min. Carefully aspirate the supernatant. Repeat the washing three times.

2   Add 0·5 ml of packed, washed cells to 20 ml of pH 7·2 buffered saline. Mix thoroughly.

3   Add 9 ml of this cell suspension to 9 ml of dilute tannic acid solution. Mix thoroughly using a Pasteur pipette and place in a water bath at 37°C for 10 min.

4   Centrifuge the suspension for 5 min at 500*g*. Decant supernatant by pouring. Resuspend in 9 ml of pH 7·2 buffered saline. Mix thoroughly. Re-centrifuge and decant supernatant. Resuspend cells in 9 ml of pH 7·2 buffered saline. Mix thoroughly.

5   To 12 ml of pH 6·4 buffered saline add 3 ml of antigen solution and 3 ml of tanned cell suspension from step 4. Mix thoroughly and allow to stand at room temperature for 10 min.

6   Prepare control cells as in 5, substituting 3 ml of saline for 3 ml of antigen solution.

7   Centrifuge for 5 min at 500*g*. Decant supernatants and resuspend cells in 6 ml of rabbit serum diluent. Mix thoroughly. Centrifuge again and decant supernatants.

8   Resuspend cells in 3 ml of rabbit serum diluent.

9   Prepare two series of two-fold dilutions of antiserum in rabbit serum diluent. The test may be carried out in test tubes (13 × 100 mm) or MRC Perspex agglutination trays. In either case, 0·5 ml of the dilution is used. To each tube of the first series add 0·05 ml of antigen coated cells, and to each tube of the second series 0·05 ml of control cells. Set up two control tubes containing 0·5 ml of rabbit serum diluent and 0·05 ml of either antigen coated cells or control cells.

10   Allow the tubes to stand at room temperature and examine at 3 hours and/or 20 hours. Score according to the following settling pattern.

+ Compact granular agglutination or diffuse film of agglutinated cells covering the bottom of the tube; edges of film either folded or somewhat ragged.

± Narrow ring of cells surrounding a diffuse film of agglutinated cells.

− Heavy ring of cells or discrete smooth button in centre of tube.

The haemagglutining titre of the antibody is the highest dilution causing ± agglutination.

Passive Cutaneous Anaphylaxis (Ovary, 1958)

Passive cutaneous anaphylaxis utilizes the local increase in vascular permeability which occurs when antigen reacts with antibody which has become 'fixed' to the tissues of the skin. Visualization of this reaction is made much easier by the use of a dye, which, when injected intravenously, is absorbed on serum albumin so that the plasma exuding in an area of increased permeability stains an area of skin and the intensity of staining is proportional to the degree of increased permeability. Although the technique has numerous applications (Ovary, 1958) only its use for the detection and estimation of antibodies will be dealt with in any detail.

The method consists in the intradermal injection of dilutions of antibody, followed, after an appropriate interval by an intravenous injection of dye mixed with antigen. The size and intensity of the blue spot at the site of the intradermal injection is a measure of the amount of antibody injected.

Albino guinea-pigs of about 250 g body weight are the most suitable. Only healthy animals, free from scars or other skin blemishes should be used. The animals are shaved with electric clippers, care being taken not to scratch the skin in the process. Intradermal injections are made on both sides of the back, about 10 cm from the mid-line and about 1·5–2 cm from each other. Three injections on each side are practicable. Antiserum, diluted in saline, is injected intradermally with the aid of a 0·5 or 1 ml all-glass tuberculin syringe fitted with a 20 or 26 gauge needle. The needle should be introduced as superficially as possible with the bevel turned downwards: a slight twist, applied as the needle is withdrawn will help to avoid back-leakage. A volume of 0·1 ml injected should immediately raise a bleb of about 8mm in diameter. Intravenous injections may be made into a marginal ear vein. The animal, wrapped in a cloth, is held by an assistant and the ear veins transilluminated by applying a light to the end of a bent Perspex rod. Up to 1 ml may be injected, and no vasodilator or anaesthetic is needed. Antigen is dissolved in 5% solution of Pontamine sky blue or 1% Evans blue and 0·5 ml of the mixture injected through a 26 gauge needle. Since a great excess of antigen does not inhibit the reaction a dose of 1 mg will often be found suitable although some pilot experiments may be necessary. A certain latent period is required for 'fixation' of antibody; for routine use an interval of 3–6 hours between intradermal injection of antibody and intravenous injection of antigen/dye mixture will often be satisfactory. Reactions are read 30–45 min after the intravenous injection. Strong reactions can be read on the outer skin of the living animal but it is preferable to kill the animal and pin the skins, inside uppermost, on a cork mat. The diameters of the blue spots can then be measured. This measurement should be made without delay as the colour tends to diffuse somewhat if the skins are allowed to stand. At least four animals should be used for each experiment.

Although this technique requires a little practice, it is an invaluable adjunct to the techniques for estimating antibodies. Interpretation of the results presents little difficulty but there are some possible sources of error which must be taken into account. Only non-toxic doses of antigen may be used and although sterility is not essential, dye and antigen solutions must be filtered before use. Certain samples of antisera may produce non-specific reactions, especially if the antibody level is low, necessitating the use of neat serum or of low dilutions. If such use appears essential, or if the serum is being used for the first time, the dye should be injected 30 min before the intravenous injection of antigen and the animals used only if no reaction is evident at this time. Although passive cutaneous anaphylaxis can be produced with as little as a 0·003 µg of antibody nitrogen, this is so only when the antiserum is rich in antibodies so that high dilutions can be used. Relatively more antibody is needed when the antiserum is weaker because the fixation of antibody to the skin is inhibited by non-antibody globulin.

REFERENCES

ACKROYD J.F. (1962) The immunological basis of purpura due to drug hypersensitivity. *Proc. roy. Soc. Med.* **55**, 30–6.

ACKROYD J.F. (Editor) (1964) *Immunological Methods.* CIOMS Symposium. Oxford, Blackwell Scientific Publications.

BOYDEN S.V. (1951) The adsorption of proteins on erythrocytes treated with tannic acid and subsequent haemagglutination by antiprotein sera. *J. exp. Med.* **93**, 107–20.

BINACHI R.A., BENACERRAF B., BLOCK K.F. & KOURILSKY F.M. (1964) Properties of rat anaphylactic antibody. *J. Immunol.* **92**, 927–33.

CAMPBELL D.H., GARVEY J.S., CREMER N.E. & SUSSDORF D.H. (1963) *Methods in Immunology.* New York & Amsterdam, W. A. Benjamin Inc.

DAVIES G.E. (1964) Some problems associated with the testing of drugs for allergenicity. *Proc. Eur. Soc. Study Drug Toxicity* **4**, 198–204.

DE WECK A.L. & BLUM G. (1965) Recent clinical and immunological aspects of penicillin allergy. *Int. Arch. Allergy* **27**, 221–56.

GELL P.G.H. & COOMBS R.R.A. (1963) *Clinical Aspects of Immunology*, p. 317. Oxford, Blackwell Scientific Publications.

HUMPHREY J.H. & WHITE R.G. (1964) *Immunology for Students of Medicine.* 2nd edition. Oxford, Blackwell Scientific Publications.

ISHIZAKA K., ISHIZAKA T. & HOLBROOK M.M. (1966) Physicochemical properties of human reaginic activity. *J. Immunol.* **97**, 75.

KABAT E.A. (1961) *Kabat and Mayer's Experimental Immunochemistry*, 2nd edition. Springfield, Charles C. Thomas.

LAYTON L.L., LEED S. & DE EDS F. (1961) Diagnosis of human allergy utilizing passive skin-sensitization in the monkey *Macaca irus. Proc. Soc. exp. Biol. (N.Y.)* **108**, 623–6.

LEVINE B.B. (1960) Studies on the mechanisms of the formation of the penicillin antigen. I. Delayed allergic cross-reactions among penicillin G and its degradation products. *J. exp. Med.* **112**, 1131–54.

NUSSENZWEIG R.S., MERRYMAN C. & BENACERRAF B. (1964) Electrophoretic separation and properties of mouse anti-hapten antibodies involved in passive cutaneous anaphylaxis and passive haemolysis. *J. exp. Med.* **120**, 315–27.

OUCHTERLONY O. (1962) Diffusion-in-gel methods for immunological analysis II. *Progr. Allergy,* **6**, 30–154.

OVARY Z., BENACERRAF B. & BLOCH K.J. (1963) Properties of guinea-pig. 7S antibodies. II. Identification of antibodies involved in passive cutaneous and systemic anaphylaxis. *J. exp. Med.* **117**, 951–64.

ROSENHEIM M.L. & MOULTON R. (eds) (1958) *Sensitivity Reactions to Drugs.* CIOMS Symposium. Oxford, Blackwell Scientific Publications.

ROWE D.S. & FAHEY J.L. (1965). A new class of immunoglobulins. II. Normal serum IgD. *J. exp. Med.* **11**, 185.

SALVIN S.B. (1965) Contact hypersensitivity, circulating antibody and immunologic unresponsiveness. *Fed. Proc.* **24**, 40–44.

SHULMAN N.R. (1964) A mechanism of cell destruction in individuals sensitized to foreign antigens and its implications in auto-immunity. *Am. int. Med.* **60**, 506–21.

STAVITSKY A.N. & ARQUILLA E.R. (1958) Studies of proteins and antibodies by specific haemagglutination and haemolysis of protein-conjugated erythrocytes. *Int. Arch. Allergy,* **13**, 1–38.

TURK J.L. (1964) Studies on the mechanism of action of methotrexate and Cyclophosphamide on contact sensitivity in the guinea-pig. *Int. Arch. Allergy,* **24**, 191–200.

CHAPTER 8

Detection of Potential to Produce Drug Dependence

R.E. LISTER

INTRODUCTION

Without doubt the oldest and most extensively documented form of drug toxicity is that which deals with the adverse effects produced in man as a result of the chronic administration of the so called 'drugs of addiction'. Some of the toxic properties of opium were mentioned by Dioscorides in the first century A.D. and in 1821 De Quincy in a chapter headed 'The Pains of Opium' in *Confessions of an English Opium Eater* described some of the psychotoxic effects accompanying prolonged abuse of opium. The increasing psycho-social pressures in modern society and the multiplicity of drugs now available that modify the psyche have led to a marked increase in drug abuse commonly referred to as addiction. For centuries the few available drugs of abuse were of natural origin and of these opium and its derivatives were the most widely employed. The medical profession soon recognized that the opiate type of abuse or addiction was different in nature to that found with other drugs such as alcohol and tobacco which were taken to produce altera-tions in mood. The opiates were capable of inducing dependence of both physical or physiological and of a psychic nature. The term addiction was often used to describe both states and the term habituation was sometimes used to describe psychic dependence alone. Both terms describe a clinical situation of multifactorial aetiology in man involving physical, psychological, and social factors.

Definitions

Drug abuse is a complex phenomenon and considerable confusion has arisen as a result of attempts to find simple definitions for the syndromes concerned.

In 1957 the Expert Committee on Addiction Producing Drugs of the World Health Organization defined the terms addiction and habituation. This was an attempt to clarify the terminology in the field but it soon became apparent that these definitions were inadequate to cover all situations and all drugs.

Many authors used the terms addiction and habituation interchangeably often leading to widespread misunderstanding. Recently another attempt to clarify the situation has been made by a WHO Expert Committee. In 1964 it recommended that the term *drug dependence* should replace both the term *drug addiction* and *drug habituation*. It was argued that dependence was a common component in all types of drug abuse whether of a physical or a psychic nature. It was further suggested that the term drug dependence should be modified by the addition of a phrase describing the particular type of drug concerned. For a fuller discussion of the definitions concerned the recent definitive paper by Eddy *et al.* (1965) should be consulted. These authors describe drug dependence as 'a state of psychic or physical dependence or both, on a drug, arising in a person following administration of that drug on a periodic or continuous basis. The characteristics of such a state will vary with the agent involved and these characteristics must always be made clear by designating the particular type of drug dependence in each specific case for example, drug dependence of morphine type, of amphetamine type, etc.'

The earlier definition attempted to include the psychosocial aspects of drug abuse but the many variables involved with such definitions tended to produce confusion rather than provide the clarification intended.

Psychic dependence is a state of mind occurring in susceptible individuals in which there is an overwhelming psychic drive for the periodic or continuous administration of a drug to produce pleasure or avoid mental discomfort.

Physical dependence is a type of pharmacological adaptation to a drug occurring at a cellular level that can only be recognized when the concentration of the drug falls below a critical threshold or

216

when a similar condition is precipitated by a specific antagonist. When this occurs a withdrawal or abstinence syndrome develops which is characterized by a pattern of signs and symptoms of both a physiological and psychological nature which tend to be specific for each drug type and each animal species.

Physical and psychic dependence may develop independently but in man it is unusual for physical dependence to occur without some accompanying psychic dependence although psychic dependence, especially on those drugs of a stimulant type, may develop without any evidence of physical dependence. Both types are pharmacologically induced but the degree and quality of psychic dependence developing in an individual varies with his psychological make-up and social relationships.

Tolerance to the pharmacological effects of centrally acting drugs frequently accompanies both forms of dependence. This is a state of adaptation to a pharmacological stimulus in which a given quantity of the drug produces a diminished response with time, or a larger dose is required to produce the same effects as previously. Drug dependence can develop without tolerance and conversely many drugs are capable of inducing tolerance without producing dependence.

Psychotoxicity is a characteristic common to all dependence producing drugs. This may be either acute or chronic or develop as one characteristic of the abstinence syndrome. The psychotoxic effects are manifested as disturbances in the normal behaviour pattern of the animal and the type and degree of these effects vary with the type of drug and the species being studied. These effects are more readily characterized in species other than man.

Types of Drug Dependence

Seven types of drug dependence have been recognized and their characteristics have been described in detail by Eddy *et al.* (1965). Each type shows consistent pharmacological and psychological characteristics and, although the range of individual variation is often wide, sufficient information is now available to allow accurate classification.

The seven types of drug dependence are recognized as:

1 Morphine type
2 Barbiturate-Alcohol type

3 Cocaine type
4 Cannabis type
5 Amphetamine type
6 Khat type
7 Hallucinogen type

Well-documented evidence for each of these types exists in the literature and in addition drug-dependence of varying degrees has been described for many other drugs including caffeine-containing beverages, tobacco, aspirin-based analgesics, but to date these have not been sufficiently well characterized for them to be included. Most work on the mechanism and detection of drug dependence has been concentrated on the two types of drug dependence which involve the greatest dangers to the individual and to society, namely the morphine type and the barbiturate-alcohol type. The recognition of the dangers posed by the other types of drug dependence has stimulated interest in the less well studied classes of dependence and this is now proving to be a fertile area of research.

Recognition and detection of the liability of new drugs to produce dependence frequently concerns the toxicologist who is principally involved in the study of the effects of chronic administration of drugs to laboratory animals. Physical dependence can be demonstrated readily in a variety of animal species but it is only with the development of modern techniques of behavioural pharmacology that any success has been achieved in demonstrating psychic dependence in laboratory animals. Little evidence of the detrimental effects of drug dependence on social behaviour of animal groups has been produced, but this may prove to be a useful technique in the future.

Psychotoxic reactions to drugs may be recognized by the alteration in behaviour of animals in standard psychopharmacological tests following single doses of centrally acting drugs or by changes in the normal behaviour patterns of the animals exposed to their chronic administration during a prolonged toxicity test.

The recent classification of drug dependence into the seven types described post-dates the development of most of the tests to be described here. The majority of the techniques developed are for the detection of the physical dependence producing properties of the morphine type of drugs and it is only recently that tests for psychic dependence have been developed. Both physical and psychic dependence will be dealt with and methods used for the detection of each type will be described, where they exist.

TESTS FOR PHYSICAL DEPENDENCE

A. Morphine Type

Dependence on morphine and the morphine-like drugs is well recognized clinically because of its distinctive characteristics and widespread occurrence. The extensive social problems produced by this form of drug dependence and the legal and social sanctions directed against the abuse of this type of drug have stimulated a great deal of research into the physiological, psychological, and social aspects of this phenomenon. This type of drug is classified in law as a narcotic but this term is capable of misinterpretation and will be avoided in this discussion. Many other terms have appeared in the literature to describe drugs with a spectrum of pharmacological actions similar to that of morphine but none have received general acceptance. To avoid confusion the term morphine-like will be used to describe drugs which have similar pharmacological profiles to morphine although they may differ widely in potency and in some minor characteristics.

Dependence on morphine-like drugs follows a characteristic, well-defined pattern in man and in the higher animals tested. In man it is characterized by the development of physical dependence, strong psychic dependence and the rapid development of tolerance to the depressant effects of the drug on the central nervous system. The physiological and pharmacological aspects of drug dependence especially that of the morphine-like drugs has been reviewed (Seevers & Deneau, 1963; Deneau & Seevers, 1964a) and a detailed survey of the tests for morphine-like dependence was made by Halbach & Eddy (1964) and Deneau & Seevers (1964b).

Two types of test are available for the detection of physical dependence in laboratory animals; the first type depends upon the ability of the drug to produce primary physical dependence after repeated administration, and the second relies on the ability of a test drug to substitute for morphine or a similar drug in animals previously made physically dependent and stabilized on a fixed-dose regimen. Primary physical dependence can be detected only on withdrawal of the drug when a characteristic abstinence syndrome develops; this syndrome results from a disturbance of the whole nervous system and tends to show specific characteristics for each species. The abstinence syndrome can be assessed quantitatively and the degree to which the syndrome can be suppressed by substitute drugs is used to obtain a quantitative assessment of morphine-like physical dependence.

A wide variety of tests for the detection of the physical dependence capacity of morphine-like drugs has been devised using a range of test subjects ranging from micro-organisms to man. In practice organisms low in the evolutionary scale make unreliable subjects and the majority of studies has been confined to the higher mammals. It is outside the scope of this review to deal in detail with all the techniques which have been used in an attempt to develop simple tests for the detection of morphine-like physical dependence. For a detailed description of the methods developed in this field the comprehensive review of Halbach & Eddy (1963) should be consulted.

ISOLATED TISSUES AND ORGANS

In the 1930's a number of Japanese workers (Semura, 1933; Sanjo, 1934; Kubo, 1939) demonstrated that cells, principally chicken heart fibroblasts, were capable of thriving in solutions of morphine. On withdrawal growth was inhibited and was restored only when morphine was added again. These authors considered this to be addiction at the cellular level. Their studies were largely neglected but recent work by Corssen (1964) and Takemori (1961) confirmed these observations.

Other studies have shown that isolated organs can develop tolerance to the effects of morphine in the bathing fluid and can show a pharmacological response when the drug is withdrawn (Paton, 1957; Kaymakcalan & Temelli, 1964). These studies indicate that tissues other than neuronal tissue can be made dependent on morphine and develop a condition in some ways analogous to a withdrawal syndrome. At present these techniques are still experimental and cannot be used as predictive tests for morphine-like dependence.

MICE

The mouse is a desirable species for biological testing because it is cheap and easy to handle, but unlike man and other primates the mouse shows a stimulant rather than a depressant response to the injection of morphine-like analgesics. Tolerance to this stimulant effect develops much less rapidly and with less regularity than to the depressant effect. The high metabolic rate of the mouse results in rapid detoxication of the drug. Because of these factors it was believed (Fichtenberg, 1951; Mercier & Mercier, 1957) that the development of physical dependence in this species was unlikely. However, by the use of morphine implants Huidobro and his colleagues (Huidobro *et al.*, 1963; Huidobro & Contreras, 1963; Huidobro, 1964) managed to induce a state of primary physical dependence in mice. A characteristic abstinence syndrome was induced in the animals following the injection of the morphine antagonists nalorphine or levallorphan. A number of factors make this technique unreliable for accurate quantitative studies of new drugs.

In an attempt to establish suitable conditions for the development of physical dependence in mice, Shuster *et al.* (1963) fed animals on a diet of evaporated milk in which was dissolved 1% of dihydromorphinone hydrochloride. This drug is a powerful morphine-like analgesic with a potency in mice approximately seven times that of morphine. Rapid tolerance to the analgesic and stimulant effects of injected dihydromorphine developed in these mice and when plain milk was substituted the animals lost weight and their spontaneous motor activity decreased markedly. This contrasts with the findings of Huidobro *et al.* (1963) that tolerant mice of their strain usually showed increased activity during the nalorphine-induced withdrawal syndrome. Shuster *et al.* also reported pilo-erection, tremors, and instability during the withdrawal period but failed to observe other signs such as convulsions, hyperpnoea, and lachrymation reported by Huidobro *et al.* Shuster *et al.* also showed that the dihydromorphinone treated mice showed cross tolerance to the analgesic effects of morphine, codeine, and pethidine but they made no attempt to substitute other morphine-like drugs for the dihydromorphinone.

Hano *et al.* (1963) have also produced evidence for the development of physical dependence in mice chronically exposed to morphine. The marked variation in the responses of mice and the evident strain differences makes the value of predictive tests using this species questionable. The overall qualitative differences between the action of morphine on this species and man would also point to possible erroneous conclusions being drawn from results in mice. However, the work of Shuster *et al.* and the development of many highly potent analgesics such as the benzimidazoles and the oripavine derivatives may lead to this species being more widely used for initial screening tests prior to the more reliable tests to be described later.

RATS

Unlike mice, rats show a predominantly depressant response to morphine and similar analgesics and the pharmacological response is well-defined and consistent. Their convenient size and strain purity have led to their frequent use in studies of experimentally induced drug dependence of the morphine type.

Himmelsbach and his colleagues (Himmelsbach *et al.*, 1935; Eddy & Himmelsbach, 1936) first demonstrated that a form of withdrawal syndrome could be demonstrated and assessed semi-quantitatively following the withdrawal of morphine from rats chronically treated with this drug. This study extended earlier qualitative studies in rats described by Joel & Ettinger in 1926.

The nalorphine induced withdrawal syndrome was studied by Kaymakcalan & Woods (1956) and later by Hanna (1960). However very large initial doses of morphine have to be used, and even so the results are variable and uncertain. This method is unsuitable for routine work in rats. In an attempt to overcome these difficulties Ettles and I (1963) tried to induce morphine-like physical dependence by giving a new morphine-like drug by mouth. Morphine is poorly absorbed orally and in the concentration necessary to produce any pharmacological effects in rats has an extremely bitter taste which makes voluntary intake of this drug impossible. The development of the very highly potent morphine-like drugs derived from thebaine by my former colleague K. W. Bentley (Bentley & Hardy, 1963; Lister, 1964) overcame these disadvantages. We used the compound etorphine M99, (6,14,*endo*-etheno-7-(2-hydroxy-2-pentyl) tetrahydro-oripavine HC1) which is a highly potent analgesic with a potency approximately 2,000 times that of morphine when tested in the rat by subcutaneous administration; it is less potent given orally but still sufficiently potent to produce well marked analgesia in doses of approximately 75 µg in a 50 g rat. Rats were given access to a 1·5 µg/ml solution of M99 which gave a calculated daily intake of approximately 10 µg/rat/day; the concentration of drug was increased daily over 2 weeks to a level at which the animals were receiving about 5 mg/rat/day, i.e. approximately 30 times the oral ED_{50} for analgesia, and the animals were stabilized at this level for a further week. At the end of this period it was found that a well-marked and readily characterized withdrawal syndrome could be precipitated by the intraperitoneal injection of 3 mg/kg levallorphan HBr. A less intense withdrawal syndrome developed on withdrawal of the drug but this was less readily characterized than the precipitated syndrome. The withdrawal syndrome produced was similar to that described by previous authors in that the overall pattern in the animal was one of central excitation but a previously undescribed feature of the syndrome was a stretching or writhing response similar to that produced in mice following the injection of phenyl-*p*-quinone or other irritants (Hendershot & Forsaith, 1959) or in rats after oxytocin (Murray & Miller, 1960). In order to obtain a quantitative assessment of the severity of the abstinence syndrome a scoring system analagous to that described by Himmelsbach (Kolb &

Table 8.1 Score chart of withdrawal signs.

Characteristic signs	Score
'Stretching'	5
Squealing	4
'Wet dog'	4
Teeth chattering	3
Hypersensitivity to noise	2
Diarrhoea	2
Chewing	1
Pinna reflex exaggerated	1
Spontaneous ear twitch	1
Excessive piloerection 'staring coat'	1
Marked scratching	1
	25

Himmelsbach, 1938; Himmelsbach, 1939) was used. Writhing or stretching was the most characteristic symptom which was never observed in control rats and this was given the highest score; other observations were scored according to their frequency and intensity as shown in Table 8.1. The intensity of the abstinence syndrome produced following precipitation by levallorphan and withdrawal of M99 in orally dosed animals is shown in Table 8.2 which also

Table 8.2 Physical dependence scores produced by Morphine and M99.

Agent	Route of administration	Abstinence produced by	No. of animals	Mean score ± s.e.
Saline	s.c.	precipitation	6	0·8±0·31
Morphine	s.c.	withdrawal	6	11·2±0·95
Morphine	s.c.	precipitation	6	8·3±0·76
M99	s.c.	precipitation	6	2·17±0·17
Water	oral	precipitation	10	1·8±0·12
M99	oral	withdrawal	10	1·0
M99	oral	precipitation	10	13·5±1·3

includes for comparative purposes some data from rats made physically dependent on M99 and morphine given by parenteral administration.

The intensity of both the spontaneous and precipitated withdrawal syndromes was reduced by the parenteral administration of drugs capable of supporting morphine-like physical dependence. Some typical results are shown in Table 8.3.

Table 8.3 Suppression of withdrawal signs.
All rats stabilized on 5 mg/rat/day of M99 orally.
Withdrawal precipitated with 3 mg/kg Levallorphan.

Suppressing agent	Dose mg/kg	Mean score for 15 min before suppression	Post suppression score	Percentage reduction
Saline	5 ml	19·5	12·3	37
Morphine	50	16·5	8	52
M183	0·05	17·6	5·0	71·5
M183	0·10	18·0	1	95
Atropine	10	15·6	7·9	43
M99	0·1	15·0	0	100

These studies have been extended by Kuhn & Friebel (1962) who obtained a similar withdrawal profile in rats made physically dependent on the much weaker analgesic codeine. They dosed their rats by subcutaneous injection thrice daily on an increasing dose schedule and precipitated the withdrawal syndrome with nalorphine.

Although the oral administration of M99 is the most convenient method of administration it suffered from the disadvantage that the abstinence syndrome on withdrawal alone was less clearly defined than when it was precipitated by an antagonist. Drugs to be tested for their ability to suppress the withdrawal signs precipitated by the levallorphan thus had to be given in sufficiently high doses to overcome any residual antagonist. In an attempt to overcome this disadvantage Buckett (1964) extended these observations by using a similar scoring system for quantitating the intensity of the withdrawal syndrome but used parenterally administered morphine to produce a state of physical dependence. He gave rats twice daily injections of morphine starting at 20 mg/kg i.p. building up to a stabilizing dose of 400 mg/kg twice daily. Withholding the morphine injection led to the development of a spontaneous withdrawal syndrome which could be suppressed by drugs of the morphine type. The incidence of the writhing response could be reduced on a quantitative basis by a single dose of morphine, diamorphine or codeine, all of which gave a straight line log relationship between dose of the drug and the reduction in the frequency of writhing. Buckett tested a number of other agents including acetylsalicylic acid, amiphenazole, atropine, BOL 148, LSD 25, and noscapine, none of which produced any significant suppression of the withdrawal syndrome indicating that neither bradykinin, acetylcholine, nor 5-hydroxytryptamine were involved in the development of the syndrome. On the other hand the antihistamine mepyramine produced a significant reduction in the frequency of the writhing responses observed suggesting that histamine may be involved in the production of at least part of the withdrawal syndrome in rats made dependent on morphine by this means.

In a similar study Martin *et al.* (1963) produced physical dependence on morphine and evaluated the abstinence syndrome produced by withdrawal. They measured both spontaneous motor activity and the frequency of spontaneous shaking episodes ('wet dog') and the metabolic and physiological changes occurring during the withdrawal period. These authors recognized both a primary and a secondary abstinence syndrome in rats but did not make any attempts to suppress it with other agents. Wikler *et al.* (1963) extended these studies, giving the animals etonitazine in the drinking water. Morphine dependent animals consumed more etonitazine solution than control animals. However this technique has not been used for the examination of new potential drugs of dependence.

DOGS

The morphine-like analgesics produce in dogs a pattern of CNS depression qualitatively similar to that of rat, monkey, and man. Plant & Pierce (1928) first described the abstinence syndrome in dogs; as with rats this is characterized by well-marked CNS stimulation. Wikler (1946, 1948) has described the abstinence syndrome in dogs and shown that this can be intensified by nalorphine precipitation in dogs made dependent on 5–10 mg/kg morphine given 6-hourly for 7 days. Carter & Wikler (1954) described the signs of the syndrome as restlessness, tremor, rhinorrhoea, salivation, lachrymation, and urination, often accompanied by yawning and vomiting. Other behavioural disturbances such as digging and persistent gnawing were observed. This compulsive gnawing is similar to that frequently observed after morphine withdrawal in dependent rats.

Dogs have been made physically dependent upon a number of other potent morphine-like analgesics, including methadone (Wikler & Frank, 1957; Winter & Flataker, 1950), piminodine, and a related derivative (Woods *et al.*, 1961). Attempts to produce primary physical dependence to pethidine itself however have proved less successful and Carter & Wikler (1954) were unable to demonstrate either a spontaneous or a precipitated withdrawal syndrome. This situation contrasts with the situation in rhesus monkeys which have been found to develop well-marked physical dependence to pethidine and its congeners.

The pattern and intensity of the withdrawal syndrome in morphine dependent dogs tends to show a marked between-animal variation and generally the reproducibility is poor. A large number of animals is required to obtain reasonably accurate data for screening for the capacity to produce physical dependence and makes the use of the dog economically unsuitable.

In an attempt to overcome the twin drawbacks of individual variation and the necessity for repeated administration of morphine Martin & Eades (1961) demonstrated that tolerance to the depressant effects of morphine on a number of physiological parameters developed rapidly following the slow intravenous infusion of morphine. The depressant effect of morphine on the respiratory, cardiovascular, and thermoregulatory centres rapidly disappeared and the analgesic effect as tested by pinching the skin of the back or squeezing of the digits of the hind limbs was soon lost. After infusion for 8 hours the injection of a large dose of nalorphine 20 mg/kg produced a pattern of effects similar to the withdrawal syndrome described by Wikler (1948). These authors considered that because of the ease and reproducibility of this method, their technique could serve as a preliminary screen for the detection of morphine-like physical dependence but to date they have not provided sufficient evidence of correlation between their method and more established methods over a range of drugs to justify this claim. More work however may establish this as a useful technique for the preliminary screening of morphine-like drugs but to date it does not appear to offer sufficient advantages over other techniques using the rat and monkey to justify recommending it as a method of choice.

In order to quantify the intensity of the withdrawal syndrome in dogs Desmarez (1960) measured the increase in spontaneous motor activity following the withdrawal of morphine from chronically treated dogs. The dogs were treated with relatively low doses for an extended period, followed by gradual increase in the dose to a level of 50 mg/kg, administered twice daily for a month before withdrawal. The increased motor activity found on withdrawal was measured in a motor activity cage, and its diminution following re-administration of morphine, or effective substitutes, was regarded as a measure of the capacity of the new drug to produce dependence.

The technique has two major disadvantages. The preliminary dosage regime is time-consuming in the extreme. More important, only one parameter of the withdrawal syndrome is measured. It is possible that further work may remove both these disadvantages. A direct test of addiction production would also be needed.

Another approach has been used by Wikler and his colleagues (Wikler & Frank, 1948; Wikler & Carter, 1953; Carter & Wikler, 1955; Martin & Eades, 1964) to develop a quantitative method of assessing the abstinence syndrome in dogs. They used dogs which had previously been chordectomized by section of the spinal cord between D10 and D12. After recovery, the intensity of the ipsilateral and crossed exterior reflexes in the hind limbs was measured. Initially morphine depressed the reflex responses to stimulation but during chronic administration these reflexes gradually became re-established. Withdrawal of the morphine was followed by an exaggerated response to the stimuli and 24–36 hours after withdrawal the animals showed spontaneous hind-limb movements, and then developed signs of CNS stimulation similar to those observed during the withdrawal syndrome in normal morphine-dependent animals. As with other species studied, precipitation with 15 mg/kg of nalorphine led to a more clearly defined withdrawal syndrome. With this technique a well-defined syndrome was observed after only 2 days, which was comparable in intensity with that produced on withdrawal after 3 months chronic administration of morphine to similar animals.

This test in spinal dogs has been shown to give similar results with methadone but no physical dependence on pethidine could be demonstrated with this technique (Carter & Wikler, 1955).

The dog can be made dependent on morphine and other strong analgesics and a well-marked withdrawal syndrome can be demonstrated following prolonged administration of the drug but the failure of the techniques to detect other potent drugs of abuse as exemplified by the less potent pethidine makes it unsuitable in its present form for routine screening purposes.

SUB-HUMAN PRIMATES

Monkeys were among the earliest laboratory species to be examined for their ability to develop physical dependence to morphine-like drugs (Tatum *et al.*, 1929; Kolb & Du Mez, 1931). These early workers described the typical abstinence signs which developed after withdrawal in monkeys which had been made physically dependent on morphine given in a dose of up to 200 mg/kg daily for periods of up to 10 months. The signs observed during the withdrawal syndrome were similar in many respects to those described for other animals and showed a characteristic pattern of CNS stimulation and in an experiment described by Kolb and Du Mez, one animal died during the withdrawal period; this was believed to be directly attributable to the withdrawal of the drug. Cross tolerance to other analgesics was also demonstrated by these early workers. The majority of studies with primates have been carried out using the rhesus monkey (*Maccaca mulatta*) but other primates are equally susceptible and Spragg (1940) reported on the successful induction of physical dependence to morphine in chimpanzees (*Pan troglodytes*).

Seevers has extended his early work on morphine dependence in monkeys and he and his school, stimulated by the increase in synthetic morphine-like analgesics after the end of the Second World War, have developed a series of tests in rhesus monkeys which have become the standard procedure for the detection of the production of physical dependence of the morphine type by new analgesic drugs. They have shown (Seevers, 1936, 1948; Deneau & Seevers, 1962, 1964b; Seevers and Deneau, 1963) that the physical dependence capacity of morphine-like drugs can be determined in rhesus monkeys using methods based on the development of primary physical dependence or upon the suppression of the withdrawal syndrome by the substitution of a morphine-like test drug.

The development of primary physical dependence and the recognition of a withdrawal syndrome is the ultimate test of the ability of a drug to induce physical dependence but this test is costly and time-consuming and unsuitable for the screening of large numbers of new drugs. However it provides valuable confirmatory evidence in borderline cases. There is ample evidence that drugs which are capable of suppressing the morphine abstinence syndrome in morphine-dependent men or animals are equally able to induce physical dependence when given by chronic administration. Seevers and his colleagues have used this observation to develop an elegant technique whereby the ability of drug to suppress the withdrawal syndrome in morphine-dependent monkeys can be assessed quantitatively. Experience has shown that the rhesus monkey and man react in a qualitatively similar manner to these drugs and that this test can be used to predict the production of physical dependence and hence to give some indication of liability to abuse in man.

In practice the test is conducted in two parts: the first part of the test is designed to ascertain whether or not the new drug is capable of suppressing the withdrawal syndrome in morphine-dependent monkeys and if so to what extent. If the drug only provides incomplete suppression the extent to which the drug suppresses the total spectrum of signs is assessed. The extent to which the abstinence syndrome is suppressed is known as the physical dependence capacity (PDC). The PDC is a qualitative function but if the test drug is found to have the ability to suppress markedly the abstinence syndrome it is assessed quantitatively relative to morphine in the second part of the test.

The physical dependence capacity of a drug is graded by Deneau and Seevers (1962) as:

(i) *High*—when the drug produces complete suppression of all abstinence signs with doses which reveal no other overt pharmacological effects.

(ii) *Intermediate*—when complete suppression of all abstinence signs is obtainable but only with doses which elicit other pharmacological actions manifested by such signs as stupor, ataxia, etc.

(iii) *Low*—when some suppression of abstinence signs is induced but attempts to produce more or complete suppression with larger doses is prevented by the intervention of toxic effects, e.g. convulsions, coma, etc.

(iv) *None*—when the drug fails to produce any specific suppression of the morphine abstinence signs. Non-specific depressants may obscure individual signs.

The technique has been described in detail by these authors (Deneau & Seevers, 1962, 1964; Seevers & Deneau, 1963) and by Halbach & Eddy (1963). For this test a group of monkeys are maintained on a stabilized dose regimen of 3 mg/kg of morphine sulphate subcutaneously every 6 hours for 60 days. At the end of this period the animals are ready for use. The morphine injections are discontinued and when abstinence signs develop, these are allowed to increase to intermediate intensity which generally occurs within 12–14 hours after withdrawal. If untreated the intensity of the withdrawal syndrome increases but if the animals are given morphine or a similar agent the withdrawal signs are reduced or suppressed completely depending upon the nature and dose of the drug. In assessing the capacity of a new drug to produce physical dependence four monkeys showing the abstinence syndrome are used; two are given 3 mg/kg morphine and two a predetermined dose of the test agent subcutaneously The intensity of the withdrawal syndrome is graded prior to, and at fixed intervals after the injection and continued until the monkeys have returned to the pre-injection state. The test is repeated with varying doses of the test agent until a degree of suppression similar to that produced by 3 mg/kg morphine is reached or until other pharmacological effects make further testing undesirable. From this study the capacity to produce physical dependence can be estimated as high, intermediate, low, or absent according to the criteria already described. This information is qualitative and provides predictive evidence of the liability of the agent to be abused. Quantitative evidence of the potency of a test drug relative to morphine may be obtained in an extended experiment in which the test drug is given at two dose levels and compared with morphine at 3 mg/kg and a dummy treatment. Time-effect curves for each treatment are obtained and the maximum effect score is plotted against the log dose. From the resulting line the dose which produces a suppressant effect equivalent to 3 mg/kg morphine can be calculated. These two studies will provide evidence of the degree of dependence and an estimate of potency relative to morphine but for confirmation of the physical dependence potential of a new morphine-like agent a primary physical dependence study should be performed. As its name implies this is an attempt to produce physical dependence directly by the chronic administration of the test agents to monkeys. In the technique used by Deneau & Seevers the dose found to be equivalent to 3 mg/kg morphine in the single dose suppression technique is given subcutaneously to monkeys at regular intervals determined by the duration of action of the drugs for a period of 31 days. On the 14th and 28th days 2 mg/kg nalorphine is given to ensure that physical dependence is developing. On the 31st day the injections are stopped and the animals observed for 7–16 days. The intensity of the abstinence syndrome is graded according to Seevers' (1963) classification.

This classification is used to grade the syndrome produced by either withdrawal or nalorphine precipitation. Four grades are recognized. They are:

(i) *Mild*—Apprehension, continual yawning, rhinorrhoea, lachrymation, hiccup, shivering, perspiration on face, chattering, quarrelling, and fighting.

(ii) *Moderate*—intention tremor, anorexia, pilomotor activity, muscular twitching and rigidity, and abdominal cramps.

(iii) *Severe*—Extreme restlessness, assumption of peculiar attitudes, vomiting, severe diarrhoea, erection and masturbation, inflammation of the eyelids, vocalization, lying on one side with eyes closed, and spasticity.

(iv) *Very Severe*—Docility in a normally excitable animal, dyspnoea, pallor, stabismus, dehydration, weight loss, prostration, circulatory collapse, or death.

All these signs indicate a hyper-irritable condition and all may be suppressed by morphine in a direct dose-related manner. On the other hand such drugs as codeine and propoxyphene are only capable of suppressing some of the signs. The effects of abstinence following drug administration are assessed according to the behavioural signs.

To date this technique developed by Seevers and his colleagues has been the most widely employed for its ability to detect drugs liable to produce morphine-like physical dependence in man. Many hundreds of substances have been tested using this technique and a great deal of background information exists which makes it possible to compare new agents suspected of showing similar properties to morphine with many well established drugs. Although the qualitative predictive capacity of the method is high, quantitative predictions may be misleading. In the monkey pethidine and its congeners show up in the single dose suppression test as considerably more potent than they actually appear in man. On the other hand the benzomorphan derivatives, e.g. phenazocine, show a converse effect and early results with this drug in the monkey suppression test led to some unjustifiable optimism about the liability to abuse this agent when it was first studied.

MAN

The detailed description of methods used in man to determine the ability of drugs to produce physical dependence of the morphine-like drugs is outside the scope of this review. These methods which use former addicts have been developed at the Addiction Research Centre, Lexington, Kentucky, USA by Drs Isbell and Fraser and their associates. The subjects are fit, male inmates of the Centre who are serving prison sentences for violation of the narcotic laws and who volunteer for the studies.

Testing of new drugs is carried out at Lexington in three stages, which run roughly parallel to the types of test described for monkeys. Before testing new drugs in post-addicts a full pharmacological and toxicological profile of the drug must be made available to the investigators and evidence that it can produce physical dependence in experimental animals should be provided.

Initially single-dose studies are carried out to establish the dose-levels and the type of effects produced by the drug. Both objective and subjective evidence is obtained on the new drug and compared with a standard drug of a similar type and a placebo. The results obtained from the single-dose study are used in an extended double-blind study in which the drug under investigation is substituted for morphine in a group of subjects previously made dependent on morphine and stabilized on a daily dose of 240 mg/day. The new drug is compared with a placebo and a morphine standard for its ability to suppress the withdrawal syndrome. The intensity of the abstinence syndrome which develops over a 24 hour period is compared for each treatment and an indication is obtained of the ability of the new drug to substitute for morphine.

If these and other clinical results justify further studies a direct addiction study may be undertaken in a group of post-addicts in which the new drug is given on a double-blind basis using an ascending dose schedule starting with a dose equivalent in effectiveness to morphine. A placebo and a standard drug other than morphine may be given in addition. After 19 or 20 days a placebo tablet or injection is substituted for the drug and controls and subjects are observed three times daily by trained observers. Rectal temperature, heart and respiratory rate, and blood pressure are recorded and the signs of abstinence scored using the Kolb & Himmelsbach (1938) scoring system. The subject's own observations as to his behaviour, degree of liking of the medication etc. are also assessed. The response to the new drug is compared to that for morphine and the placebo. Although a direct quantitative evaluation of the potential for the production of physical dependence of the new drug cannot be determined by this method it can give indications of both physical and psychic dependence and hence a very good indication of the likelihood that the new drug will be abused.

For a more detailed description of the techniques involved the reader is referred to the original work of the Lexington group (Isbell, 1948; Fraser *et al.*, 1961; Fraser, 1964) and to the paper by Halbach & Eddy (1963) which summarizes much of this work.

OTHER SPECIES

The evidence indicates that under the right conditions all animals with a functional nervous system may develop physical dependence.

A wide variety of species in addition to those mentioned here have been used by various workers in a search for simple models but the evidence to date indicates that the greater the degree of cerebral development the greater is the ease of development of physical dependence.

Krueger *et al.* (1941) showed that the rabbit develops a tolerance to the hyperglycaemic effects of morphine, and withdrawal after the development of tolerance results in a transitory secondary hyperglycaemia. Phatak & David (1953) after studying a number of morphine-like analgesics suggested that this phenomena might be used to predict addiction potential of new drugs. However, a direct relationship between tolerance and liability to produce dependence has not been demonstrated (Seevers & Deneau, 1963).

Ettles and I attempted to produce physical dependence on the potent morphine-like drug, M99 (etorphine) in goldfish. We found that the fish became tolerant to the sedative effects of the drug added to the water in which they swam. When placed back into fresh water they frequently showed disturbed swimming behaviour but the changes observed were not sufficiently consistent to enable us to use this as a basis for a test.

INDIRECT METHODS

The time-consuming and expensive methods for determining the liability of new drugs to produce dependence, have induced many workers to try to develop indirect methods to achieve the same objective. All the major morphine-like analgesics produce a typical 'Straub Tail' response in mice when injected intravenously. Shemano & Wendel (1964) described a technique which depends on this phenomenon. They determined the ratio between the ED_{50} for the Straub tail response and the acute LD_{50} and called it the Straub Index (LD_{50}/ED_{50}). A high index was found for compounds thought likely to produce physical dependence, and others with a low index were thought unlikely to be abused.

They showed a significant rank order correlation between the Straub Index and the estimated addiction hazard in man with a wide range of analgesics from the potent drugs phenazocine and heroin to the much weaker dextropropoxyphene. They also obtained a similar correlation between the analgesic index determined as the ratio between ED_{50} for analgesia determined by the Hafner method in mice and the addiction liability. However, apomorphine which is apparently devoid of both analgesic and addictive properties was a potent inducer of the Straub tail phenomenon and this finding casts doubt on its value as a predictive test.

Cullumbine & Konop (1959) suggested that the cat might be used for the indirect assessment of addictive potential. They demonstrated that all morphine-like drugs tested induced mania in cats and that tolerance developed rapidly to this stimulant effect. These authors felt that the development of this form of tolerance may be used to predict the danger of possible addiction. Until direct relationship between tolerance and physical dependence is demonstrated the same objections must be raised to this test as to the rabbit tests described earlier.

B. Barbiturate-Alcohol Type

In their definitive paper describing the types of drug dependence Eddy *et al.* (1965) classify drug dependence to barbiturates and to alcohol under the same heading. The acute and chronic effects following overdosage of both agents are virtually indistinguishable and the pattern of dependence on both drugs shows a striking similarity. Both drugs are capable of substituting for each other during chronic intoxication. Cross-dependence is well established; barbiturates can suppress the abstinence syndrome following alcohol withdrawal in alcohol-dependent subjects and to a large extent alcohol will suppress the symptoms of barbiturate withdrawal.

Although alcohol is the most widely abused drug in the world today and there are thought to be more people physically dependent on alcohol than any other drug, methods for assessing physical dependence to this class of agent have only recently been developed. The barbiturates are capable of inducing physical dependence in man and animals and there is a growing body of evidence which suggests that all sedative drugs from the old-established chloral to the more recently introduced tranquillizers such as chlordiazepoxide are capable of producing physical dependence of the same basic type (Essig, 1964d).

Tests for assessing the propensity of the barbiturate-alcohol type of drugs to produce physical dependence have proved much more difficult to devise because of the relatively long period of time required for physical dependence to develop to this class of drug when compared with the morphine-type drugs. Physical dependence of this latter type can be demonstrated after a single dose of morphine (Martin & Eades, 1961) but with the barbiturate-alcohol type of drug physical dependence develops only after a much longer period of psychic dependence.

RODENTS

Early attempts to demonstrate physical dependence in rats and mice were often unsuccessful (Stanton, 1936) and many workers believed that physical dependence of the barbiturate-alcohol type could not be demonstrated in rodents. However, recent studies have shown that given the right conditions this is possible.

Mice have been used by McQuarrie & Fingl (1958) to study the influence of acute and chronic administration of alcohol on electroshock thresholds. They demonstrated that following withdrawal from either a large single dose or a period of chronic alcohol administration the convulsive threshold to electroshock was lowered within 8 hours of a large single dose or on the second and third day after chronic intoxication when compared with controls. Increased susceptibility to audiogenic seizures has also been demonstrated in rats following withdrawal of barbitone from chronically treated rats (Bentley, 1961). Swinyard et al. (1957) have also demonstrated hyperexcitability in mice during the withdrawal from chronically administered barbiturates and meprobamate.

Crossland & Leonard (1963) reported similar studies in albino rats. They forced the animals to drink solutions of barbitone sodium by severely restricting their fluid intake. By using progressively more concentrated solutions starting with 50 mg/kg/day and increasing to 400 mg/kg/day over a period of 4–5 weeks they were able to produce physical dependence. On withdrawal of the drug many of the animals developed spontaneous convulsive seizures and auditory stimulation induced further convulsions.

These observations in rats have been confirmed and extended by Essig (1966). He demonstrated that the rate of intoxication to sodium barbital influenced the degree of physical dependence produced. Animals forced to drink to a final level of 396 mg/kg/day all developed convulsions after 111 days but those made to drink at a lower level of 313 mg/kg/day had a lower incidence of convulsions when given the drug over a longer period, viz. 159 days. In addition to developing convulsions during the withdrawal period the animals tended to lose weight and reduce their food and water intake during the initial withdrawal period. Evidence of depressed fluid intake during barbiturate withdrawal has also been provided by Schmidt & Klainman (1964), but the relationship between hypodipsia and physical dependence has not been established.

It is evident from these studies that, if the right conditions are chosen, rats and mice can be made physically dependent on drugs of the barbiturate-alcohol type but the techniques are still experimental and no evidence has been produced of the predictive ability of any of these tests with new drugs and reliable substitution studies have not yet been reported in rodents. As with the tests described for rodents with the morphine-like drugs much research is still needed before a reliable and practical method for predicting physical dependence of the barbiturate-alcohol type can be developed.

CATS

Unlike the morphine-like drugs, the barbiturates and alcohol depress the CNS of the cat and this species has been used for physical dependence studies on this group of drugs. Essig & Flanary (1959, 1961) reported the development of convulsions following the withdrawal of barbitone sodium from chronically treated cats. Recently Jaffe & Sharpless (1965) have shown that in cats physical dependence on the shorter acting barbiturates can develop in a relatively short period. They gave intravenous injections of anaesthetic doses of pentobarbitone sodium three to four times daily and demonstrated that a significant reduction of the convulsive threshold to metrazole developed after a period of intoxication of as little as 26 hours. A greater reduction in the threshold was seen after longer periods although there was little difference between readings taken after a period of 5 days and 20 days. Spontaneous seizures were also observed on withdrawal after only two weeks' chronic administration; other behavioural signs reflecting a hyperexcitable state were also noticed during the withdrawal period.

DOGS

As early as 1931 Seevers & Tatum (1931) made attempts to produce evidence of physical dependence in dogs treated with barbitone. They were partly successful but the technique used was time-consuming and the results not clear cut. They reported signs of excitation after withdrawal in animals given 100 mg/kg daily on 6 days per week for 2 months. This early study aroused little interest but the growing awareness of the problems of barbiturate abuse has stimulated further work during the past decade. Fraser & Isbell (1954) extended these early studies and confirmed the earlier observations of Seevers & Tatum. They described behavioural changes and hyperexcitability in dogs on withdrawal after chronic administration of doses of various barbiturates in excess of 100 mg/kg per day for periods of up to 11 months.

Withdrawal of long acting barbiturates, e.g. barbitone, was followed by excitation and delirium but withdrawal of shorter acting drugs, e.g. pentobarbitone, produced increased irritability but no signs of delirium. This is in contrast to results obtained by Jaffe & Sharpless (1965) previously referred to. Essig (1964b) has demonstrated convulsions following withdrawal of barbitone sodium from chronically treated dogs and he has demonstrated that convulsions occur with similar frequency in dogs which were decerebellated prior to the start of the experiment. The same worker has also demonstrated similar withdrawal syndromes characterized by hyperexcitation and convulsions in dogs chronically treated with the non-barbiturate sedatives meprobamate (Essig, 1958) and glutethimide (Essig, 1963). There were minor qualitative differences in the withdrawal syndromes following barbiturates, glutethimide, and meprobamate but they all showed typical excitatory patterns; in the meprobamate-treated animals severe and sometimes fatal epileptiform convulsions developed approximately a day after withdrawal of the drug.

There is little experimental evidence of physical dependence on alcohol in dogs; some authors have failed to observe any evidence of dependence in tolerant chronically treated dogs (Newman & Card, 1937) but evidence of physical dependence on alcohol in dogs has been reported recently by Goldenberg & Korolenko (1963). These authors fed large doses of alcohol, 6–8 ml of 4% ethanol/kg/day, to dogs with their food. Although this study was not aimed at studying physical dependence the authors reported acute excitation, irritability, aggression, increased sensitivity to sounds, tremor, and unusual behavioural patterns suggesting hallucinations and two animals developed convulsions. These signs developed after 4–6 months of chronic administration and although they developed during the dosing period they are suggestive of a withdrawal syndrome.

The dog has also proved to be a suitable animal for demonstrating physical dependence of the barbiturate-alcohol type but the techniques have not yet been developed to the same degree of refinement as has been the case with the morphine-like drugs. Deneau and his colleagues (personal communication) have used a single dose suppression technique in dogs analogous to that used in monkeys for predicting morphine-like physical dependence. They have shown that a wide range of sedative drugs is capable of sustaining physical dependence in dogs made physically dependent on barbitone sodium. These authors have produced physical dependence in dogs by the daily oral administration of one dose of 100 mg/kg barbitone sodium for 6 weeks. Physical dependence is checked by withdrawing the barbitone and observing signs of abstinence over a 5 day period. The drug is then continued for a further 4 weeks after which period the drug to be tested is substituted for the barbitone. The dose of the test drug is chosen by determining the dose required to produce equivalent sedation to 30 mg/kg phenobarbitone sodium and the frequency of administration is chosen by reference to its duration of action. The test drug is given in the pre-determined dose to the barbitone dependent dogs for a period of 5 days and then withdrawn. Observations are made over the whole of the 10 day period and the abstinence syndrome compared in intensity and frequency with that produced in control animals.

Deneau has classified the intensity of the barbiturate abstinence syndrome in a manner analogous to that of the morphine-like analgesics as:

(i) *Mild*—tachycardia, hyperpnoea, weight loss, and tremors.

(ii) *Intermediate*—anorexia, nervousness, restlessness, insomnia, and fighting.

(iii) *Severe*—hyperthermia, muscle fasciculations, convulsions, and delirium.

They have shown that, if a suitable dose and frequency of administration is chosen, the following can all substitute for barbitone sodium: pentobarbitone sodium, phenobarbitone sodium, paraldehyde, chloral hydrate, glutethimide, methyprylon, bromural, chlordiazepoxide, carisoprodol, and meprobamate. On the other hand the sedative phenothiazine promethazine was incapable of substituting for barbitone sodium despite its high potency as a sedative in man.

These studies are being extended to other sedative hypnotic agents but the results to date are sufficient to suggest that if the right conditions are chosen physical dependence of the barbiturate-alcohol type may develop to all the drugs which have been shown to be capable of substituting for barbitone sodium in this test. The validity of these observations is supported and confirmed by the increasing number of reports in the clinical literature describing cases of physical dependence on glutethimide, meprobamate, and other sedative agents (Essig, 1964a). This method promises to be an extremely valuable one allowing the ability of new sedative drugs to produce physical dependence to be predicted without the time-consuming study frequently required for the demonstration of primary physical dependence.

MAN

Dependence on barbiturates and alcohol is well-known and a vast clinical literature exists on these phenomena. In many cases the authors have not differentiated between physical and psychic dependence. Evidence for physical dependence on alcohol in man was provided by Isbell *et al.* (1955) in their classic paper on the aetiology of 'rum fits'. Other workers had observed convulsions and signs of excitation in patients following withdrawal of barbiturate therapy (Kalinowsky, 1942; Brownstein & Pacella, 1943; Dunning, 1940; Fraser *et al.*, 1953; Westgate & Stiebler, 1964).

These clinical results have been confirmed and extended by Fraser and his colleagues at Lexington in experiments with human volunteers. In clinically controlled studies they have given various barbiturates on different dose regimens to volunteers and have shown that there is a wide variation between subjects in the intensity and the quality of the abstinence syndrome but in general the intensity of the withdrawal syndrome varies directly with the dose and the duration of administration (Fraser *et al.*, 1954, 1958).

The barbiturate abstinence syndrome in man shows characteristic signs which are qualitatively similar to many of those observed in the dog and in order of appearance include apprehension, muscular weakness and fasciculations, tremor, hyperactive reflexes, insomnia, nausea and vomiting, cramps, dehydration and weight loss, hypoglycaemia, tachycardia, hyperpnoea, chronic convulsion of a grandmal type, delirium, and visual and auditory hallucinations (Seevers & Deneau, 1963).

Similar evidence of withdrawal signs after alcohol withdrawal under controlled conditions has been provided by Mello & Mendelson (1965) using volunteers. Fraser *et al.* (1957) provided evidence of cross-dependence between barbiturates and alcohol by showing that alcohol could prevent the development of withdrawal signs when substituted for barbiturates in subjects chronically intoxicated with barbiturates.

There is growing evidence to support the contention that under suitable conditions physical dependence can develop with the majority of non-barbiturate sedatives used in therapy. Withdrawal signs of varying severity, even including death, but all showing a qualitatively similar pattern to that of the barbiturate-alcohol abstinence syndrome have been reported after chronic intoxication with paraldehyde (Mendelson *et al.*, 1957), chloral (Margetts, 1950), meprobamate (Ewing & Haizlip, 1958; Swanson & Okada, 1963), glutethimide (Lloyd & Clark, 1959), methyprylon (Berger, 1961), and chlordiazepoxide (Hollister *et al.*, 1961). Aspects of dependence to the non-barbiturate sedatives have been reviewed recently by Essig (1964d).

Techniques using human subjects for the detection and quantitation of physical dependence of the barbiturate-alcohol type have not been developed as fully as with the morphine-like drugs and there is as yet no recognized technique that will accurately predict the physical dependence potential of new drugs of this type. There are a number of factors which inhibit further developments in this field; because of the severe abstinence syndrome there is a real possibility of a fatal outcome to the study, in addition there is at present no drug capable of precipitating the abstinence syndrome which tends to make controlled studies difficult. If the findings in dogs of evidence of physical dependence to certain barbiturates after only short periods of intoxication cited earlier can be extended to man this may prove to be a more valuable technique than the time-consuming studies reported to date.

Other Types

MORPHINE-ANTAGONIST TYPE

Morphine antagonists such as nalorphine and levallorphan are capable of precipitating an abstinence syndrome in morphine-dependent persons and thus they will not substitute for morphine. In direct addiction studies in moneys no evidence of any liability to produce dependence was found (Seevers & Deneau, 1963). Evidence of physical dependence on nalorphine in man was provided by Schrappe (1958) from studies in psychotic patients, but these studies have not yet been confirmed. However, evidence for the development of physical dependence to the morphine-antagonist cyclazocine   (2-cyclopropylmethyl-2'-hydroxy-5,9-dimethyl-6,7-benzomorphan) has been presented by Martin *et al.* (1965). These authors described an abstinence syndrome which was qualitatively different from that seen following morphine dependence. The syndrome was described as mild and there would appear to be no strong motivation for patients to continue taking the drug.

This particular type of physical dependence developed following a direct addiction study in volunteers showing that the technique used for the detection of morphine-like physical dependence is capable of detecting substances producing physical dependence of a qualitatively different type. Although physical dependence to cyclazocine has been demonstrated this type is not recognized by the WHO in the classification of dependence-producing drugs because to date this drug has not been available commercially and the question of abuse does not yet arise, but these observations support the viewpoint that all drugs which have a chemical or pharmacological affinity with morphine should be evaluated by this direct addiction technique before general release.

AMPHETAMINE TYPE

Animal experiments have failed to reveal any conclusive evidence of physical dependence to drugs of the amphetamine type although their abuse is widespread both alone and in combination with barbiturates.

Oswald & Thacore (1963) have provided evidence of physical dependence in patients dependent on dexamphetamine, phenmetrazine, and a dexamphetamine-amylobarbitone mixture. These authors studied the neurophysiological changes developing in patients following withdrawal of the drug upon which they had become dependent. They studied the EEG patterns and eye movements during sleep of patients before and after withdrawal and showed that the amount of hind brain sleep (paradoxical) as measured by the period of rapid eye movement (REM time), which was normal whilst the patients continued taking the drug, rose rapidly on withdrawal. In normal patients hind brain sleep begins about 70 min after the onset of sleep and occupies about 10 min of the first 2 hours of the sleeping period. The values for the amphetamine-dependent subjects were within normal limits but when the drugs were withdrawn the hind brain sleep began within

4 min and occupied up to 70 min of the time period and as much as 48% of a normal night's sleep compared with 22% in control patients. In the abstinent patients the normal sleep pattern could be restored by further administration of the drug suggesting true physical dependence. These results have yet to be confirmed. Oswald & Thacore have provided evidence in support of their claim that amphetamine-type drugs may produce physical dependence but that it may only be detected by the use of sophisticated techniques to detect complex neurophysiological changes which may well not develop in laboratory animals. This is the only evidence to date to suggest that physical dependence can develop to the stimulant drugs but further work in this field may disprove the hypothesis that physical dependence can only develop to those drugs which produce overt depression (Seevers & Deneau, 1963).

TESTS FOR PSYCHIC DEPENDENCE

Drugs of each of the seven types described earlier are capable of inducing some degree of psychic dependence in susceptible individuals. They are all capable of producing a pharmacological disturbance of the central nervous system resulting in an elevation of mood, euphoria, or the prevention of dysphoria. The preference of certain psychologically inadequate individuals for the drugged rather than the normal mental state is the most potent stimulus to drug abuse. In the individual dependent on drugs of the morphine or barbiturate-alcohol type the picture is complicated by the presence of physical dependence but in the other five types there is as yet little or no evidence for the development of physical dependence either in man or laboratory animals. Psychic dependence has been recognized clinically in man for many years and there is a vast amount of clinical literature describing the syndromes resulting from the various types of drug abuse, but until recently it was considered that these phenomena were confined to man. The development of the science of animal behaviour and the realization that behavioural patterns in animals can be assessed quantitatively and be modified by drugs has led many workers to attempt to study psychic dependence in laboratory animals.

The importance of the morphine-like compounds as drugs of abuse has resulted in many investigators using this class of drug for studying possible drug-seeking behaviour in laboratory animals. These studies have been complicated by the development of physical dependence and it was found impossible to decide whether the animals sought the drug to relieve or prevent the development of the abstinence syndrome or for a possible euphoriant effect. Spragg (1940) showed that chimpanzees made physically dependent on morphine would choose morphine rather than food during a period of abstinence. The work of Skinner on conditioning has led a number of workers to apply these principles to the study of psychogenic dependence. The rat has been used frequently; Nichols and his colleagues (Nichols *et al.*, 1956; Nichols & Davis, 1959; Davis & Nichols, 1962) have shown that rats can be trained to drink a solution of morphine in preference to water despite its bitter taste. Morphine is not well absorbed from the gut and Wikler *et al.* (1963) used a combination of morphine injections and etonitazine in the drinking water to demonstrate opiate-seeking behaviour in rats. Weeks (1961, 1964) has developed an elegant method for the administration of morphine directly into the blood streams of conscious rats via an indwelling cannula in the jugular vein. Using operant conditioning techniques he has also shown that rats will work for the drug on a lever pressing schedule and that pethidine and codeine can partially substitute for morphine in this situation. Other workers have used similar conditioning techniques with rhesus monkeys either fully restrained (Thompson & Schuster, 1963) or partially restrained (Yanagita *et al.*, 1965).

All these studies have demonstrated that animals can show drug-seeking behaviour of the escape-avoidance or negative reinforcement type when made dependent upon morphine-type drugs. Beach (1957) suggested that there may be a positive reinforcement component in this behaviour and that rats may receive a pleasurable stimulus but he could provide no conclusive evidence in support of his hypothesis. The demonstration by Olds & Milner (1954) of the existence in the rat of so-called 'pleasure centre' in the hypothalamus supports Beach's suggestion that morphine-dependent rats may show positive reinforcement behaviour. Psychic dependence in man invariably involves a learned behaviour pattern following the active, rather than the passive, administration of a euphoriant drug by an individual to himself. This active participation in the drug taking process can only take place in animals when they can have some control over the process of administration. The development of sophisticated techniques of self-administration in animals, especially primates, has made this possible. Yanagita *et al.* (1965) have studied the self-administration by rhesus monkeys of a number of drugs known to induce psychic dependence in man. In this technique the animals were trained to tolerate a harness attached via a swivelling arm to a giving system. A catheter was passed along an arm over and through the jugular vein into the right heart. Drugs were administered through the catheter in response to the depression of a bar by the animal. Untrained animals were used which eventually pressed the lever during their normal exploratory behaviour. If the effects of the drug gave rise to a desirable effect (positive conditioning) the animal repeated the bar pressing or if negatively rewarding bar-pressing was avoided. Continued bar-pressing by the animal indicated either positive reward as during psychic dependence or negative reinforcement as expected in response to physical dependence. In order to distinguish between the two types of dependence the animal was removed from the apparatus for several weeks to allow for possible physical dependence to be eliminated and then connected back to the apparatus. Further self-administration on reconnection was taken to be indicative of psychic dependence. Although these studies are still in their early stages preliminary results indicate that drugs known to produce both psychic dependence alone and combined with physical dependence in man can induce drug seeking behaviour in monkeys. With the stimulants cocaine and amphetamine, all the animals tested on each drug developed spontaneous self-administration of the drugs. When morphine was given alone 8 out of 11 monkeys tested showed positive responses and when morphine was mixed with cocaine, a mixture frequently abused in man, four out of four animals showed psychic dependence. Four out of five monkeys given codeine responded positively as did four out of five given alcohol and five out of five given pentobarbital.

Signs of psychotoxicity developed in animals taking cocaine and amphetamine and with both drugs animals showed periods of spontaneous abstinence. Periodic voluntary abstinence was also seen in the animals taking alcohol. During these periods the animals showed apprehension, tremor, dysmetria, convulsions, and apparent hallucinations. With morphine self-administration no extended periods of abstinence were seen and with pentobarbital there were no periods of voluntary abstinence at all. The animals maintained themselves with sufficient barbiturate to produce an almost continuous state of light anaesthesia. The only period of abstinence observed was for a period of 45 min each day when the animal consumed enough food to maintain its normal body weight.

No evidence of psychic dependence would be obtained with nalorphine, nalorphine-morphine mixtures, chlorpromazine, or mescaline (Seevers, 1966—personal communication).

Drugs of the cannabis or of the khat type are not believed to induce physical dependence in man (Eddy *et al.*, 1965) and to date no evidence for experimental psychic dependence has been published although there is an extensive literature on the clinical aspects of dependence of drugs of these two types. Psychic dependence is of a lower grade than with cocaine and the harm to the individual is more marked by its effects on his social behaviour than by any psychotoxic effects. Studies on the effects of these drugs on the social behaviour of animals using a combination of self-administration of drugs to unrestrained animals in a social group might provide valuable information for drugs of this type. Suitable techniques have been developed by Delgado (1962) and their application in this field should prove rewarding. The studies by MacDonald & Heimstra (1965) on the changes in social behaviour in rats induced by drugs may provide valuable information on possible mechanisms involved in social aspects of drug taking. These workers have shown that drugged rats can alter the behaviour patterns of non-drugged rats in the same social group. Amphetamine and chlorpromazine when given to one rat of a pair affected the behaviour pattern of its partner. The amphetamine-treated animal stimulated its untreated partner to mimic its own behaviour but with chlorpromazine the increase in passive social behaviour by the treated animal induced an increase in active behaviour in its partner. It is believed that drugs such as amphetamine, cannabis, and khat are frequently taken to alter social behaviour and these newly developed behavioural techniques may provide valuable tools for the study of psychic dependence.

PSYCHOTOXICITY

All the drugs which are capable of inducing dependence in susceptible individuals are capable of producing behavioural disturbances in man and often in animals. These disturbances may follow a single dose or may only develop after repeated administration or on withdrawal of the drug after a period of chronic intoxication.

Each of the drug types described earlier are capable of producing characteristic alterations of normal behaviour patterns and although the disturbances produced show marked quantitative variations between individuals, each type of drug produces qualitatively similar pharmacological effects in individuals of the same species. Evidence of psychotoxicity is not in itself sufficient to warrant classifying a drug as capable of inducing dependence. Many drugs which are capable of producing behavioural changes in normal individuals, e.g. phenothiazine tranquillizers and the monoamine oxidise inhibitors, do not induce drug dependence. Thus tests for psychotoxicity alone cannot be used to predict potential production of drug dependence but may provide additional evidence for possible liability to abuse.

Drugs which produce behavioural disturbances in animals will normally be recognized during the pharmacological evaluations which precede trials of new drugs in man. The commonly applied screening methods (Nodine & Siegler, 1964; Laurence & Bacharach, 1964) will indicate which type of activity a drug possesses and if it is found to influence the central nervous system the type and intensity of effect produced may be more clearly defined following more specific pharmacological evaluation. The animal pharmacology of the morphine-like drugs, barbiturates, and similar sedatives and stimulants of the amphetamine type is well documented and substances found to fall into these pharmacological classifications should be assessed for their dependence capacity using the techniques outlined earlier. Pharmacological technique for detecting the psychotoxic effects of drugs of the cocaine, cannabis, khat, and hallucinogen types are much less well defined.

Cocaine is capable of producing psychotoxic effects in dogs (Tatum & Seevers, 1929) and behavioural and neurophysiological disturbances have been reported in monkeys and cats following injection of relatively large doses of lysergic acid diethylamide and bufotenine (Evarts, 1956; Evarts & Marshall, 1956; Evarts *et al.*, 1955; Key & Bradley, 1963).

Cannabis (Bose *et al.*, 1963; Valle *et al.*, 1966) and mescaline (Krueger *et al.*, 1960; Downing, 1964) can also produce charac-

9—M.T.

teristic behavioural changes in experimental animals but none of these changes have been shown to be specific for any one type of drug and no direct relationship between the psychopharmacological effects produced in animals by centrally acting drugs and their potential for producing dependence has been established. For further information on psychopharmacological testing techniques in animals the reader is referred to a number of reviews dealing with this aspect of the drug dependence problem (Hunt, 1961; Votava *et al.*, 1963; Cook & Kelleher, 1963; Steinberg, 1964; Gollub & Brady, 1965).

Wikler (1957) has reviewed the behavioural disturbance produced by psychoactive drugs in man and workers at the Addiction Research Centre at Lexington (Haertzen *et al.*, 1963; Hill *et al.*, 1963a, b) have developed an inventory for evaluating the subjective effects of morphine, amphetamine, pentobarbital, alcohol, LSD 25, pyrahexyl, and chlorpromazine. This test, developed from the Minnesota multiphasic personality inventory (MMPI), promises to be of value in defining and classifying centrally acting drugs according to behavioural effects produced in human volunteers. The effect of drug abuse on social behaviour is an important aspect of the problem of drug dependence. Recent work has shown that a number of dependence-producing drugs can influence conflict behaviour in animals; morphine-like compounds, barbiturates, meprobamate, and chlordiazepoxide can all normalize conflict behaviour (Jacobsen, 1962). Delgado (1962) has shown that social behaviour patterns amongst primate groups can be modified by centrally-acting drugs but the relationship between these effects and liability of drugs to be abused by man has still to be established.

CONCLUSIONS

All new drugs which during the course of routine pharmacological testing are found to possess marked CNS depressant or stimulant activity should be regarded as potential drugs of dependence. If the pharmacological spectrum obtained during the early investigation indicates that the drug might be classed as either morphine-like or barbiturate-alcohol-like, tests to assess possible dependence producing properties should be instigated. Evidence for this may be found during the normal prolonged toxicity testing when tolerance to the central effects may be obvious and withdrawal signs may become apparent during the normal dosing schedule. These tests, however, cannot be substituted for a more detailed investigation aimed at detecting and measuring the liability of the new drug to produce dependence.

A new drug showing suspected morphine-like properties should be investigated to determine its capacity to produce physical dependence. For this purpose the tests which use rodents may be used for initial screening purposes but at present these are not sufficiently well established for reliable predictions to be made. Of the tests available to date, the techniques described by Buckett (1964) or Martin *et al.* (1963) are capable of providing qualitative evidence of physical dependence but for a quantitative assessment of a new morphine-like drug the technique of Deneau & Seevers (1962) using rhesus monkeys must be the method of choice. The establishment of a colony of morphine-dependent monkeys is an expensive and time-consuming operation. As a public service the facilities and experience of the Department of Pharmacology of the University of Michigan Medical School under Dr Seevers are made available for the testing of new drugs with possible morphine-like dependence potential. Requests for testing of drugs of this type should be submitted to the Executive Secretary of the Committee on Problems of Drug Dependence (formerly the Committee on Drug Addiction and Narcotics) of the National Research Council, Washington, USA, giving details of the chemical nature, pharmacological properties, and the reason for wanting the compound evaluated. The drug is then submitted under a code number to the laboratory for testing, the results are reported back to the Executive Secretary who will pass on the information to the producer of the drug. Should the drug prove to have a high physical dependence capacity and no compensating advantages it is unlikely that further studies will be performed but should these initial studies reveal interesting properties, e.g. high analgesic potency with a marked qualitative or quantitative separation of physical dependence capacity the drug may be submitted to further direct substitution studies in the monkey. Should these results provide evidence of a potentially valuable drug showing definite advantages over established drugs in this class the drug may be sent to the workers at Lexington for evaluation of its potential to produce dependence in man. On the basis of all the accumulated evidence the Committee on Problems of

Drug Dependence may make recommendations to the appropriate national and international agencies as to whether the drug should or should not be submitted to control.

The dog appears to be the animal of choice for the assessment of the dependence properties of drugs of the barbiturate-alcohol type as the tests using rodents have not yet been evaluated on a sufficiently wide range of drugs to make them reliable. Even with the dog, experience is strictly limited and no one method has been found to satisfy all the criteria but the technique of Weiss & Deneau (1964) promises the nearest approach to a satisfactory test and further results using this technique are awaited.

As the techniques for detecting psychic dependence are even less well established than those for physical dependence no method can be recommended but the increasing tempo of work in this field holds out promises for the development of reliable techniques for studying this most difficult aspect of drug abuse.

Drug dependence is a complex phenomenon involving the interplay of physiological, psychic, and social factors. No tests relying on animal experiments alone can be expected to predict the eventual response of man to a drug but the work described and that at present being undertaken in many centres throughout the world can reduce the area of uncertainty which faces the physician when he prescribes a new drug to a patient for the first time.

REFERENCES

BEACH H.D. (1957) Morphine addiction in rats. *Canad. J. Psychol* **11**, 104–12.

BENTLEY G.A. (1961) The susceptibility of rats to audiogenic seizures following acute and prolonged medication with narcotic drugs. *Arch. int. Pharmacodyn* **132**, 378–91.

BENTLEY K.W. & HARDY D.G. (1963) New potent analgesics in the morphine series. *Proc. Chem. Soc.* July, p. 220.

BERGER, H. (1961) Addiction to methyprylon. *J. Am. med. Ass.* **117**, 63–5.

BOSE B.C., VIJAYVARGIYA, R., SAIFI A.Q. & BHAGWAT A.W. (1963) Chemical & Pharmacological investigation of Cannabis indica (Linn.) Part I. *Arch. int. Pharmacodyn.* **146**, 99–105.

BROWNSTEIN S.R. & PACELLA B.C. (1943) Convulsions following abrupt withdrawal of barbiturates—Clinical and electroencephalographic studies. *Psychiat. Q.* **17**, 112–22.

BUCKETT W.R. (1964) A new test for morphine-like physical dependence (addiction liability) in rats. *Psychopharmacologia* **6**, 410–16.

CARTER R.L. & WIKLER A. (1954) Use of N-allyl normorphine in early demonstration of physical dependence on potent analgesics in dog. *Fedn. Proc. Fedn Am. Socs, exp. Biol.* **13**, 342.

CARTER R.L. and WIKLER A. (1955) Chronic meperidine intoxication in intact and chronic spinal dogs. *Fedn. Proc. Fedn. Am. Socs. exp. Biol.* **14**, 325.

COOK L. & KELLEHER R.T. (1963) Effects of drugs on behaviour, *Ann. Rev. Pharmac.* **3**, 205–22.

CORSSEN G. (1964) Addiction reaction in cultured human cells. *J. Am. med. Ass.* **187**, 328–32.

CROSSLAND J. & LEONARD B.E. (1963) Barbiturate withdrawal convulsions in the rat. *Biochem. Pharmac. Suppl.*, **12**, 103.

CULLUMBINE H. & KONOP T.S. (1959) The relation between drug induced excitation in the cat and addiction liability. *Can. J. Biochem.* **37**, 1075–9.

DAVIS W.M. & NICHOLS J.R. (1962) Physical dependence and sustained opiate directed behaviour in the rat. *Psychopharmacologia*, **3**, 139–45.

DELGADO J.M.R. (1962) Pharmacological modifications of social behaviour. *Proc. 1st int. Pharmac. Meet.* **8**, 265–92.

DENEAU G.A. & SEEVERS M.H. (1962) Evaluation of morphine-like physical dependence in the rhesus monkey (Macaca mulata). *Minutes of the Committee on Drug Addiction and Narcotics*, Addendum 2, pp. 1–11, National Academy of Sciences, National Research Council, Washington.

DENEAU G.A. & SEEVERS M.H. (1964a) Pharmacological aspects of drug dependence. *Adv. Pharmac.* **3**, 267–83.

DENEAU G.A. & SEEVERS M.H. (1964b) *Drug Dependence in Evaluation of Drug Activities, in Pharmacometrics*, Ed. Laurence D.R. & Bacharach A.L., pp. 167–79. London, Academic Press.

DESMAREZ J.J. (1960) Contribution to the study of body fluids during pain. Effects of pain on the acid-base equilibrium of the blood and its ascorbic content. *Ann. soc. roy. sci. med. et nat. Bruxelles*, **13**, 73–124.

DOWNING D.F. (1964) Psychotomimetic compounds, in *Psychopharmacological Agents*, ed. Gordon M., Vol. I, p. 576, New York, Academic Press.

DUNNING H.S. (1940) Convulsions following withdrawal of sedative medication. *Int. Clin.* **3**, 255–64.

EDDY N.B. & HIMMELSBACH C.K. (1936) Experiments on the tolerance and addiction potentialities of dihydrodesoxymorphine D (desomorphine). *Pub. Hlth. Rep. W.S. Suppl.* **118**, 1–14.

EDDY N.B., HALBACH H., IBSELL H. & SEEVERS M.H. (1965) Drug dependence: its significance and characteristics. *Bull. Wld Hlth Org.* **32**, 721–33.

ESSIG C.F. (1958) Withdrawal convulsions in dogs following meprobamate intoxication. *Arch. Neurol & Psychiat.* **80**, 414–17.

ESSIG C.F. & FLANARY H.T. (1959) Convulsions in cats following withdrawal of barbital sodium. *Exptl Neurol.* **1**, 529–33.

ESSIG C.F. (1963), Additive and possible toxic properties of glutethimide. *Am. J. Psychiat.* **119**, 993.

Essig C.F. (1964a) Addiction to non-barbiturate sedative and tranquilizing drugs. *Clin. Pharmac. Ther.* **5,** 334–43.

Essig C.F. (1964b) Barbiturate withdrawal convulsions in decerebellate dogs. *Int. J. Neuropharmacol.* **3,** 453–6.

Essig C.F. (1966) Barbiturate withdrawal in white rat*s. Int. J. Neuropharmacol.* **5,** 103–7.

Essig C.F. & Flanary H.G. (1961) Convulsive aspects of barbital sodium withdrawal in the cat. *Exptl Neurol.* **3,** 149–59.

Ettles M. & Lister R.E. (1963) The assessment of withdrawal symptoms in narcotic dependent rats. Communication to British Pharmacological Society, Dublin.

Evarts E.V., Landau W., Freygang W. & Marshall W.H. (1955) Some effects of lysergic acid diethylamide and bufotenine on electrical activity in the cat's visual system. *Amer. J. Physiol.* **182,** 594–8.

Evarts E.V. (1956) Some effects of bufotenine and lysergic acid diethylamide on the monkey. *Arch. Neurol. & Psychiat.* **75,** 49–53.

Evarts E.V. & Marshall W.H. (1956) The effects of lysergic acid diethylamide on the excitability cycle of the lateral geniculate nucleus. *Trans. Am. Neurol. Ass.* pp. 58–60. Byrd, Richmond.

Ewing J.A. & Haizlip T.M. (1958) A controlled study of the habit forming propensities of meprobamate. *Am. J. Psychiat.* **114,** 835.

Fichtenberg D.G. (1951) Study of experimental habituation to morphine. I. Review of morphine habituation in the rat. *Bull. Narcot.* **3,** 19–42.

Fraser H.F., Shaver M.R.. Maxwell E.S. & Isbell H. (1953) Death due to withdrawal of barbiturates. *Ann. int. Med.* **38,** 1319–25.

Fraser H.F. & Isbell H. (1954) Abstinence syndrome in dogs after chronic barbiturate medication. *J. Pharmac. exp. Ther.* **112,** 261–7.

Fraser H.F., Isbell H., Eisenman A.J., Wikler A. & Pescor F.T. (1954) Chronic Barbiturate Intoxication. *AMA Arch. internal. Med.* **94,** 34–41.

Fraser H.F., Wikler A., Isbell H. & Johnson H.K. (1957) Partial equivalence of chronic alcohol and barbiturate intoxications. *Q. Jl. Stud. Alcohol* **18,** 541–51.

Fraser H.F., Wikler A., Essig C.F. & Isbell H. (1958) Degree of Physical dependence induced by secobarbital or pentobarbital. *J. Am. med Ass.* **166,** 126–9.

Fraser H.F., van Horn, Martin W.R., Wolbach A.B. & Isbell H. (1961) Methods for evaluation addiction liability. (A) Attitude of opiate addicts toward opiate-like drugs, (B) A short term direct addiction test. *J. Pharmac. exp. Ther.* **133,** 371–87.

Fraser H.F. (1964) Clinical techniques for evaluating addiction liability of drugs, in *Pharmacologic Techniques in Drug Evaluation,* eds. Nodine J.H. & Siegler P.E., pp. 411–17. Chicago, Year Book Medical Publishers.

Goldenberg M.A. & Korolenko T.P. (1963) Alcoholic 'psychopathological' syndrome in experimental animals. *Zh. Neuropat. Psikhiat.* **63,** 1861–6.

Gollub L.R. & Brady J.V. (1965) Behavioural Pharmacology. *Ann. Rev. Pharmac.* **5,** 235–62.

HAERTZEN C.A., HILL H.E. & BELLEVILLE R.E. (1963) Development of the addiction research centre inventory (ARCI). Selection of items that are sensitive to the effects of various drugs. *Psychopharmacologia* 4, 155–66.

HALBACH H. & EDDY N.B. (1963) Tests for addiction (Chronic Intoxication) of morphine type. *Bull. Wld Hlth Org.* 28, 139–73.

HANNA C. (1960), Demonstration of morphine tolerance and physical dependence in the rat. *Arch. int. Pharmacodyn.* 124, 326–9.

HANO K., KANETO H. & KAKUNAGU T. (1963) Pharmacological studies on analgesics: Report 5—Development of physical dependence in morphinized mice. *Jap. J. Pharmac.* 13/2, 207–14.

HENDERSHOT L.C. & FORSAITH, J. (1959) Antagonism of the frequency of phenylquinone-induced writhing in the mouse by weak analgesics and non-analgesics. *J. Pharmac. exp. Ther.* 125, 237–40.

HILL H.E., HAERTZEN C.A., WOLBACH A.B. & MINER E.J. (1963a) The Addiction Research Center Inventory; Standardization of scales which evaluate subjective effects of morphine, amphetamine, pentobarbital, alcohol, LSD-25, pyrahexyl and chloropromazine. *Psychopharmacologia* 4, 167–83.

HILL H.E., HAERTZEN C.A., WOLBACH A.B. & MINER E.J. (1963b) The Addiction Research Center Inventory; Appendix I—Items comprising empirical scales for seven drugs. II—Items which do not differentiate placebo from any drug condition. *Psychopharmacologia* 4, 184–205.

HIMMELSBACH C.K. (1939) Studies of certain addition characteristics of dihydromorphine (paramorphan), dihydrodesoxymorphine-D (desmorphine), dihydrodesoxycodeine-D (desocodeine) and methydihydromorphinone ('metopon'). *J. Pharmac. exp. Ther.* 67, 239–49.

HIMMELSBACH C.K., GERLACH G.H. & STANTON E.J. (1935) A method for testing addiction tolerance and abstinence in the rat. Results of its application to several morphine alkaloids. *J. Pharmac. exp. Ther.* 53, 179–88.

HOLLISTER L.E., MOTZENBECKER F.P. & DEGAN R.O. (1961) Withdrawal reactions from chloridiazepoxide. *Psychopharmacologia* 2, 63–8.

HUIDOBRO F. (1964) Studies on Morphine. VI. Injection of morphine solutions in normal mice and rats and in animals with chronic morphinism. *Arch. int. Pharmacodyn.* 151, 299–312.

HUIDOBRO F. & CONTRERAS E. (1963) Studies on morphine. II. Repeated administration of nalorphine to white mice chronically treated with pellets of morphine. *Arch. int. Pharmacodyn.* 144, 206–13.

HUIDOBRO F., MAGGIOLO C. & CONTRERAS E. (1963) Studies on morphine I. Effects of nalorphine and levallorphan in mice implanted with pellets of morphine. *Arch. int. Pharmacodyn.* 144, 196–205.

HUNT H.F. (1961) Methods for studying the behavioural effects of drugs. *Ann. Rev. Pharmac.* 1, 125–44.

ISBELL H. (1948) Methods and results of studying experimental human addiction to the newer synthetic analgesics. *Ann. N.Y. Acad. Sci.* 51, 108–22.

ISBELL H., FRASER H.F., WIKLER A., BELLEVILLE R.E. & EISENMAN A.J. (1955) An experimental study of the etiology of 'rum fits' and delirium tremors. *Q.J. Studies Alcohol* 16, 1–33.

JACOBSEN E. (1962) Drug induced changes in behaviour. *Proc. 1st int. Pharmac. Meet.* **8,** 251–63.

JAFFE J.H. & SHARPLESS S.K. (1965) The rapid development of physical dependence on barbiturates. *J. Pharmac.* **150,** 140–5.

JOEL E. & ETTINGER A. (1926) Zur Pathologie der Gewohnung III Mitteilong; Experimentelle Studien ulser Morphingewohnung. *Arch. exp. Path. u. Pharmak.* **115,** 334–50.

KALINOWSKY L.B. (1942) Convulsions in nonepileptic patients on withdrawal of barbiturates, alcohol and other drugs. *Arch. Neurol. & Psychiat.* **48,** 946–56.

KAYMAKCALAN S. & WOODS L.A. (1956) Nalorphine-induced abstinence syndrome in morphine tolerant albino rats. *J. Pharmac. exp. Ther.* **117,** 112–16.

KAYMAKCALAN S. & TEMELLI S. (1964) Response of the isolated intestine of normal and morphine-tolerant rats to morphine and nalorphine. *Arch. int. Pharmacodyn.* **151,** 136–41.

KEY, B.J. & BRADLEY P.B. (1960) The effects of drugs on conditioning and habituation to arousal stimuli in animals. *Psychopharmacologia* **1,** 450–62.

KOLB L. & DU MEZ A.G. (1931) Experimental addiction of animals to opiates. *Publ. Hlth Rep. (U.S.)* 46, 698–726.

KOLB L. & HIMMELSBACH C.K. (1938) Clinical studies of drug addiction; critical review of withdrawal treatments with method of evaluating abstinence syndromes. *Amer. J. Psychiat.* **94,** 759–99.

KRUEGER H., EDDY N.B. & SUMWALT M. (1941) The pharmacology of the opium alkaloids. *Publ. Hlth Rep. (U.S.) Suppl.* **165,** 741–2.

KRUEGER R.F., LAUCK D.E., MOFFAT E. & GREEN D.M. (1960) Effects of analgesics on the mescaline scratch response in mice. *Fedn. Proc. Fedn. Am. Soc. exp. Biol.* **19,** 271.

KUBO T. (1939) Studien uber die Gewohnung an opiumalkaloide k2w. die entwohnung von denselben beim kulturgewebe. *Arch. F. exp. Zellforsch.* **23,** 253–68.

KUHN H.F. & FRIEBEL H. (1962) Uber den nachweis von 'Physical Dependence' bei codeine-behandeltern ratten. *Med. Exp.* **6,** 301–6.

LAURENCE D.R. & BACHARACH A.L. (1964) Evaluation of drug activities. *Pharmacometrics.* London, Academic Press.

LISTER R.E. (1964) Structure-activity requirements in some novel thebaine derived analgesics. *J. Pharm. Pharmac.* **16,** 364–6.

LLOYD E.A. & CLARK L.D. (1959) Convulsions and delirium incident to glutethimide. *Dis. nerv. system* **20,** 1–3.

MACDONALD A.L. & HEIMSTRA N.W. (1965) Social influence on the response to drugs. V. Modification of behaviour of non-drugged rats by drugged. *Psychopharmacologia* **8,** 174–81.

MCQUARRIE D.G. & FINGL E. (1958) Effects of single doses and chronic administration of ethanol on experimental seizures in mice. *J. Pharmac. exp. Ther.* **13,** 264–71.

MARGETTS E.L. (1950) Chloral delirium. *Psychiat. Quart.* **24,** 278–80.

MARTIN W.R. & EADES C.G. (1961) Demonstration of tolerance and physical dependence in the dog following a short-term infusion of morphine. *J. Pharmac. exp. Ther.* **133**, 262–70.

MARTIN W.R., WIKLER A., EADES C.G. & PESCOR F.T. (1963) Tolerance and Physical Dependence on Morphine in Rats. *Psychopharmacologia* **4**, 247–60.

MARTIN W.R. & EADES C.G. (1964) A comparison between acute and chronic physical dependence in the chronic spinal dog. *J. Pharmac. exp. Ther.* **146**, 385–95.

MARTIN W.R., FRASER H.F., GORODETSKY C.W. & ROSENBERG D.E. (1965) Studies on the addiction potential of the narcotic antagonist 2-cyclopropymethyl-2-hydroxy-5,9-dimethyl-6,7 benzomorphan (cyclazocine, Win 20, 740, ARC II-C-3). *J. Pharmac. exp. Ther.* **150**, 437–42.

MELLO N.K. & MENDELSON J.H. (1965) Operant Analysis of Drinking Patterns of Chronic Alcoholics. *Nature* **206**, 43.

MENDELSON J., WEXLER D., LIEDERMAN P.H. & SOLOMON P. (1957) A study of addiction to non-ethyl alcohols and other poisonous compounds. *Q. Jl Stud. Alcohol* **18**, 561–9.

MERCIER J. & MERCIER E. (1957) Etude de l'accoumatumance experimentale per une methode psycho-physiologique II Etude de quelques analgesique centraux de synthese. *Ann. pharm. franc.* **15**, 106–18.

MURRAY W.J. & MILLER J.W. (1960) Oxytocin induced cramping in the rat. *J. Pharmac. exp. Ther.* **128**, 372–9.

NEWMAN H. & CARD J. (1937) The nature of tolerance to ethyl alcohol. *J. nerv. ment. Dis.* **86**, 428–40.

NICHOLS J.R., HEADLEE C.P. & COPPOCK H.W. (1956) Drug Addiction I. Addiction by escape training. *J. Am. Pharm. Ass. (Sci. Ed.)* **45**, 788–91.

NICHOLS J.R. & DAVIS W.M. (1959) Drug Addiction II. Variation of Addiction. *J. Am. Pharm. Ass. (Sci. Ed.)* **48**, 259–62.

NODINE J.H. & SIEGLER P.E. (eds.) (1964) *Pharmacologic Techniques in Drug Evaluation.* Chicago, Year Book Medical Publishers.

OLDS J. & MILNER P. (1954) Positive reinforcement produced by electrical stimulation of septal area and other regions of rat brain. *J. comp. physiol. Psychol.* **47**, 419–27.

OSWALD I. & THACORE V.R. (1963) Amphetamine and phenmetrazine addiction. *Brit. Med. J.* **2**, 427–31.

PATON W.D.M. (1957) The action of morphine and related substances on contraction and on acetylcholine output of coaxially stimulated guinea pig ileum. *Brit. J. Pharmac. Chemother.* **12**, 119–27.

PHATAK N.M. & DAVID W.A. (1953) Effects of hydergine on the modification of tolerance to morphine and 1-isomethadone hyperglycemia in rabbits. *J. Pharmac. exp. Ther.* **109**, 139–47.

PLANT O.H. & PIERCE I.H. (1928) Studies of chronic morphine poisoning in dogs. I. General symptoms and behaviour during addiction and withdrawal. *J. Pharmac. exp. Ther.* **33**, 329–57.

SANJO K. (1934). Experimentelle untersuchungen ulser die Gewohnung der Inisepithelkulturen am morphin. *Folia Pharmac. jap.* **17**, 14.

SCHMIDT H. Jr. & KLAINMAN K.M. (1964) Effect of chronic administration and withdrawal of barbiturates upon drinking in the rat. *Arch. int. Pharmacodyn.* **151,** 142–9.

SCHRAPPE O. (1959) Physical dependence following chronic application of N-allyl normorphine. *Arzneimittel-Forsch.* **9,** 130–2.

SEEVERS M.H. & TATUM A.L. (1931) Chronic experimental barbital poisoning. *J. Pharmac. exp. Ther.* **42,** 217–31.

SEEVERS M.H. (1936) Opiate addiction in the monkey. I. Methods of study. *J. Pharmac. exp. Ther.* **56,** 147–56.

SEEVERS M.H. (1948) Animal experimentation in studying addiction to the newer synthetic analgesics. *Ann. N.Y. Acad. Sci.* **51,** 98–107.

SEEVERS M.H. & DENEAU G.A. (1963) Physiological Aspects of Tolerance and Physical Dependence, in *Physiological Pharmacology,* eds. Root W.S. & Hofmann F.G., Vol. IA, pp. 565–640. New York, Academic Press.

SEMURA S. (1933) Uber den Einfluss verschiedener Pharmaka der Morphingruppe auf des Wachstum der in vitro Kulturen von Fibroblasten. *Folia Pharmac. jap.* 16, 5–6.

SHEMANO I. & WENDEL H. (1964) A rapid screening test for potential addiction liability of new analgesic agents. *Toxicol. appl. Pharmac.* **6,** 334–9.

SHUSTER L., HANNAM R.V. & BOYLE W.E. (1963) A simple method of producing tolerance to dihydromorphinone in mice. *J. Pharmac. exp. Ther.* **140,** 149–54.

SPRAGG S.D.S. (1940) Morphine addiction in chimpanzees. *Comp. Psychol. Monogr.* **15,** 132–8.

STANTON E.J. (1936) Addiction and tolerance to barbiturates. Effects of daily administration and abrupt withdrawal of phenobarbital sodium and pentobarbital sodium in the albino rat. *J. Pharmac. exp. Ther.* **57,** 245–52.

STEINBERG H. (ed.) (1964) *Animal Behaviour and Drug Action.* London, Churchill.

SWANSON L.A. & OKADA T. (1963) Death after withdrawal of Meprobamate. *J. Am. med. Ass.* **184,** 780–1.

SWINYARD E.A., CHIN L. & FINGL E. (1957) Withdrawal hyperexcitability following chronic administration of meprobamate to mice. *Science, N.Y.* **125,** 739–41.

TAKEMORI A.E. (1961) Cellular adaptation to morphine in rats. *Science. N.Y.* **133,** 1018–19.

TATUM A.L. & SEEVERS M.H. (1929) Experimental cocaine addiction. *J. Pharmac. exp. Ther.* **36,** 401–10.

TATUM A.L., SEEVERS M.H. & COLLINS K.H. (1929) Morphine addiction and its physiological interpretation based on experimental evidence. *J. Pharmac. exp. Ther.* **36,** 447–75.

THOMPSON T. & SCHUSTER C.R. (1964) Morphine self administration, food reinforced and avoidance behaviours in rhesus monkeys. *Psychopharmacologia* **5,** 87–94.

VALLE J.R., SOUZA J.A. & HYPPOLITO N. (1966) Rabbit reactivity to cannabis preparations pyrahexyl and tetrahydrocannabinol. *J. Pharm. Pharmac.* **18,** 476–7.

VOTAVA Z., HORVATH M. & VINAR O. (eds.) (1963) *Psychopharmacological Methods.* Oxford, Pergamon Press.

WEEKS J.R. (1961) Self-maintained morphine addiction; a method for chronic programmed i.v. injections in unrestrained rats. *Fedn. Proc. Fedn. Am. Socs. exp. Biol.* **20,** 397.

WEEKS, J.R. (1964) Experimental Narcotic addiction. *Sci. Am.* **210,** 46–52.

WESTGATE H.D. & STIEBLER H.J. (1964) Barbiturate Abstinence Syndrome *Anesthesiology* **25,** 403–6.

WIKLER A. (1946) Effects of a cycle of morphine addiction on conditioned responses and experimental neuroses in dogs. *Fedn. Proc. Fedn. Am. Socs. exp. Biol.* **5,** 213.

WIKLER A. (1948) Recent progress in research on neurophysiological basis of morphine addiction. *Am. J. Psychiat.* **105,** 329–38.

WIKLER A. & FRANK K. (1948) Hindlimb reflexes of chronic spinal dogs during cycles of addiction to morphine and methadone. *J. Pharmac. exp. Ther.* **94,** 382–400.

WIKLER A. (1957) *The Relation of Psychiatry to Pharmacology.* Baltimore, Williams & Williams.

WIKLER A., MARTIN W.R., PESCOR F.T. & EADES C.G. (1963) Factors regulating oral consumption of an Opioid (Etonitazene) by Morphine-Addicted Rats. *Psychopharmacologia* **5,** 55–78.

WINTER C.A. & FLATAKER L. (1950) Studies on Heptazone (6-morpholino-4, 4-diphenyl-3-heptanone hydrochloride) in comparison with other analgesic drugs. *J. Pharmac. exp. Ther.* **98,** 305–17.

WOODS L.A., DENEAU G.A., BENNETT D.R., DOMINO E.F. & SEEVERS M.H. (1961) A comparison of the pharmacology of two potent analgesic agents Piminodine and Win 13·797 with morphine and meperidine. *Tox. appl. Pharmac.* **3,** 358–79.

YANAGITA T., DENEAU G.A. & SEEVERS M.H. (1965) Evaluation of pharmacologic agents in the monkey by long term intravenous, self or programmed administration. *Proc. 23rd Int. Congr. Physiol. Sci.* pp. 453–57.

CHAPTER 9

Experimental Inhalation Toxicity

J.C. GAGE

The procedures which will be described in this chapter are those suitable for laboratories concerned with the toxicity of chemicals which may contaminate industrial or agricultural atmospheres, or which may give rise to a community air pollution problem. They may also find application in the study of the effects of volatile or air-borne drugs, or of the gases and smokes used in chemical warfare.

The questions which must be asked when it is proposed to expose men to a chemical substance for occupational or other reasons are in the following form: can the substance be used without any special precautions being taken? What effects are likely to be observed if men are exposed to excessive concentrations for short or long periods and what treatment is appropriate in cases of poisoning? Is there a daily intake which can be regarded as safe for occupational exposure? In the study of toxicity by inhalation, this last consideration leads to the establishment of a threshold limit value or maximal allowable concentration to act as a guide in the maintenance of satisfactory working conditions (American Conference of Government Industrial Hygienists, 1966). The experimental work on which such limiting values are based usually involves the establishment of a 'no-effect level' on one or more species and in this respect resembles the investigations undertaken to determine tolerances for pesticides and other additives in food for human consumption. The scale of such experiments varies from brief 'range-finding tests' on rats to extended tests lasting 6 months or more on a variety of species, and, in the unique case of lead dust, to exposures lasting several years on man.

In all inhalation studies there are a number of factors to be considered; the design of the exposure chamber for housing the animals during the experiment, the generation and control of the atmospheric concentration of the material to be investigated; the maintenance of the animals in the exposure chamber, the design of the experiment and, finally, the assessment of the effects produced on the animals.

The Design of the Exposure Chamber

It is very seldom that published work nowadays refers to the exposure of animals to static atmospheres, that is, the insertion of animals into an enclosed chamber into which a known amount of the material to be investigated is dispersed. Such experiments must be of limited duration on account of the progressive deterioration in the environment from the accumulation of moisture and carbon dioxide, and because the atmospheric concentration tends to decrease due to adsorption on surfaces and absorption by the animals. Dynamic exposures, in which the animals are placed in a chamber through which passes an atmosphere containing the substance to be investigated, are much more satisfactory and only chambers of this type will be considered in this chapter.

As air must flow through the chamber during the experimental period, the design will be influenced to some extent by aerodynamic considerations. The flow of air should be sufficient to maintain the concentration of water vapour and carbon dioxide, and frequently also the temperature, within suitable limits, and also to ensure that the animals are exposed to a constant concentration of the substance under investigation. With volatile and stable materials, the aerodynamic factors are of minor importance; provided that there are not excessive dead spaces within the chamber, the convection arising from the heat dissipation and movement of the animals is usually sufficient to ensure adequate mixing of the. air. In small-scale experiments of this type a glass desiccator may conveniently be used; the animals, usually rats or mice, are placed on a wire mesh of galvanized iron or stainless steel suitable to permit passage of the excreta. Holes are bored in the desiccator wall, diametrically opposite one another, to take the air entry and exit tubes, and a water bottle may be introduced through the lid. An example of a chamber used for large-scale investigations is that operated by the Dow Chemical Company; this is a cubical metal box with an edge of 1·5 m and double doors to permit the introduction

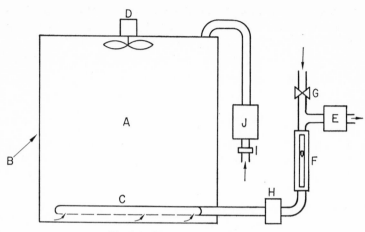

Fig. 9.1 Dow exposure chamber

A, chamber; B, double doors; C, exhaust manifold; D, fan; E, exhaust pump;
F, flowmeter; G, air leak; H, filter; I, charcoal filter; J, constant temperature
apparatus for injection of volatile substance.

of racks of animal cages (Fig. 9.1). Air enters at the top and
out through an exhaust manifold at the bottom, and a fan is
provided to facilitate mixing of the air. In the author's laboratory
the chamber, which, in its simplest form, is constructed from a
length of wide glass tube 12 in. in diameter surmounted by a well
fitting glass plate, is housed in an outer shell under exhaust ventilation to prevent contamination of the laboratory when very toxic or
otherwise unpleasant substances are under investigation; the test
atmosphere enters the chamber from below through a glass tube
which passes through the tray and wire grid at the base and reaches
nearly to the top. The air leaks out of the chamber through a gap
at the base and is removed by the exhaust duct. The chamber is
divided by radial partitions to keep the animals separated. The
apparatus for generating the atmosphere is located under the
chamber in order to save space (Fig. 9.2) (Gage, 1959).

If the material under investigation is in the form of a particulate
air contaminant, or is a vapour or gas which is unstable in air,
then more attention must be directed to the design of the chamber
to ensure that the linear flow of air across the chamber is approximately uniform. An excellent review of the earlier literature has
been published (Fraser *et al.*, 1959), which gives an indication of

the various approaches to chamber design. An intensive study of this subject was undertaken at the Department of Radiation Medicine of the University of Rochester in connection with the toxicity of radioactive dusts, and this led to the development of

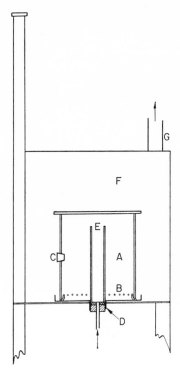

Fig. 9.2 Small ICI chamber

A, chamber; B, grid; C, sampling port; D, rubber stopper surmounted by sponge rubber pad; E, glass tube; F, outer chamber with rising door; G, duct to exhaust fan.

what is now generally known as the Rochester chamber (Leach *et al.*, 1958). These chambers are hexagonal in section, this being regarded as the nearest practical approximation to the ideal cylinder, with a stainless steel pyramidal top and bottom (Fig. 9.3). Each of the six sides is 110 cm high and 60 cm wide, and is constructed of polymethyl methacrylate sheet in a stainless steel frame. Two adjacent sides are hinged to form doors, carefully constructed to give a tight seal when closed. The total volume is about

2 m³, and it is claimed that it can house 16 monkeys, 32 beagles, or 160 rats, and that it is possible to house together 4 monkeys, 8 beagles, and 40 rats in one chamber.

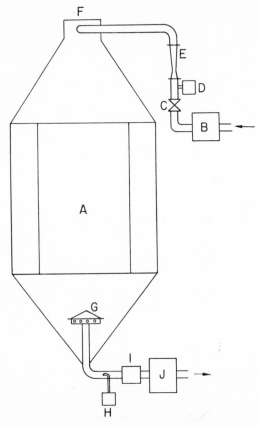

Fig. 9.3 Rochester chamber

A, chamber; B, pump; C, valve; D, injection point for substance; E, venturi throat for mixing; F, tangential entry of air into chamber; G, filter; H, pitot tube for flow measurement; I, filter; J, exhaust fan.

Extensive experiments with dust are also undertaken at the United States Public Health Service Toxicology Laboratory at Cincinnati (Fraser *et al.*, 1959). The chambers here differ in several respects from the Rochester pattern; they are cubical and larger, ranging between 2·5 and 6·5 m³ capacity, and although they have

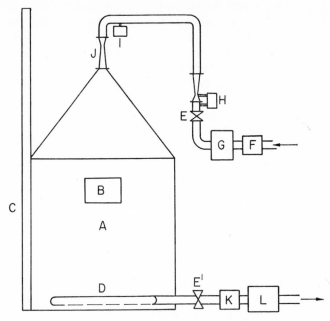

Fig. 9.4 USPHS chamber

A, chamber; B, window; C, rising door; D, exhaust manifold; E, E^1, control valves; F, pump; G, air conditioning unit; H, venturimeter; I, injection of substance under investigation; J, venturi throat air inlet; K, filter; L, exhaust fan.

a pyramidal top, the base is only slightly dished, sufficient to allow drainage during washing down (Fig. 9.4). Various construction materials are used, but aluminium sheet on an angle iron frame is preferred. Rather small inspection windows are inserted in each side, and there is top illumination. The larger chambers have counterbalanced, vertically rising doors. Chambers of this same shape have also been described by Wright (1957); these include the valuable feature of a safety hatch which opens if the air pressure fails, to prevent loss of the experimental animals by asphyxiation.

In these chambers careful attention has been directed to the prevention of contamination of the general laboratory atmosphere by the materials under investigation. In the Rochester chamber, air is pumped in at the top and exhausted from the bottom, the two flows being balanced to maintain a slight negative pressure in the chamber to prevent leakage to the outside air. A similar system is in operation in the chambers at Cincinnati. In the Dow chamber (Fig. 9.1) air is exhausted from the base through a manifold and enters at the top without assistance from a pump; the pressure drop in this air entry duct is kept low to avoid an excessive negative pressure in the chamber. Wright (1957) exhausts the air from the base of the chamber at a rate greater than that of the input air; leaks are provided near the exhaust to let in the surplus air. Small chambers may for safety be placed in a fume cupboard. The chambers illustrated in Figs. 9.2 and 9.5 are provided with their own outer casing under exhaust ventilation; the medium-sized

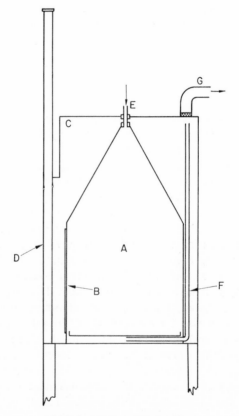

Fig. 9.5 Medium ICI chamber
A, chamber; B, door; C, outer casing; D, rising door; E, air inlet; F, air outlet; G, duct to exhaust fan.

chamber shown in Fig. 9.5 is in use in the author's laboratory for exposing animals to particulate contaminants. This type of chamber appears to be rather more complicated than those illustrated in Figs. 9.1, 9.3, and 9.4, but it is somewhat easier to construct as the materials and specifications are less critical. Moreover, there is no need for careful balancing of the rates of input and exhaust air; the only requirement is that the latter should be in excess of the former.

The Test Atmosphere

The air supplied to the chamber should be clean and conditioned to a suitable humidity and temperature. In order to maintain the concentration of the substance under investigation, both the flow of air and the rate of addition of the substance to the air stream should be known and constant.

With small chambers these conditions are not difficult to attain. Air from a compressor is filtered to remove dust and oil mist and is cleaned if necessary by means of a charcoal filter. The air may be dried by a silica gel or some other desiccant. The air then preferably passes through a reducing valve to maintain a constant line pressure, usually 10–15 lb/in.^{2}, and the flow is controlled by means of a suitable valve and flowmeter.

The most convenient means of measuring the flow of air in a small apparatus is undoubtedly the variable aperture flowmeter (for example, the Rotameter). In the author's laboratory a series of chambers of the type shown in Fig. 9.2 has been operated without a separate flowmeter on each chamber. The chambers are attached to a common air line which is kept at constant pressure by means of a reducing valve of adequate capacity, and the line leading to each chamber bears a needle valve and a pressure gauge to measure the line pressure beyond the valve. Before an experiment is undertaken, a flowmeter is attached by a length of tubing to the outlet of the air-line into the chamber, and the pressure gauge is calibrated in units of air flow. During the experiment the pressure gauge is adjusted if necessary by means of the needle valve to maintain the required flow; a check on the calibration of the pressure gauge is made each morning.

Procedures which have been used for the control and measurement of air flow in large exposure chambers are shown diagrammatically in Figs. 9.1, 9.3, and 9.4. The variable aperture flowmeter is available for such installations, though in some designs the pitot tube and the venturi meter may be more suitable. Details of such measuring equipment are given in a British Standard Specification (1964), but in general it is preferable to obtain special advice in the selection of pumps, valves and flowmeters, particularly if air is to be moved along large ducts with a low pressure drop.

The flow of air through the chamber is selected to maintain satisfactory concentrations of oxygen, carbon dioxide and moisture, and an adequate dissipation of the heat generated by the animals. The humidity and temperature in the chamber are probably the most critical considerations; they are a complex function of the humidity and temperature of the input air, of the air flow and of the load of animals. Fraser *et al.* (1959) have outlined the calculation which defines the performance of an air-conditioning unit to ensure that the temperature in the chamber is $26 \pm 1\,^\circ C$ and that the relative humidity does not exceed 55%, conditions which are regarded to be suitable for most laboratory animals. Such a unit is essential for large exposure chambers, and its installation requires the advice of a heating and ventilation engineer.

With smaller chambers in laboratories where conditioned air is not available it is usually simpler to dry the air with a desiccant; a self-regenerating column is convenient for this purpose. The minimal flow of air for a given load of animals may be determined directly by measurement of the temperature in the chamber and of the humidity of the exit air, and adjusting the air flow so that the conditions quoted above are achieved. Direct reading hygrometers, based on the change in dimensions of a membrane or fibre, are not suitable for this purpose, as such instruments may be subject to error by interference from the substance in the atmosphere under investigation. A simple aspiration hygrometer, based on the wet and dry bulb principle, is shown in Fig. 9.6. This is inserted through a sampling port in the chamber and air is drawn through until equilibrium is reached. By such means it has been found in the author's laboratory that for rats a supply of dry air at a rate of 0·5 1/min/rat recommended by Wright (1957) is adequate; when 4 1/min were supplied to a group of eight rats in the chamber shown in Fig. 9.2, a temperature rise of $2\,^\circ C$ and a relative humidity of 42% was recorded.

The removal of carbon dioxide is usually regarded as a factor less critical in the control of air flow, than is the limitation of the

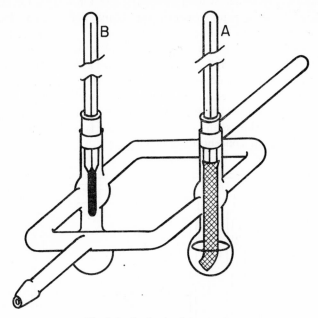

Fig. 9.6 Aspiration hygrometer
A, wet bulb thermometer; B, dry bulb thermometer.

rise in humidity and temperature. The flow of 0·5 l/min/rat quoted above would lead to a carbon dioxide concentration in the region of 0·5% by volume, which can be regarded as without effect on animals in the quiescent state normally encountered in the exposure chamber. If, however, the effect of atmospheres is being studied on animals undergoing enforced activity, it might be desirable to maintain the carbon dioxide concentration at a lower figure.

The Introduction of the Toxic Substance

VAPOURS

Unlike gaseous and particulate contaminants, vapours cannot be introduced into an air stream in excess of a limiting concentration determined by the vapour pressure of the substance at the temperature concerned. A concentration approaching that of the saturated vapour can readily be achieved by bubbling air through the liquid, usually in a bubbler with a sintered glass air distributor which accelerates equilibrium between the liquid and vapour by increasing the air–liquid interface and decreasing the rate of rise of the bubbles through the liquid. Complete saturation can be achieved by passing the air up a tower packed with rings down which trickles the liquid, or, if the liquid is stable to heat, by passing air over the heated liquid and then passing it through a filter to remove condensed particles after it has cooled to room temperature. Fig. 9.7 shows an apparatus of this type for preparing a saturated vapour concentration of mercury.

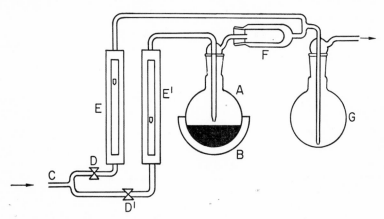

Fig. 9.7 Apparatus for preparing concentrations of mercury vapour
A, flask containing liquid mercury; B, heating mantle; C, air inlet; D, D^1, needle valves; E, E^1, flowmeters; F, filter; G, mixing flask.

The production of a saturated vapour concentration by blowing air through a liquid can only be undertaken if the liquid is pure and if it is stable to continual aeration. Moreover, in order to calculate the concentration the vapour pressure must be known with accuracy. With impure liquids, containing components with varying volatilities, the atmosphere produced will change qualitatively and quantitatively throughout the duration of an experiment.

A range of vapour concentrations may be prepared by diluting the saturated vapour with clean air, but in general it is preferable to use procedures which are free from the above drawbacks. Vapour concentrations of mercury metal are frequently prepared by diluting the saturated concentration as no satisfactory alternative exists (Fig. 9.7). It will be seen that the saturated vapour and diluting air are mixed by passage through a jet sufficiently fine to cause turbulence. There is a tendency in publications nowadays to depart from these earlier procedures and to prepare atmospheric concentrations by direct injection of the substance at a known rate into a metered air stream. Atmospheric concentrations of the vapour from volatile liquids are readily prepared by this procedure as the liquid can be filled into a syringe from which it is delivered at a constant rate into a vaporising device. The Palmer Slow Injection Apparatus (C. F. Palmer Ltd) is a convenient means of operating the syringe; it has a ram operated by a set of gears to give six speeds ranging between 0·003 and 0·1 in./min, and which can be obtained both in a horizontal and vertical design. The liquid delivery rate of such a system, expressed in milligrams per cubic metre (mg/m^3) is given by the expression $10^3\, \rho ab/v$, where ρ is the density of the liquid, a is the rate of travel of the piston in cm/min, b is the volume of the syringe in ml/cm along the barrel, and v is the air flow in l/min. To convert the concentration in mg/m^3 to parts per million by volume (p.p.m. v/v), this expression is multiplied by the factor $22\cdot4\times760(273+t)/273Mp$, where M is the molecular weight of the vapour, t is the temperature (°C) and p is the barometric pressure (mm Hg). At 20°C and 760 mm pressure this factor is almost exactly $24/M$. This conversion to p.p.m. cannot, of course, be undertaken for particulate dispersions; the concentration of these is always reported as mg/m^3. With such a system liquid delivery rates range between 6 ml/min with a 50 ml syringe and 0·0025 ml/min with a 1 ml syringe. Even lower delivery rates can be obtained with smaller syringes, thus with a 40 µl Hamilton syringe, 10^{-4} ml/min can be achieved. This system is not very suitable for high flow rates; at 6 ml/min a 50 ml syringe will have to be refilled every 8 min. Liquid delivery rates above 0·25 ml/min can more conveniently be achieved by a continuous pump such as the Watson-Marlow peristaltic pump.

The vaporization of a highly volatile liquid presents no difficulties; a needle attached to the syringe may be passed through a stopper in a short side arm on the air line, and the tip of the needle may touch on a roll of filter paper to spread the liquid and facilitate evaporation. This procedure is not suitable for liquids of lower volatility unless the syringe delivers the liquid on to a heated surface in the air stream, which is a procedure which can be operated only if the liquid is stable to heat. In the author's laboratory the liquid is volatilized by means of a controlled fluid-feed atomizer as shown in Fig. 9.8; the syringe delivers into a concentric air jet atomizer and the efficiency of subdivision of the liquid depends on the linear flow of air through the annular space around the jet (Gage, 1953). With low-boiling liquids the gap should be large, otherwise the venturi effect would cause the liquid to boil in the jet, while with higher boiling liquids smaller gaps are used. The construction of atomizers of this type has been described by Rosebury (1947). Lubricants for the syringe, taps, or joints which are soluble in the liquid must be avoided, as they might form a non-volatile mist. For many organic solvents, the grease described by Meloche & Fredrick (1932) may be recommended.

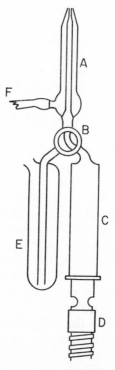

Fig. 9.8 Controlled fluid-feed atomizer

A, concentric air-jet atomizer; B, three-way tap; C, glass syringe; D, ram of slow injection apparatus; E, reservoir; F, air supply.

Direct atomization is not suitable for low concentrations of high-boiling liquids, and in some cases it is preferable to dilute the sample with an inert volatile solvent, such as water or, in certain cases, organic solvents such as propanol or petroleum ether. Low atmospheric concentrations of more volatile liquids, or also of volatile solids, may be prepared in a similar manner. The saturated vapour concentration of a volatile solid may be obtained by passage of air up a column of the material in a granular form. If the sample can only be obtained as a fine powder it may be dispersed on the surface of granules of an inert material such as kieselguhr.

GASES

Atmospheric concentrations of gases, or of the vapours of low-boiling liquids, may be readily prepared by direct admixture with air, if the sample is supplied under pressure in a cylinder. The gas is passed through a reducing valve to bring the pressure to a constant value, usually in the region of 10–20 lb/in², and then through a needle valve or suitable length of capillary tubing to control the flow. The gas is then mixed with a metered stream of clean air by passage through a jet to produce turbulence. The gas stream may be measured by a variable aperture flowmeter, and meters of this type are available which will measure down to about 10 cm³/min. Flowmeters of the moving soap film variety are available for rates less than this, but in general the preparation of atmospheric concentrations by a single stage dilution with air is not usually suitable for concentrations much less than 1,000 p.p.m. For lower concentrations the dilution of gas in air may be further diluted with air by a similar process, but such an operation is somewhat complicated to operate and subject to appreciable error. In a more satisfactory procedure for concentrations down to about 100 p.p.m., the gas is filled into a collapsible impermeable bag at a pressure not much above atmospheric, and from there it is fed at a known rate by means of a peristaltic or other suitable pump into an air stream. Very low concentrations of gases, of the order of 1 p.p.m. or less, may be prepared by direct injection of the gas from a syringe into the air stream, but this method is subject to error if changes in the line pressure cause air to be forced in or gas to be drawn out of the syringe. If a volatile and toxicologically inert solvent is available for the gas, it is much simpler to prepare a solution and inject this by syringe as described above for volatile liquids.

AEROSOLS

Special difficulties attend the generation of test atmospheres containing particulate matter. In addition to the requirement of a constant and known concentration, the particle size distribution must receive careful consideration as this will determine the regions of the respiratory tract in which the particles are deposited (Hatch & Gross, 1964), and this will affect toxicity. Coarser particles, which are trapped in the nose and upper respiratory tract, may cause local damage, or they may be absorbed systemically through the mucous membranes, or swallowed with mucus. The more serious lung diseases, however—and to investigate the possibility of these is usually the aim of the study of inhalation toxicity— derive from the inhalation of those particles which are sufficiently small to penetrate to the alveolar regions of the lungs, and sufficiently large to be to an appreciable extent retained there. It is considered that in man particles in the range 1–2 μ are most likely to be deposited in the alveolar regions, and particles of this size present, therefore, the greatest hazard. In animals the nasal cavity is regarded as being a more efficient filter for the coarser particles and few of these penetrate deep into the lungs. However, the dimensions of the alveolar regions are approximately the same in animals and in man, and the conditions for deposition there are much the same. It has been suggested that an assessment of the toxicity to man from experiments on animals will be most reliable if the animals are exposed to an aerosol in the size range 1–2 μ, although there is some evidence that the optimal size is rather larger than this for the rat (Gage, 1968).

The establishment of a known, constant concentration of a dust or mist within a narrow size range presents technical difficulties, and many procedures for tackling this problem have been described. The Wright dust feed mechanism (Wright, 1950) has been widely used for mineral dusts, provided that these are obtainable in a fine enough powder. The powder, which must be well dried, is compressed into a capsule and the surface is scraped off at a constant rate and blown into an air stream. More reliable results are obtained if the powder is compressed by a hydraulic ram at a controlled pressure. This apparatus can be used for some organic powders but most of these tend to cake and a uniform delivery of fine particles cannot be achieved. The United States Bureau of Mines apparatus may be more suitable for such materials (Schrenk, 1937); in this device the powder is loosely packed in a vertical cylinder which is slowly raised to bring the surface of the powder into contact with a static head, through which it is sucked up into an air stream. A modification has been described (Byers & Gage, 1961) in which the delivery of the dust is made more uniform by giving the vertical container an oscillatory motion, and passing a measured flow of air through the static head to pick up the dust and inject it into the main air stream.

Atmospheric concentrations of mists are somewhat easier to prepare. Droplets of a uniform size can be obtained with the spinning disc atomizer (Green & Lane, 1957), but this has rarely been used in toxicological investigations. More conventional atomizers are usually employed; these give a wide range of droplet size, and it is customary to remove the coarser particles, usually by directing the jet on to a surface with which the larger particles collide while the finer particles are carried on with the air stream. A simple atomizer for this purpose has been described and is sometimes termed the Collison's spray (Green & Lane, 1957); it is used for the preparation of methylene blue particles to test air filters (British Standard Specification, 1957). Commercial atomizers designed for aerosol therapy may also be used. An atomizer has recently been described (Gage, 1968) in which droplets fine enough to be drawn into the lungs are selected by a cyclone, and the coarser droplets are collected and returned to the atomizer; from the rate of decrease of liquid level in the reservoir the atmospheric concentration of fine droplets can be estimated.

If an aqueous solution of a solid is atomized, and if the vapour pressure of the saturated solution is greater than the vapour pressure due to moisture in the chamber, then the droplets will dry to give solid crystals. This is the easiest way to prepare an aerosol from a solid sample, but it is only practicable if the material is freely water-soluble. However, the preparation of an aerosol from an aqueous suspension of an insoluble solid has been described (Wilson *et al.*, 1953), using an atomizer somewhat similar to the Collison's spray. When aqueous solutions or suspensions are atomized in this manner, the air should first be saturated with water as otherwise there will be a progressive enrichment due to evaporation of water; the mist produced is then mixed with dry air to reduce the humidity to a suitable figure.

The Analytical Control of the Atmospheric Concentration

It is an excellent practice to check the concentration in the chamber atmosphere at least once a day. Analytical methods have been described for the determination of many substances of toxicological interest (Hanson *et al.*, 1965; American Conference of Governmental Industrial Hygienists, 1958; International Union of Pure and Applied Chemistry, 1962); there can be little doubt that gas chromatography provides the most convenient method for a laboratory investigating a range of gases and vapours. Most manufacturers of this apparatus provide a gas sampling valve which may be suitable for air analysis, and other sampling methods have been described in which a syringe or an absorption tube are used (Hanson *et al.*, 1965). With aerosols the analysis is more complex as not only must the total weight concentration be determined but also it is desirable to study, at any rate initially, the size distribution of the particles. The total mass concentration in the atmosphere may be determined by drawing a measured volume through a membrane filter and by determining the amount collected either by weighing or, if this is practicable, preferably by a specific chemical determination. The size distribution of the aerosol may be investigated by microscopical examination of the deposit on a membrane filter, but it is preferable to use a device such as the Cascade Impactor (Lippman, 1961), as this not only indicates the fraction of the total weight in each size range rather than the fraction of the total number, but the size range as determined by an aerodynamic method is more toxicologically relevant than an estimate derived from inspection of the dimensions under a microscope.

The Maintenance of the Experimental Animals

Apart from theoretical studies into absorption and excretion, there are few investigations in which it is advantageous to expose the animals continuously in the chamber for extended periods, and there are considerable practical difficulties in the provision of food and water, and in keeping the cage clean, unless the internal structure of the chamber has been designed with this in mind. It is the usual practice to keep animals in the chamber for periods up to 8 hours, and if repeated daily exposures are to be made, to remove them to other accommodation for the overnight period. In such experiments there is no need to feed and water the animals while they are in the chamber, and at the end of the exposure period there is an opportunity to examine and weigh the animals if required, and to clean the chamber. It is rare that any attempt is made to collect the excreta during exposure, though a metabolism cage has been described in which rats may be continuously exposed 24 hours a day, with provision for access to food and water and for the separate collection of urine and faeces (Gage, 1961). When several cages containing animals of different species are stacked into a chamber for exposure to an atmosphere containing particulate matter, it has been recommended that the base of each cage should not be a solid tray, as this would interfere with the flow of the aerosol through the chamber. This practice implies that the excreta from the animals placed in the upper part of the chamber will fall on those below, and it is customary to place the larger animals at the bottom of the chamber. Exercise cages have been described, in which animals may be placed during exposure, in order to study the effects of the increased respiratory rate on the toxicity of the substance under investigation (Fraser *et al.*, 1935).

When an atmosphere is passed into a chamber, there is a delay until the concentration reaches its calculated value. If rapid mixing of the air in the chamber is assumed, the concentration C_t at time t is given by the following expression:

$$t = \frac{V}{n} \log_e \left(\frac{C}{C - C_t} \right)$$

where C is the calculated concentration, n is the flow of air in litres per minute, and V is the volume of the chamber in litres. According to this expression, the time taken for an atmosphere to reach 90% of its final value is $2 \cdot 3 V / n$, and when a small rate of air flow is used in a large chamber, this period may amount to more than one hour. To overcome this, air-locks or other means have been recommended whereby animals may be introduced into the chamber after the concentration has been established. If possible, however, it is preferable to select a chamber just large enough for the group of animals under investigation.

The Design of the Experiment

The selection of the number and species of experimental animals, of the duration of the experiment, and of the range of concentrations to which the animals are exposed, will depend upon the purpose of the investigation. In experiments concerned with industrial toxicology, it is customary initially to study the effects of high concentrations on relatively small groups of animals in order to assess the likely effects on man if there is an industrial accident. The acute toxicity may be expressed as the LD_{50}, the concentration required to kill 50% of the animals, the time of exposure being stated. A more prolonged series of exposures is necessary to establish the conditions for the safe use of the substance; if, in such experiments, no toxic effects are observed at the saturated vapour concentration of a volatile liquid, it may be assumed that, under normal circumstances, this liquid will not present an inhalation hazard. If toxic effects are observed, the concentration is progressively reduced and the numbers of animals increased, until a 'no-effect' level is reached. With a substance of considerable commercial importance, and to which a large number of individuals may be exposed, experiments may be continued for six months or more, and a range of animal species may be used, including mice, rats, guinea-pigs, rabbits, dogs, and even monkeys. With substances of minor importance with fewer individuals at risk, experiments may be continued for shorter periods, though it seems desirable to expose animals for at least 15 daily periods spread over 3 weeks, as with shorter experiments there seems to be a real risk of missing some major toxic effect.

In all experiments it is very desirable to maintain a group of control animals under identical conditions but without the addition of the toxic substance to the atmosphere, and which at the end of the experiment are subjected to an examination similar to that used for the test animals. This is particularly important when "no-effect" levels of a chemical are being sought, as otherwise minor changes may be attributed to the chemical when they are, in fact, due to the environment of the animals, or to some intercurrent disease.

The Assessment of Results

The examination of animals during and subsequent to an experiment to ascertain the nature of any toxic effects produced by the exposure, will follow those procedures customary after administration of chemicals by other routes, though more attention may be paid to the effects on the lungs. Records should be kept of growth, behaviour, food and water consumption, the nature and time of appearance of toxic effects, and mortality, bearing in mind that, after animals have been exposed to materials with an irritant action on the lungs, severe toxic effects may be first observed up to several days after the termination of the exposure. Towards the end of the exposure period it is desirable to perform a complete haematological examination, and also to apply any appropriate diagnostic bichemical tests. At post-mortem examination, formol saline may be injected into the lungs through the trachea until the pleura is just distended; the trachea is then tied off and the lungs removed and dropped into formol saline, when the ligature is removed. Toxic effects on the lungs may not be uniformly distributed; some parts may be severely affected while others may remain normal, and it is desirable that the pathologist should inspect the lungs and select the portion to be processed for histopathological examination.

REFERENCES

AMERICAN CONFERENCE OF GOVERNMENTAL INDUSTRIAL HYGIENISTS (1958) *Manual of Analytical Methods Recommended for the Sampling and Analysis of Atmospheric Concentrations*. Cincinatti.

AMERICAN CONFERENCE OF GOVERNMENTAL INDUSTRIAL HYGIENISTS (1966) *Documentation of Threshold Limit Values*. Cincinnati.

BRITISH STANDARD SPECIFICATION (1957) B.S.2831.

BRITISH STANDARD SPECIFICATION (1964) B.S.1042.

BYERS P.D. & GAGE J.C. (1961) *Br. J. industr. Med.* **18**, 295.

FRASER D.A., BALES R.E., LIPPMAN M. & STOKINGER H.E. (1959) Exposure Chambers for Research in Animal Inhalation. *U.S. Dept. of Hlth, Educ. & Welf., Pub. Hlth. Monogr. No. 57*. Washington, D.C., U.S. Government Printing Office.

GAGE J.C. (1953) *J. sci. Instr.* **30**, 25.

GAGE J.C. (1959) *Br. J. industr. Med.* **16**, 11.

GAGE J.C.(1961) *Br. J. industr. Med.* **18**, 287.

GAGE J.C. (1968) *Br. J. industr. Med.* **25**, 304.

GREEN H.L. & LANE W.R. (1957) *Particulate Clouds: Dusts, Smokes and Mists*. London, E. & F.N. Spon Ltd.

HANSON N.W., REILLY D.A. & STAGG H.E. (eds.) (1965) *The Determination of Toxic Substances in Air*. Cambridge, W. Heffer & Sons Ltd.

HATCH T.F. & GROSS P. (1964) *Pulmonary Deposition and Retention of Inhaled Particles.* New York, Academic Press.

INTERNATIONAL UNION OF PURE AND APPLIED CHEMISTRY (1962) *Methods for the Determination of Toxic Substances in Air.* London, Butterworths.

LEACH L.J., SPIEGL C.J., WILSON R.H., SYLVESTER G.E. & LANTERBACH K.E. (1958) *Univ. Rochester Rept.* UR-534.

LIPPMAN M. (1961) *Am. industr. Hyg. Ass. J.* **22,** 341.

MELOCHE C.C. & FREDRICK W.G. (1932) *J. Am. chem. Soc.* **54,** 3264.

ROSEBURY T. (1947) *Experimental Air-borne Infection: Section III.* Baltimore, The Williams & Wilkins Co.

SCHRENK H.H. (1937) *U.S. Bureau Mines I.C.* 7086.

SILVERMAN L. & BILLINGS C.E. (1959) *J. Air Pollut. Control Ass.* **6,** 76.

WILSON H.B., SYLVESTER G.E., LASKIN S. & LABELLE C.W. (1953) Pharmacology and Toxicology of Uranium Compounds VI-1, eds. VOEGTLIN C. & HODGE H.C., p. 1700. New York, McGraw Hill Book Co. Inc.

WRIGHT B.M. (1950) *J. sci. Instr.* **27,** 12.

WRIGHT B.M. (1957) *Br. J. industr. Med.* **14,** 219.

CHAPTER 10

Methods of Detecting Drug Interaction

M.W. PARKES

THE IMPORTANCE OF DRUG INTERACTIONS

The safety of a drug depends upon two properties: its therapeutic efficacy and its toxicity. Their relationship determines how well the therapeutically effective doses used in practice will be tolerated. Each of the determining factors may be altered by different circumstances, the age and clinical condition of the patient, his diet, habits, and any other drug taken during treatment, with consequent effects on the safety of the drug. It is with the last of these that we are concerned here, for if the effectiveness of one drug is diminished, or its toxicity enhanced, in the presence of another then its safety is thereby reduced. Numerous instances that are known of drug interactions may be found in several recent reviews (Cohen, 1965; McIver, 1965; Hussar, 1967).

We may recognize three ways in which such interactions can affect safety. One drug may increase the effectiveness of another, by exerting a similar action concurrently or by one of several other means of potentiation and, by so doing, render an otherwise tolerated level of dosage harmful. This is particularly important when the therapeutic effect of a treatment itself can endanger life when exerted beyond the required level. Examples of this are the cardio-active glycosides and the anticoagulants, where the safe therapeutic dose, once found for the individual patient, should not be exceeded.

Alternatively, one drug may reduce the effectiveness of another, by direct antagonism of its action or otherwise, resulting in a lower intensity or shorter duration of effect. If this results in an inadequate therapeutic effect of the dose used in a treatment essential for life, as for example by anticoagulants, antibiotics or cardioactive glycosides, then the patient may be endangered. Lastly, although the processes involved here may not really differ from those just mentioned in the previous classes, one drug may alter the action of another by enhancing a previously sub-threshold side effect and thus allow unwanted consequences to appear, which may result in hazard. Many examples of synergism are given in a review by Veldstra (1956).

It will be clear, on reflection, that where interactions may occur between a drug intended for treatment and any others taken during that treatment, it will contribute to the safety with which the drug is used if the nature and extent of these interactions are known.

THE SCOPE OF INVESTIGATIONS

It also becomes immediately apparent that an investigation cannot be undertaken of the interactions between a proposed drug and all others which may conceivably be taken by a patient under treatment. These could comprise all listed drugs and proprietary products, besides many constituents of food and drink, some of which have been shown to interact dangerously with prescribed drugs.

Informed common sense has to be applied here and this directs that two principal practical approaches be made to the problem.

1 For any proposed drug, it should be possible to list those drugs which are likely to be administered additionally to the patient during treatment, either as part of that treatment or for other reasons, or which the patient may take of his own volition, and with which interaction could have serious consequences. The drugs prescribed concurrently will depend upon the condition; for instance, cardio-active glycosides and anticoagulants with drugs used in cardio-vascular disorders; anaesthetics for conditions which may involve surgical intervention. The list will also include barbiturates and other central depressants, given to or taken by the patient to aid sleep and should also include alcohol unless it can be certain that the drug is only to be used by patients in hospital.

It has to be recognized that this policy entails the possibility of an unforeseen interaction arising, particularly with agents not prescribed medically, as occurred recently with monoamine oxidase inhibitors and certain foodstuffs (see refs. in Natoff, 1964). Contrary to what has been implied in some quarters (Laurence, 1964; Macgregor, 1965), it is not reasonable to expect that investigations should have been made, before the incidents which drew attention to the matter, of interactions between these drugs and constituents later found to be present in the implicated foodstuffs, certain cheeses, broad beans, and a yeast product.

2   Such possibilities may be anticipated, however, by examining the drug for properties which are known to be generally responsible for interactions between drugs. Many such properties are now recognized, from comparatively recent studies of the mechanism of drug action, a field which is still vigorously developing. They include actions influencing the absorption, distribution, metabolism, and excretion of other drugs. Of these the most important concern protein binding, the inhibition and stimulation of enzyme activity and effects on renal function; other effects which may be important are those on gastro-intestinal absorption, or that from a parenteral site, or upon mechanism for transport across tissue membranes (for reviews, see Brodie, 1964a, b; Binns, 1964; Schanker, 1964; Cohen, 1965).

Again, however, the extent to which it may be necessary to examine a proposed drug for these properties must be judged according to its intended use, and account taken of the anticipated frequency and duration of dosing and the circumstances in which it is to be used. It will be clear, for example, that there will be relatively few possibilities that a drug, used on a single occasion in the course of surgical anaesthesia, may affect adversely the actions of others concerned in concurrent treatment of the patient, though the alternative possibility, that other drugs may interact to the detriment of a drug used in anaethesia, ought to be examined. At the other end of the scale, a drug intended for prolonged treatment, possibly prophylactic, of relatively healthy, ambulant patients will have maximum opportunity for interaction with others and its relevant properties ought certainly to be investigated.

These two approaches to investigating drug interactions are also recommended by the Association of Food & Drug Officials of the US (Goldenthal, 1959).

PRINCIPLES OF INVESTIGATION

1 Specific Interactions

The general principle of investigating interactions will direct that a definitive action of one of the drugs, which can readily be measured quantitatively, be evaluated in the presence and absence of the other drug. The conditions under which such investigations must be made impose certain limitations. They must usually be made in laboratory animals, for instance, and it will hardly be necessary here to emphasize that the degree of interaction observed in the test species may not be that which will occur in man. It can, however, indicate where caution may have to be exercised and the predictive value of such observations can be increased by support from general investigations of mechanisms, described below, where these can be shown to apply to man as well as the laboratory species.

Then again, it will be feasible to examine only certain doses and frequency of repetition of one drug, and intervals between doses of the two drugs, in determining the effect of one drug upon the other. In such situations, where the most informative conditions must be judged according to the case concerned, recommendations are a poor substitute for experience. A great deal of work has been done by Loewe and others in determining the activity of a drug over a range of doses and proportion of admixture with another, or even two others (Loewe, 1955a, b, 1957, 1958; Chen, 1957). The complexities of the relationships revealed have theoretical interest but little bearing on our present purposes.

It is necessary, however, that the examination be made on a quantitative basis, so that comparisons are valid. The effect selected as appropriate for assessing the activity of the drug, on which the interaction of another is to be tested, could be mortality or reaction time or duration of sedation, to give only a few examples. The variability of such effects between animals entails, not only that sufficient numbers of animals be used to enable representative assessments to be obtained, as is well recognized, but that estimates of the variance also be available so that the activity of the one drug in the presence of the other may be validly compared with that in its absence. Although a pilot-scale experiment might reveal a very marked interaction, one that is less well marked might still be of significance, though it might not be detected using small groups. It is salutary to refer to Trevan's (1927) figures to see the difference in proportions of small groups that the incidence of an effect must represent before a real difference in activity can be deduced with certainty. Adequate numbers will also be necessary to prove the absence of interaction, which can be equally important information for a proposed drug.

For similar reasons, it is rarely adequate to give a single active dose of a drug and compare its effects with those after it is given to animals pre-treated with a second drug; still less, of course, to observe only the effects of the combination, comparing this with previous records of the effects of the first drug alone, no matter how extensive. Preferably, a comparative test should be set up, according to well-established principles for biological assay, comprising sufficient doses of one drug in the presence and absence of the other to enable dose-response curves, or a parameter derivative from such curves, to be obtained from each situation, from which a statistical estimate of probability can be attached to any difference, or lack of difference; this could take the form of a potency ratio with confidence limits to the required probability level (Emmens, 1948; Rümke & de Jonge, 1964).

Drugs causing the same effects may be expected to act additively, but frequently an enhanced effect of a drug may be observed when it is given together with another that causes only a generally similar effect, e.g. the action of various central depressants in potentiating the hypnotic action of barbiturates or alcohol. True potentiation, as distinguished from addition, always indicates that the two drugs act differently, the action of one amplifying that of the other (Veldstra, 1956), and examples of mechanisms responsible for such effects are to be found in a later section. Although the distinction between addition and potentiation (or synergism) is theoretically interesting it is often difficult to establish and it is of practical importance only if knowledge of the mechanism of synergism permits prediction of further interactions.

Antagonism of one drug by another also occurs, sometimes by direct competition for the sites of action, but also by other mechanisms, some of which are dealt with in a later section. Drugs exerting pharmacologically opposite effects may also be expected to antagonize each other and physicians are familiar with such principles as that of centrally stimulant drugs counteracting the effects of central depressants. Where a new drug is concerned, however, it should not be assumed that a simple algebra applies and a predicted interaction should always be tested, a watch being kept for the unexpected emergence of distinct effects of the combination. The interesting effects of combining amphetamine and barbiturates make an instructive example here (Steinberg *et al.*, 1961; Legge & Steinberg, 1962; Rushton & Steinberg, 1963a, b); the combination has unexpected properties that make it clinically useful and also liable to misuse to the point of constituting a social problem.

METHODS

Because, as stated earlier, the interactions to be investigated must be selected according to the uses intended for any proposed drug, it is not possible to outline here all the procedures that might, at any time, become necessary. Descriptions will be limited to some that may be particularly likely or important, and which serve to illustrate the principles involved.

Barbiturates, alcohol, and other hypnotics

The examination of drugs for effects on the activity of hypnotics is a familiar procedure in pharmacological laboratories (Winter, 1948; Holten & Larsen, 1956). Mice, or more rarely rats, are employed; the animals are pre-treated with an appropriate dose of the test drug followed, after a suitable interval for absorption, by challenge doses of the hypnotic to be examined. This may be a barbiturate such as pentobarbital or hexobarbital, given by intravenous or intraperitoneal injection, or ethyl alcohol in 20% aqueous solution, injected intraperitoneally. If potentiation is expected, the doses chosen include one which puts the animals to sleep for a moderate time and another which is a submultiple of this. The test drug may be given by intraperitoneal, subcutaneous, or oral routes and corresponding groups of unpre-treated animals are also given the challenge doses of hypnotic. Sleeping time may be recorded as the interval between the instant when the animal first remains on its back and that when it refuses to remain in that posture although returned to it. Sufficient numbers of animals should be used for each dose of hypnotic to provide data for the construction of dose-response relations for test and control groups, capable of ascertaining the probability that any difference observed is a real one (see p. 283). Should it be possible to arrange that the examination is carried out on a sequential basis, this may ensure that only sufficient animals are used to establish with confidence any difference that exists.

Central depressants may potentiate the action of hypnotics by direct action, depressing the central nervous system so that it is more susceptible to the further depression caused by the hypnotic; or by an indirect action, if they happen to inhibit, or to compete as substrate for, an enzyme system which inactivates the hypnotic, and limits its duration of action. Such effects may well occur in species other than that in which they are experimentally established. In mice, however, and to a lesser extent in rats, many agents including central depressants may also impair the already barely adequate mechanism for body temperature regulation, so that in the temperatures prevailing on most laboratory benches, the body temperature of the animal falls (Lessin & Parkes, 1957a). At the lower body temperature, enzymic inactivation of the hypnotic will be reduced and the duration of hypnotic action prolonged (Fuhrman, 1947). This consequence of the action of the drug will not necessarily occur in other species whose body temperatures are not so drastically affected and it may be necessary to establish that any potentiation of a hypnotic observed in small rodents is not due to this cause. For this purpose, the procedure described above should be performed at an ambient temperature in which body temperature cannot fall significantly, the animals being kept in a warm cupboard, or the work being carried out in a small room, kept at 32°C. Larger doses of the hypnotic may be necessary than at room temperature, as under these conditions it will not hinder its own enzymic inactivation by causing hypothermia as it does at lower temperatures, so that this experiment, too, must include its own control groups.

Cardioactive glycosides
Examination of a proposed drug for alteration of the action of cardioactive agents involves estimation of the effects of the drug on the potency of a suitable glycoside, such as digitoxin or ouabain. Of the methods recommended for determination of the potency of such agents (see Holland & Briggs, 1964; Dipalma, 1964) only those involving the use of intact mammals can really be regarded as relevant for the purpose. Others, though quite reliable for assessment of the potency of the cardioactive agents, are unlikely

to inspire confidence as reflecting a relevant contribution of the proposed drug to the interaction; this applies to the assay methods using frogs or pigeons and even more to those using isolated hearts or strips of heart muscle.

The procedure will entail establishing the dose of glycoside which just stops the heart when injected intravenously in anaesthetized cats, or possibly guinea-pigs, with or without pretreatment with the drug under trial. Since only one value can be obtained from each animal, and since sufficient values will be necessary to allow valid comparisons of the activity in each group, it is clear that such examinations will involve considerable effort and expenditure. As indicated above, they will be necessary, particularly for those drugs intended for cardiovascular indications, but in only a proportion of others.

Anticoagulants
The activity of anticoagulants of the coumarin type may be affected by a variety of other drugs in a number of ways, depending on properties that are discussed below; including interactions due to binding with plasma proteins (p. 288) or alterations of the rate of enzymic inactivation (pp. 291 *et seq.*). In view of the potential importance of any effects on anticoagulant activity exerted by drugs that could be given concurrently, it might be advisable to examine a proposed drug specifically for this possible interaction.

The anticoagulants now in use interfere with the extrinsic clotting system and may be detected by the one-stage prothrombin test (Biggs & Macfarlane, 1962). The effect of a given dose of anticoagulant, say warfarin, upon the coagulability of rabbit blood may be assessed with sufficient sensitivity to detect any alteration of this by concurrent treatment with the drug under investigation if the test is performed on serially diluted samples of plasma.

Rabbits, preferably male, are injected intravenously with a suitable dose of anticoagulant and samples of blood withdrawn after an interval. Anticoagulant activity is determined so as to obtain serial dilution—prothrombin time curves and a sufficient number of animals used to provide a reasonable estimate of the curve for that dose of anticoagulant. Further groups of rabbits, pre-treated with the drug under investigation and given the same dose of anticoagulant after a suitable interval, are used to make similar determinations to establish if anticoagulant activity has been altered by the pre-treatment. It may be necessary to investigate the effect of a course of repeated dosage with the test drug as well as that of a single dose. Alternatively, the same animals that were used for the baseline determination may be used, after an interval of not less than one week, to determine the effect of the test drug, each animal then acting as its own control. In this case, it would be advisable to establish that such successive dosage with anticoagulant in the absence of the test drug, gives similar values for prothrombin time.

2 Properties of Drugs Responsible for Interactions

Even though it is not possible to examine all the specific interactions that could occur, it may be possible, as stated earlier (p. 281), to predict interactions from certain properties of the proposed drug, once these are known. The principal mechanisms responsible for interactions between drugs may be broadly classified as follows (Macgregor, 1965):

Physical or chemical interactions, e.g. between heparin and protamine.

Pharmacological interactions: Competition for active receptor sites, resulting in antagonism, e.g. atropine and methacoline.

Competition for inactive and storage receptor sites, resulting in potentiation, e.g. imipramine and noradrenaline.

Action on receptor sites for different systems resulting in physiological interactions, e.g. choline esters and sympathomimetic amines.

Biochemical interactions. Alteration by one drug of the absorption of another, e.g. by alteration of gastric pH.

Competition for non-specific binding with protein, e.g. sulphonamides and hypoglycaemic agents, phenylbutazone, and anticoagulants.

Competition for non-specific binding with protein, e.g. sulphona-gastro-intestinal absorption, passage from plasma into tissues and absorption or excretion at the renal tubules, e.g. effect of probenecid on penicillin excretion.

Alteration by one drug of the metabolism of another: by competition for metabolizing enzymes for which both drugs are substrates; by inhibition of metabolizing enzymes, e.g. by monoamine oxidase inhibitors; by facilitation or induction of metabolizing enzyme activity, e.g. phenylbutazone, barbiturates.

Alteration by one drug of the renal excretion of another, e.g. by altering urinary pH.

Pharmacological interactions may be predictable from the properties established by the appropriate studies which have supported the proposal of the drug for trial, in the light of the knowledge of the properties of other drugs which may also be taken by the patient. It is now gradually becoming realized that biochemical investigation of a proposed drug is an equally proper accompaniment of pharmacological and toxicological studies, in its preparation for clinical examination (Paget, 1963; Hennessey, 1964). Indeed, it may be held that the validity of pharmacological and toxicological findings in animals for the utility and safety of a drug in man depends on interpretation in the light of information on its absorption, metabolism, and excretion in both man and the animal species (Scholz, 1963; Duncan, 1963; Brodie, 1964a; Williams, 1964).

In the course of these biochemical studies, and also in association with prolonged toxicity examinations, certain properties of the drug should be established, many of which may lead to prediction of possible interaction with other drugs. Such interactions may then be directly investigated if they are considered potentially important, but the knowledge of the relevant properties is particularly valuable as a basis for general predictions.

ABSORPTION

Studies of effects upon gastrointestinal absorption are perhaps not particularly likely to yield results of predictive value. The recommendations of the Association of Food and Drug Officials of the US (Goldenthal, 1959), include, among those pertaining to interactions between drugs, that examination should be made of the effects of a proposed drug upon the absorption of essential minerals and vitamins from the gastrointestinal tract. Such effects could, in the opinion of the author, most readily be suspected from observations of growth and other findings of prolonged toxicity studies.

PLASMA PROTEIN BINDING

Many drugs are bound by proteins in body fluids and circulate in this form, in equilibrium with a certain fraction in the unbound state. Only the latter is able to exert activity or to be metabolized or excreted and as this active form is removed from circulation it is replaced by release of the bound form in accord with the equilibrium requirements (Goldstein, 1949; Thorp, 1964; Brodie, 1965). A drug which binds to protein will thus compete with others which bind to the same sites, to an extent determined by their amounts and binding affinities. The effects of such a drug may thus be different in the presence of other protein-bound drugs than when it acts alone. Displacement from binding will increase the intensity of action of a drug and shorten its duration. Protein-binding plays a significant part in the distribution of sulphonamides, anticoagulants, salicylates, phenylbutazone, tolbutamide, and many other drugs. The level of some of these required for clinical effect are sufficiently critical that their disturbance by another drug which can displace them from plasma proteins can seriously affect their safety.

Examples of this are provided by the anticoagulants, the effectiveness of which may be increased by many other drugs that bind with protein, including clofibrate (Oliver *et al.*, 1963) and phenylbutazone (Aggeler *et al.*, 1967). Phenylbutazone, in the same way, also affects the clinical activity of tolbutamide (Christensen *et al.*, 1963) and sulphonamide (Anton, 1960, 1961).

Studies of absorption of the proposed drug and the resulting plasma levels reached will be rendered more realistic if the degree of binding to plasma proteins is also determined. If, in addition, an estimate can be made of even the order of the affinity constant for this binding, predictions may be made of the other drugs which the proposed drug might be expected to displace from protein (and thus possibly intensify and/or shorten their action) and which other drugs, in turn, might displace it.

It is not certain, however, that determinations of plasma binding will always yield results capable of ready interpretation in this way, since the determinant factors are variable. The binding of a drug to plasma protein depends upon the affinity of the interaction, the concentration of the drug in the plasma and the temperature. The plasma of different species will not behave alike in this respect, and so human plasma must be used. Drugs may bind differently to the various binding sites in plasma proteins and so a drug which is extensively bound in plasma as a whole may not necessarily displace another which may interact with a different grouping in the proteins.

METHODS

Goldstein (1949) lists 14 means by which the extent of binding of a drug to plasma proteins may be estimated, not all quantitatively satisfactory. The favoured methods employ dialysis or ultra-filtration of plasma in equilibrium with known drug concentrations, and depend upon separating the aqueous phase containing unbound drug in solution from the protein fraction. Estimation of the unbound drug concentration will yield by difference the fraction bound. Dialysis can introduce some errors due to dilution of the protein phase and also to the Donnan effect with ionized drugs. Although ultrafiltration, on the other hand, concentrates the protein phase, the consequent errors are slight. Moreover, it is very rapid and convenient.

Human plasma, to which is added various concentrations of drug, is placed in a semipermeable bag in an apparatus such as that described by Keen (1965), in which it is maintained at body temperature, and a pressure applied. Estimations are made of the drug content of the ultrafiltrate, from which the proportion bound may be calculated. Formulae derived from the kinetics of binding (Goldstein, 1949; Thorp, 1964) permit the further calculation of an affinity constant for the interaction. Several factors affect the validity of this calculation, as mentioned above. If the binding involves more than one plasma protein, the relation of binding to concentration may not be sufficiently linear to justify the assumptions underlying the formula. For this reason, the concentrations employed should be within the limits likely to occur in plasma during therapy.

From the values obtained it may be possible to deduce likely interactions with other drugs known to be bound to plasma proteins and which might be of importance, such as sulphonamides, salicylates, phenylbutazone, tolbutamide, and anticoagulants. In the present state of knowledge, it would be wise to confirm predicted displacements experimentally, using a similar method to that just described, in which a second drug is added to plasma equilibrated with the first, the degree of displacement being derived from estimation of the amount of the first drug appearing in the ultrafiltrate.

Renal function

Among the data recorded on the urinary excretion of the proposed drug, any marked change in urinary pH may indicate that it could alter the excretion of weak electrolytes. Studies of its effects upon renal function should include those upon the excretion of phenol red or *p*-aminohippuric acid and *N'*-methylnicotinamide, which can indicate the ability of the drug to interfere with the renal tubular secretion of organic acids and strong organic bases, respectively (Beyer, 1950; Sperber, 1959; Peters, 1960).

From this information, the possibility that the proposed drug may alter the excretion of others may be evaluated.

Interactions of the drug with enzymes

(a) *As substrate.* Certain readily conducted enzyme studies can give results of considerable predictive value. If a drug is normally metabolized to a less active and more readily execreted form by a particular enzyme system, then another drug which inhibits that system will increase or prolong the action of the first. Enzymes notably involved in drug metabolism include some situated in the liver microsomes, such as glucuronidase and the system known as non-specific oxidase. The question whether a drug is itself a substrate for these enzymes may be answered biochemically, using enzyme preparations *in vitro*, or pharmacologically. Treatment of animals with known inhibitors of these enzymes may permit the activity or acute toxicity of the drug to be compared in such animals with that in untreated controls. If the drug is inactivated by the enzyme system, then the inhibition of this will result in potentiation of the activity of the drug.

It is quite possible for an enzyme inhibitor to affect more than one enzyme system; it is therefore necessary to choose carefully the inhibitors to be used in such investigations. The classification of several psychotropic drugs, many of them chemically related in being organic acid hydrazides, as monoamine oxidase inhibitors on account of their common action on this enzyme, has prevented general appreciation of the possibility that all their effects may not be due to this particular action (Pletscher *et al.*, 1960). It is, for example, the cause of their producing hypertensive crises in patients who have consumed certain foods containing pressor amines or their precursors, while being treated with these drugs. Once the presence of these amines in such foods was realized, the interaction could be predicted for all drugs which inhibited monoamine oxidase. This is not, however, the reason for the potentiation of pethidine which has been reported for some of these drugs (Sjöqvist, 1965). Pethidine is deaminated by the liver microsomal non-specific oxidase system (Brodie, 1956), which is inhibited by iproniazid (Fouts & Brodie, 1956) and other hydrazides derived from aromatic acids (Lessin & Long, unpublished). Some, such as isocarboxazid, although equal, or more potent, inhibitors of mono-amine oxidase, inhibit non-specific oxidase less strongly and do not interact with pethidine (Parkes, unpublished). The prediction that all monoamine oxidase inhibitors may interact with pethidine would thus be fallacious. Those members which do potentiate pethidine, however, also potentiate barbiturates, for the same reason (Pletscher *et al.*, 1960; Laroche & Brodie, 1960).

The finding that the effects of a proposed drug were potentiated after treatment with an inhibitor of monoamine oxidase would not necessarily mean, therefore, that the drug is metabolized by this enzyme, unless isocarboxazid or a similar unequivocal inhibitor had been used. The possibility is certainly worth examining; and even more so, that of whether its effects are potentiated by in-hibition of the liver microsomal enzyme system, for which the in-hibitor proadifen, SKF 525A, or one of its analogues, should be used.

Should enzyme inhibition potentiate the effects of the drug, in-teractions may be predicted with inhibitors or other drugs which may compete with it as substrates. There is also the possibility, in such a case, that the activity of the drug may be lessened by ad-ministration of drugs which can stimulate enzyme activity (see below).

METHODS

A suitable effect of the proposed drug in mice or rats, such as the acute toxicity, may be determined in animals 1 hour after treat-ment with a suitable enzyme inhibitor, such as proadifen, 25 mg/kg intraperitoneally, for the drug-metabolizing enzyme systems of liver microsomes or isocarboxazid, 50 or 100 mg/kg orally for monoamine oxidase. A significant increase in the potency of the drug in the treated animals compared with controls suggests that other drugs interacting with the enzyme concerned may enhance activity of the proposed drug. Alternatively, the decline in plasma levels of the drug may be followed if a suitable method of estimation is available, as inhibition of an enzyme metabolizing the drug will cause a delay in this decline.

Conversely, estimation of the activity or plasma levels of the drug in animals treated overnight with agents known to increase non-specific oxidase activity (see below), preferably a barbiturate such as pentobarbital, 50 mg/kg intraperitoneally, can give confirmation, since a significant decrease in activity or more rapid decline in levels now indicates enzymic inactivation.

(b) *As inhibitor.* A proposed drug may, alternatively, inhibit the drug-metabolizing enzyme system, and so alter the effectiveness of other drugs normally metabolized by the enzyme. These include commonly used drugs such as the barbiturates, phenacetin, aminopyrine, phenylbutazone, pethidine, chlorpromazine, codeine, and imipramine (Brodie, 1956, 1964a). Inhibition of metabolizing enzymes by a proposed drug may be detected by its effect on the activity or plasma levels of suitable substrates. These include barbiturates, the activity of which may be measured by the duration of hypnosis they produce in mice (Cook *et al.*, 1954); chlorpromazine, measured by its hypothermic activity in mice (Lessin & Parkes, 1957b); and Schradan (octamethylpyrophosphoramide, OMPA), measured by its toxicity (Davison, 1955; Lessin, 1959a). This last is a very suitable complement for one of the others, since the enzyme converts this non-toxic compound to a toxic one so that inhibition of the enzyme decreases its toxicity, while the other two examples are inactivated by the enzyme so that inhibition potentiates their effectiveness. A necessary precaution in all these cases is to ascertain that the body temperature of the animals used, usually mice or rats, is not lowered by the drug, since the activity of the enzyme is thereby reduced, giving an effect of apparent inhibition (Lessin, 1959a). Should the drug cause hypothermia, this should be prevented by keeping the animals at 32°C when chlorpromazine obviously becomes an unsuitable choice as test substrate.

METHODS

A proposed drug is not very likely to be found to inhibit monoamine oxidase unexpectedly. If an effect is suspected from observations of interference with the oxidation of a suitable substrate by a preparation of the enzyme, *in vitro*, its relevance should be checked by determining the effect of pretreatment with the drug upon the stimulant action of 5-hydroxytryptophan in mice (Lessin, 1959b; Corne *et al.*, 1963), or tryptamine in rats (Tedeschi *et al.*, 1962).

To test for an inhibitory action on drug-metabolizing systems, the hypnotic activity of a barbiturate, such as pentobarbital or hexobarbital, may be determined, as described on p. 284, in mice pretreated with the proposed drug, in comparison with mice not so pretreated, preferably in an ambient temperature of 32°C. Alternatively, the rectal temperatures of mice may be followed as a measure of the effect of chlorpromazine, 2·5 mg/kg intraperitoneally, with and without pretreatment; this must, of course, be undertaken at ordinary room temperature and is only suitable if the proposed drug itself does not lower the rectal temperature of mice at the doses to be used. In both these methods, significant increases in activity can denote inhibition of drug-metabolizing enzymes.

The acute toxicity of Schradan (OMPA) in mice or guinea-pigs is readily measured for this purpose by means of the time elapsing between the injection of each animal with 50 mg/kg intraperitoneally and its death. Mean survival times may be compared for pretreated and control groups; here, a significant decrease in toxicity of Schradan indicates enzyme inhibition, which confirms evidence from the potentiation of barbiturate or chlorpromazine (Lessin, 1959a).

(c) *As inducer of enzyme activity.* Many drugs show the converse effect, that of inducing drug-metabolizing enzyme activity, and thus reduce or shorten the action of others which are substrates for this enzyme (Fouts, 1965; Burns & Conney, 1965). Drugs causing this effect are, or are closely related to, substrates for liver microsomal enzymes (Conney, 1965). They include many barbiturates, including barbital, which is not itself metabolized by the enzyme, chlorpromazine, imipramine, and phenylbutazone, together with other agents such as chlorinated insecticides. This mechanism of increasing drug-metabolizing activity has been shown to be responsible for clinical interactions; for example, the decreased anticoagulant effectiveness, by accelerated inactivation, of warfarin during treatment with phenobarbitone (Robinson & Macdonald, 1966) or chloral hydrate (Cucinell *et al.*, 1966). A single dose of such drugs in animals may, after a suitable interval for development, show marked reduction of the activity of other drugs. If a proposed drug were found to cause this effect, it would be proper to predict the possibility of its decreasing the effectiveness of other drugs, concurrently or subsequently taken, that are metabolized by the enzyme concerned. If the proposed drug is itself so metabolized, then the possibility of developing a degree of tolerance may be predicted.

As described in the previous section, an elegant demonstration of the induction of metabolizing enzyme activity by a proposed drug may be obtained by determining the activity of a barbiturate or chlorpromazine in mice, and the toxicity of Schradan in mice or guinea-pigs, treated 24 hours earlier with the drug, in comparison with untreated animals. Induction of non-specific oxidase activity will result in reduced activity of barbiturates and chlorpromazine but increased toxicity of Schradan (Lessin, 1960).

Caution has to be exercised in interpreting the results of such investigations, however, as many anomalies are known. Drugs which are found to be affected similarly by the inhibition or stimulation of enzyme activity in one species can be affected differently by the same treatment in another. Four tests listed for detection of accelerated drug metabolism by Burns *et al.* (1963) are: Sleeping time and rate of metabolism of hexobarbital in rats and dogs; increased urinary excretion of ascorbic acid in rats; excretion of a demethylated metabolite of Novalgin in man; and rate of metabolism of phenylbutazone in dogs. Yet chlorpromazine is without effect on phenylbutazone metabolism in the dog (Burns *et al.*, 1965), although it stimulates the metabolism of barbiturates in rodents (Kato & Chiesara, 1962). Similar differences exist between the interactions of phenylbutazone or tolbutamide with the drug-metabolizing enzyme systems in the dog and man (Remmer & Merker, 1965; Burns *et al.*, 1965).

METHODS

The methods described for detection of an action of the proposed drug in inhibiting liver microsomal metabolizing activity in rodents may also be employed to detect an effect in inducing this enzyme activity. For this purpose, the hypnotic activity of a suitable barbiturate or the acute toxicity of Schradan may be determined in animals pretreated overnight with the proposed drug. Any acute effect of the drug is likely to have disappeared within 16–24 hours leaving only any increased enzyme activity that may have been induced. Repeated daily dosage with the drug for several days before challenge will favour detection of a weak effect, though it will then have to be considered how important this is likely to be.

A suitable challenge dose of barbiturate or Schradan may not be the same as that for detecting enzyme inhibition. Since induced enzyme activity will be shown by a reduced activity of barbiturate, but an increased toxicity of Schradan, larger doses will be needed of the former and smaller doses of the latter.

Because of the species variation found for this activity it will be advisable to use tests on several species. Barbiturate sleeping time may be used in mice or rats, Schradan toxicity in guinea-pigs. The same effect may be sought in dogs, using the rate of disappearance from the blood of administered phenylbutazone (Burns *et al.*, 1963). This may be followed by taking repeated blood samples 7 hours after giving 25 mg/kg phenylbutazone intraperitoneally and estimating the plasma level of this drug chemically (Werner & Wünker, 1959). Prior treatment of the dogs with the proposed drug, daily for 1 month or more, markedly lowers the plasma level found 7 hours after phenylbutazone. Few compounds interfere with the estimation of phenylbutazone, but it is advisable to use as blank a blood sample taken before its administration in order to check this for the drug under test.

REFERENCES

AGGELER P.M., O'REILLY R.A., LEONG L. & KOWITZ P.E. (1967) Potentiation of anticoagulant effect of warfarin by phenylbutazone. *New Engl. J. Med.* **276**, 496–501.

ANTON A.H. (1960) The relation between the binding of sulfonamides to albumin and their antibacterial effect. *J. Pharmac.* **129**, 282–90.

ANTON A.H. (1961) A drug-induced change in the distribution and renal excretion of sulfonamides. *J. Pharmac.* **134**, 291–303.

BEYER K.H. (1950) Functional characteristics of renal transport mechanisms. *Pharmac. Rev.* **2**, 227–80.

BIGGS R. & MACFARLANE R.G. (1962) *Human Blood Coagulation and its Disorders*, 3rd edition. Oxford, Blackwell Scientific Publications.

BINNS T.B. (1964) (ed.) *Absorption and Distribution of Drugs*. London, Livingstone.

BRODIE B.B. (1956) Pathways of drug metabolism. *J. Pharm. Pharmac.* **8**, 1–17.

BRODIE B.B. (1964a) Distribution and fate of drugs; therapeutic implications, in *Absorption and Distribution of Drugs,* ed. BINNS T.B., 199–251. London, Livingstone.

BRODIE B.B. (1964b) Kinetics of absorption, distribution, excretion and metabolism of drugs, in *Animal and Clinical Pharmacologic Techniques in Drug Evaluation,* eds. NODINE J.H. & SIEGLER P.E., pp. 69–88. Chicago, Year Book Medical Publishers.

BRODIE B.B. (1965) Displacement of one drug by another from carrier or receptor sites. *Proc. roy. Soc. Med.* **58,** 946–55.

BURNS J.J., CONNEY A.H. & KOSTER R. (1963) Stimulatory effect of chronic drug administration on drug-metabolizing enzymes in liver microsomes. *Ann. N.Y. Acad. Sci.* **104,** 881–93.

BURNS J.J. & CONNEY A.H. (1965) Enzyme stimulation and inhibition in the metabolism of drugs. *Proc. roy. Soc. Med.* **58,** 955–60.

BURNS J.J., CUCINELL S.A., KOSTER R. & CONNEY A.H. (1965) Application of drug metabolism to drug toxicity studies. *Ann. N.Y. Acad. Sci.* **123,** 273–86.

CHEN G. (1957) A graphical method for studying the joint action of three substances. *Arch. int. pharmacodyn.* **111,** 322–33.

CHRISTENSEN L.K., HANSEN J.M. & KRISTENSEN M. (1963) Sulphaphenazole-induced hypoglycaemic attacks in tolbutamide-treated diabetics. *Lancet* **ii.** 1298–1301.

COHEN LD. (Symposium chairman) (1965) Clinical effects of interactions between drugs. *Proc. roy. Soc. Med.* **58,** 943–98.

CONNEY A.H. (1965) *Enzyme induction and drug toxicity,* in *Drugs and Enzymes,* eds. BRODIE B.B. & GILLETTE J.R.. pp. 277–97. London, Pergamon.

COOK L., TONER J.J. & FELLOWS E.J. (1954) The effect of β-diethylamino-ethyldiphenylpropyl-acetate hydrochloride (SKF No. 525A) on hexobarbital. *J. Pharmac.* **111,** 131–41.

CORNE S.J., PICKERING R.W. & WARNER B.T. (1963) A method for assessing the effects of drugs on the central actions of 5-hydroxytryptamine. *Br. J. Pharmac.* **20,** 106–20.

CUCINELL S.A., ODESSKY L., WEISS M. & DAYTON P.G. (1966). The effect of chloral hydrate on bishydroxycoumarin metabolism. *J. Am. med. Ass.* **197,** 366–8.

DAVISON A.N. (1955) The conversion of Schradan (OMPA) and parathion into inhibitors of cholinesterase by mammalian liver. *Biochem. J.* **61,** 203–9.

DIPALMA J.R. (1964) Animal techniques for evaluating digitalis and its derivatives, in *Animal and Clinical Pharmacologic Techniques in Drug Evaluation,* eds. NODINE J.H. & SIEGLER P.E., pp. 154–9. Chicago, Year Book Medical Publishers.

DUNCAN W.A.M. (1963) The importance of metabolism studies in relation to drug toxicity. 2. A general review. *Proc. Eur. Soc. Study Drug Toxicity* **2,** 67–77.

EMMENS C.W. (1948) *Principles of Biological Assay*. London, Chapman & Hall.

FOUTS J.R. (1965) Impairment of drug metabolism in drug toxicity. *Drugs and Enzymes*, eds. BRODIE B.B. & GILLETTE J.R., pp. 261–76. London. Pergamon.

FOUTS J.R. & BRODIE B.B. (1956) On the mechanism of drug potentiation by iproniazid. *J. Pharmac.* **116**, 480–5.

FUHRMAN F.A. (1947) The effect of body temperature on the duration of barbiturate anaesthesia in mice. *Science* **105**, 387–8.

GOLDENTHAL E.I. (ed.) (1959) *Appraisal of the Safety of Chemicals in Foods, Drugs and Cosmetics*, p. 62. Baltimore, Association of Food & Drug Officials of the U.S.

GOLDSTEIN A. (1949) The interactions of drugs and plasma proteins. *Pharmac. Rev.* **1**, 102–65.

HENNESSEY R.S.F. (Chairman) (1964) *First Report of the Expert Committee on Drug Toxicity*. London, Association of the British Pharmaceutical Industry.

HOLLAND W.C. & BRIGGS A.H. (1964) Cardioactive Agents, in *Evaluation of Drug Activities. Pharmacometrics*, eds. LAURENCE D.R. & BACHARACH A.L., Vol. 2, 601–13. London, Academic Press.

HOLTEN C.H. & LARSEN V. (1956) The potentiating effect of benactyzine derivatives and some other compounds on evipal anaesthesia in mice. *Acta pharmac. tox.* **12**, 346–63.

HUSSAR D.A. (1967) Therapeutic incompatibilities: drug interactions. *Am. J. Pharm.* 215–33.

KATO R. & CHIESARA E. (1962) Increase of pentobarbitone metabolism induced in rats pretreated with some centrally acting compounds. *Br. J. Pharmac.* **18**, 29–38.

KEEN P.M. (1965) The binding of three penicillins in the plasma of several mammalian species as studied by ultrafiltration at body temperature. *Br. J. Pharmac.* **25**, 507–14.

LAROCHE M.J. & BRODIE B.B. (1960) Lack of relationship between inhibition of monoamine oxidase and potentiation of hexobarbital hypnosis. *J. Pharmac.* **130**, 134–7.

LAURENCE D.R. (1964) Problems of predicting unwanted clinical drug interactions. *Proc. Eur. Soc. Study Drug Toxicity* **4**, 145–52.

LEGGE D. & STEINBERG H. (1962) Actions of a mixture of amphetamine and a barbiturate in man. *Br. J. Pharmac.* **18**, 490–500.

LESSIN A.W. (1959a) Pharmacological methods of estimating inhibition of drug oxidation in the mouse. *Br. J. Pharmac.* **14**, 251–5.

LESSIN A.W. (1959b) The pharmacological evaluation of monoamine oxidase inhibitors. *Biochem. Pharmac.* **2**, 290–8.

LESSIN A.W. (1960) Species difference in the effect of barbiturate habituation on sensitivity to drugs (Title only). *Br. J. Pharmac.* **15**, 361.

LESSIN A.W. & PARKES M.W. (1957a) The relation between sedation and body temperature in the mouse. *Br. J. Pharmac.* **12**, 245–50.

LESSIN A.W. & PARKES M.W. (1957b) The hypothermic and sedative action of reserpine in the mouse. *J. Pharm. Pharmac.* **9**, 657–62.

LOEWE S. (1955a) Isobols of dose-effect relations in the combination of pentylenetetrazole and phenobarbital. *J. Pharmac.* **114**, 185–91.

LOEWE S. (1955b) Isobols of dose-effect relations in the combination of nikethamide (coramine) and phenobarbital. *J. Pharmac.* **115**, 6–15.

LOEWE S. (1957) Antagonisms and antagonists. *Pharmac. Rev.* **9**, 237–42.

LOEWE S. (1958) Isobols of combined effects of strychnine and barbiturates. *Arch. int. pharmacodyn.* **114**, 451–64.

MACGREGOR A.G. (1965) Review of points at which drugs can interact. *Proc. roy. Soc. Med.* **58**, 943–6.

MCIVER A.K. (1965) Drug incompatibilities. *Pharm. J.* **195**, 609–12.

NATOFF I.L. (1964) Toxic manifestations of foodstuffs during drug therapy. *Proc. Eur. Soc. Study Drug Toxicity* **4**, 158–66.

OLIVER M.F., ROBERTS S.D., HAYES D., PANTRIDGE J.F., SUSMAN M.M. & BERSOHN, I. (1963). Effect of Atromid and ethylchlorophenoxyisobutyrate on anticoagulant requirements. *Lancet*, **i**, 143–4.

PAGET G.E. (1963) Standards for the laboratory evaluation of the toxicity of a drug. *Proc. Eur. Soc. Study Drug Toxicity* **2**, 7–12.

PETERS L. (1960) Renal tubular excretion of organic bases. *Pharmac. Rev.* **12**, 1–35.

PLETSCHER A., GEY K.F. & ZELLER P. (1960) Monoaminoxydase-Hemmer. *Prog. Drug. Res.* **2**, 417–590.

REMMER H. & MERKER H.J. (1965) Effect of drugs on the formation of smooth endoplasmic reticulum and drug-metabolizing enzymes, *Ann. N.Y. Acad. Sci.* **123**, 79–97.

ROBINSON D.S. & MACDONALD, M.G. (1966) The effect of phenobarbital administration on the control of coagulation achieved during warfarin therapy in man. *J. Pharmac.* **153**, 250–3.

RÜMKE CHR.L. & DE JONGE H. (1964) Design, statistical analysis and interpretation, in *Evaluation of Drug Activities: Pharmacometrics*, eds. LAURENCE D.R. & BACHARACH A.L., Vol. 1, pp. 47–110. London, Academic Press.

RUSHTON R. & STEINBERG H. (1963a) Dose response relations of amphetamine-barbiturate mixtures. *Nature, Lond.* **197**, 1017–8.

RUSHTON R. & STEINBERG H. (1963b) Mutual potentiation of amphetamine and amylobarbitone measured by activity in rats. *Brit. J. Pharmac.* **21**, 295–305.

SCHANKER L.S. (1964) Physiological Transport of drugs. In *Advances in Drug Research*, eds. HARPER N.J. & SIMMONS A.B., Vol. 1, pp. 71–106. London, Academic Press.

SCHOLZ J. (1963) The importance of metabolism studies in relation to drug toxicity. 1. Introduction. *Proc. Eur. Soc. Study Drug Toxicity* **2**, 65–6.

SJÖQVIST F. (1965) Psychotropic drugs. (2) Interaction between monoamine oxidase (MAO) inhibitors and other substances. *Proc. roy. Soc. Med.* **58**, 967–78.

SPERBER I. (1959) Secretion of organic anions in the formation of urine and bile. *Pharmac. Rev.* **11**, 109–34.

STEINBERG H., RUSHTON R. & TINSON C. (1961) Modifications of the effects of an amphetamine-barbiturate mixture by the past experience of rats. *Nature, Lond.* **192**, 533–5.

TEDESCHI D.H., TEDESCHI R.E. & FELLOWS E.J. (1962) The effects of tryptamine on the central nervous system, including a pharmacological procedure for the evaluation of iproniazid-like drugs. *J. Pharmac.* **126**, 223–32.

THORP J.M. (1964) The influence of plasma proteins on the action of drugs, in *Absorption and Distribution of Drugs*, ed. BINNS T.B., pp. 64–76. London, Livingstone.

TREVAN J.W. (1927) The error of determination of toxicity. *Proc. roy. Soc.* **B.101**, 483–514.

VELDSTRA H. (1956) Synergism and potentiation. *Pharmac. Rev.* **8**, 339–87.

WERNER G. & WÜNKER R. (1959) Mydriasis in rabbits due to L-hyoscyamine. *Naturwiss.* **46**, 627.

WILLIAMS R.T. (1964) Drug metabolism in man as compared with laboratory animals. *Proc. Eur. Soc. Study Toxicity* **4**, 9–21.

WINTER C.A. (1948) The potentiating effect of antihistaminic drugs upon the sedative action of barbiturates. *J. Pharmac.* **94**, 7–11.

CHAPTER 11

Safety Testing of Biological Products (Sera and Vaccines)

F.T. PERKINS

INTRODUCTION

Although the majority of this book is concerned with the testing of chemical compounds, there is a place for the consideration of biological substances with special reference to immunological products. Millions of doses of vaccines are given each year with so few untoward reactions that the pharmaceutical industry may well feel proud of its achievement. The control of immunological products has been effective in this country since the Therapeutic Substances Act of 1925, which gave powers for the framing of regulations and for securing uniformity of standards, but more has been learnt in the last 10 than in the previous 30 years. The rapid development of virus vaccines has largely been responsible for this and some of the lessons we have learnt may well apply to the testing of any biological substance.

The safety tests applicable to a substance are determined by the potential hazards that may arise in the course of production. Although the ultracautious nature of control authorities tends to superimpose particular tests specific for any new product upon those already employed for established vaccines, such caution can be taken too far. There is little point, for example, in looking for simian viruses in a vaccine produced on tissue derived from chickens.

The safety of a vaccine may be considered under several headings.

SAFETY OF THE BACTERIAL OR VIRUS STRAINS

The bacterial diseases have been brought under control by effective immunization programmes using toxoids (diphtheria and tetanus) or whole bacterial suspensions, either living, e.g. Bacillus Calmette Guerin (BCG) for tuberculosis, or killed, e.g. whooping cough and typhoid, etc. Since toxoid production preceded the manufacture of bacterial vaccines, great stress was placed on a search for the most suitable bacterial strain and thereafter maintaining it without alteration in biological properties. Provided that no contaminants grow in the culture, which may introduce unwanted byproducts, the problems of control are reduced to a minimum. For the toxoids that are inactivated and separated from the bacterial culture the yield of toxin is most important but the inherent safety of the original bacterial strain has little significance. Even with the bacterial suspension vaccines, in which the bacteria are killed, there is much greater emphasis on the immunogenicity of the strains than on the toxicity of them and the only danger is in the quantity of protein being injected in the human dose. All the killed bacterial vaccines give some local reactions but these are more uncomfortable than dangerous.

With living bacterial vaccines such as BCG, however, the situation is much more like that of virus vaccines. Here the safety tests are applied to ensure that the vaccine strain does not differ from the original material shown to be safe in clinical trials in man (Medical Research Council 1958). Any deviation must be regarded as a danger signal. The rate of growth, bacterial size, reaction to intradermal injection in guinea-pigs are significant tests. Since the introduction of freeze-dried BCG vaccine, however, which can be stored pending satisfactory results before use, the hazards associated with this vaccine have largely been removed.

For virus vaccines the tests for identity with the seed virus shown to be safe in man are most complex. Especially is this the case when the vaccine is a living attenuated virus delicately poised in its degree of attenuation between a fully virulent and a non-infectious, non-immunogenic strain. Before live poliomyelitis vaccine was prepared the viruses were attenuated by growth in monkey kidney cell cultures at temperatures below 37°C (i.e. $34.5 \pm 0.5°C$) and not until the viruses failed to paralyse monkeys after inoculation into the thalamus were they considered suitable for tests in humans (Sabin *et al.*, 1954). Living attenuated vaccine, therefore, is subjected to a multiplicity of stringent tests to ensure that there has been no deviation in the course of production from the seed virus shown, by courageous clinical trials, to be safe in man. The same is true for live attenuated measles virus vaccine in which the virus was passaged through several cell substrates before it was adapted to grow on chick embryo fibroblast cultures. At this stage the virus failed to infect monkeys and use in humans was contemplated (Enders *et al.*, 1962). The degree of attenuation of the virus is closely followed by a decrease in the incidence and severity of reactions after inoculation into children. It is somewhat ironical that the modern developments in virus vaccines have given rise to some most elegant techniques and yet the first vaccine known to man, smallpox vaccine, is still prepared in much the same way as it was almost a century ago. Even with this vaccine, however, tests are now made to ensure that the seed strain does not differ with time. The modern principles will apply in the production of any future vaccine; if it is to be inactivated then the most immunogenic strain must be used, whereas in the production of a living vaccine great care must be taken to ensure the safety and stability of the seed virus.

SAFETY OF THE SUBSTRATE

The production of bacterial toxoids presents few difficulties from the point of view of safety of the substrate. Peptones are used as growth media and if serum is not used in the growth of the organisms there is little of the substrate present in the final purified product. Even with the bacterial vaccines the organisms are invariably washed free from culture medium before heat or chemical inactivation. The large quantity of protein present in the form of the bacterial suspension far outweighs any traces of proteins from the substrate in the final product. The only constituent that may cause concern in a bacterial suspension vaccine is an endotoxin, the concentration of which may be affected by the substrate and intradermal tests in animals can control this.

These problems are trivial compared with those encountered in virus vaccine production. Here the substrate must be a living cell and, since the rapid development of cell-culture techniques for virus growth, chick cell fibroblasts have been used on a large scale as well as kidney tissue from monkeys, dogs, cattle, and guinea-pigs. Even though oncogenic agents of simian origin have been isolated from the monkey tissues and the fowl leucosis viruses are known to contaminate egg vaccines, the absence of any immediate untoward effects in man has fostered a feeling of false security in these substrates.

By 1958, 26 simian agents had been isolated from monkey kidney (Hull, 1958) and the number is now much larger (Virology Monographs No. 2, 1968). All the early agents were recognized by giving a specific cytopathic effect (CPE) but only one, virus B, is known to be lethal to man. In 1960 vacuolating virus (SV 40) was isolated (Sweet & Hilleman, 1960) by subculture of the fluid from rhesus monkey kidney tissue on to cultures from kidneys of grivet, patas or vervet monkeys. Thus a live simian virus hitherto undetected was shown to be a contaminant of rhesus monkey kidney cultures and it appeared live in apparently killed polio-myelitis vaccines. It has now been demonstrated that SV 40 can produce tumours in hamsters (Eddy *et al.*, 1962), and transform cell cultures of human skin (Koprowski *et al.*, 1962; Girardi *et al.*, 1962) and kidney (Shein & Enders, 1962). Different monkey species differ in the extent to which they are infected with simian viruses and manufacturers have largely overcome the problem of contamination of vaccines by using the least contaminated species, transporting them in such a manner that contact with different species is avoided. Quarantine of monkeys before the kidneys are removed for vaccine production is also helpful.

A similar situation is present in the use of chicken fibroblast tissue as a substrate. Chickens are known to carry avian leucosis viruses and such viruses must be eliminated from human vaccines. Fortunately it has been possible to breed flocks free from avian leucosis viruses and tissue for measles vaccine production is derived from fertile eggs of such flocks.

Even though many millions of doses of inactivated poliomyelitis vaccine must have contained living SV 40 virus and there are no less than nine human vaccines produced on chick tissue known to contain avian leucosis virus none has been associated with onco-genesis in man (Hilleman, 1962). However, this cannot be used as an excuse for continuing the use of contaminated substrates because we do not know how long our observation period must extend before we can be certain of their harmlessness.

A more recent suggestion is that cell cultures known to be free from all detectable viruses should replace the use of primary tissue. It is traditional to refer to tissue cultures prepared directly from animal organs as 'primary cultures'. To be accurate this is incorrect terminology since a very small portion of the cells in the original trypsinized suspension take part in the initiation of a confluent cell sheet and thus the cells used for vaccine production are a population of mixed age some of which are already at the tenth to the fifteenth generation. Nevertheless, the cells have not been subcultivated and so they are referred to as 'primary'.

Hayflick has used a new terminology and has classified cells that can be subcultivated indefinitely as 'cell lines' whereas cells that undergo limited propagation are called 'cell strains'. The common property is that both 'cell lines' and 'cell strains' can be passaged. Until recently it was believed that any tissue capable of more than two or three passages must either be derived from a carcinoma or, if it had originated as normal tissue, must have been transformed. Thus it was assumed that the characteristic of continuous propagation was associated with malignancy. Today we know this to be untrue. Any tissue, normal or malignant, when propagated in suitable medium can be passaged many times and 'normal' tissue degenerating at the third or fourth passage is either in an unsuitable medium or is inherently infected. Thus the majority of monkey kidney tissue used in vaccine production today does not survive propagation because of inherent simian virus infection, which may not be detectable by a cytopathic effect. Kidneys taken from a monkey foetus having no inherent simian virus infection give cells capable of thirty to forty culture passages before degeneration. This is the critical difference between a 'cell strain' and a 'cell line'. All tissues derived from carcinomas, as well as transformed cells, can be propagated indefinitely and are 'cell lines'. HeLa cells, for example, initiated many years ago from the cancer of a cervix, must be in every virology laboratory in the world and must have given rise to several tons of tissue. All these 'cell lines' are capable of being cloned to reduce the heterogeneity of the cell population but even after repeated cloning a certain variation in chromosome numbers remains in the cell population. On the other hand, although cell strains, all of which are initiated from normal tissue, can be propagated for a finite time they maintain their normal karyotype throughout their life of active growth, only becoming slightly abnormal when entering the phase of decline.

This is a relatively new development and in some quarters even these 'cell strains' are associated with the possibility of carrying some hypothetical cancer factor. The fact remains that no virus has been isolated from healthy human foetal lung tissue cells; they maintain their normal karyotype, they do not produce a tumour when inoculated into the cheek pouch of a hamster and they are sensitive to human viruses, making them candidate substrates for virus vaccine production.

Stringent controls on the substrate used for virus growth would not only be a more logical point at which to look for extraneous viruses but would greatly strengthen our confidence in the safety of the vaccines.

SAFETY TESTING OF SERA AND VACCINES

The safety testing of sera is relatively simple compared with the more complex testing of modern virus vaccines. Provided that the serum is collected aseptically from the animals, and never becomes contaminated, then extraneous toxicity is not a problem. The protein injected into man with the antitoxic dose has been a problem in the past but today antitoxins are prepared from whole serum by separating the gamma globulins and there is an upper limit on the protein contained in the therapeutic or prophylactic dose. Apart from this the only control is to ensure that the product is free from abnormal toxicity.

The toxoids also have simple controls since animal tests to ensure both complete toxoiding and adequate potency suffice. Freedom from abnormal toxicity and bacterial sterility complete the tests.

Killed bacterial vaccines have similar tests to those of toxoids with the additional safeguard against too much protein being given in a single human dose. Thus a lower limit is placed on potency but an upper limit is placed on bacterial number. Even with the living BCG vaccine strict control of the approved strain is exercised and care taken to prevent its contamination by prohibiting other strains to be handled in the production area. Control of the bacterial count is essential as are tests to observe that the course of infection on animal inoculation is not unusual. Apart from these specific tests there are no other additional general tests.

With virus vaccines, especially those developed in the last ten years, the complexity and multiplicity of tests are such that their manufacture and control require special techniques. The scheme of such tests is set out in the figure. We have already dealt with the criteria necessary in the choice of a strain and substrate and the vaccine production is based on a seed virus system. Since the majority of tissue used is derived from monkey kidneys or chick embryos which may carry an inherent infection a portion (usually 25%) of the tissue production is set aside as controls and examined for the presence of extraneous viruses. The virus harvests from satisfactory tissue are also tested for the presence of extraneous virus in several tissues capable of detecting all viruses infectious for man. It is equally important to ensure that the test procedure both in the period of observation and the number of subcultures taken are adequate for the detection of all viruses. If an inactivated vaccine is tested, the detection of partially inactivated virus in the presence of a large mass of inactivated antigen calls for special techniques. With live vaccines prepared from attenuated viruses, tests in cell cultures are designed to match the characteristics of the vaccine virus with those of the seed virus from which all batches of vaccine are made. At this stage also tests in small laboratory animals are made for extraneous viruses.

The final vaccine in the ampoules or vials from which it is given to humans is further tested for sterility, potency and, where applicable, for identity with the seed virus.

Undoubtedly the most time consuming part of these tests is the search for extraneous viruses and even when they are completed with satisfactory results they cannot be taken as an absolute guarantee that every ampoule of the vaccine is free from these agents; the degree of confidence is similar to that given by a sterility test. The production of many batches of vaccine which consistently pass all tests is the strongest basis for confidence in a product.

The problems of discovering hitherto undetectable contaminants are very difficult, but there are three techniques worth considering:

(a) The use of an interference effect by which a known observable change in a cell culture is inhibited by the presence of the 'undetectable' virus. Such a technique is used in detecting the fowl leucosis viruses and rubella virus.

(b) The special staining of infected cell cultures especially with fluorescent antibody.

(c) The use of the electron microscope. This method has serious limitations both in interpretation and because the number of virus particles must be large before they are detected.

The greatest concern is that an undetected oncogenic virus may be present and for this reason inoculation of virus harvests into hamster cheek pouches, a route particularly sensitive to oncogenic viruses, is worth consideration, as is the use of mice treated with antilymphocytic serum (Stanbridge & Perkins).

POTENCY TESTS

Of equal importance with safety testing is potency testing since an innocuous but non-antigenic vaccine gives false security to the community and its use may eventually give rise to the reappearance of the disease. Live virus vaccines confer immunity by establishing infection in the host and the only index of potency therefore is the virus titre sufficient to establish infection in all inoculated subjects. With the inactivated vaccines, however, it is essential to measure the antibody response of an animal and important to check that the antibody responses are similar to those of humans. Where possible, attempts should be made to determine the circulating antibody titre necessary to give protection against the disease.

Since the first attempts at potency of toxoids the immune response to a particular dose of antigen, either in immunity to challenge or antibody titre has been used as an index of response. Recently it has been found more satisfactory to determine the responses to a number of different concentrations of antigen and thus giving a dose response curve. There are two advantages of this method: the one is that the determination of the 50% end point of antigen extinction is more accurate (Gard *et al.*, 1956) and the other is that a comparison of the slopes of the dose response curves obtained with a vaccine and reference preparation gives an indication of the similarity of the two products. The use of an antigen extinction limit test has also given much more reproducibility between laboratories and between countries.

It has been suggested that when once the immunizing antigen has been identified a technique involving precipitation lines after diffusion of antigen and antibody through gels is a quicker and more accurate assay of antigen concentration (Beale & Mason, 1962). This can be regarded as a most useful 'in process' control for a manufacturer but cannot replace a test for measuring the antigenic stimulus of the vaccine in the final container. For example it is possible to purify diphtheria toxoid to such an extent that it will not stimulate an antibody response in animals although *in vitro* tests show it is an excellent toxoid. This situation may also apply to other antigens and such tests cannot be relied upon to replace an antibody production test.

THE NEED FOR CLINICAL TRIALS

The development of a vaccine is greatly assisted by the discovery of a laboratory animal in which the human disease can be transmitted or simulated. Such was the case with yellow fever vaccine, but it has not been possible to assess the efficacy of either the living or inactivated poliomyelitis vaccine in the laboratory. Clinical trials on a large scale observing the epidemiological effects have been necessary to answer these questions.

The measles virus, however, was considered satisfactory for use in man when it had been attenuated to such an extent that it no longer gave measles infection in monkeys. In spite of this the number of virus particles necessary to give immunity after intradermal inoculation of man could only be determined by clinical trials.

In some countries the upper respiratory virus diseases are regarded as clinically important but their unique epidemiology and sporadic occurrence make evaluation of protection impossible by classical methods. Furthermore, the multiplicity of viruses giving similar clinical syndromes has largely been responsible for the chaos that is only just being resolved. It has been shown recently at the Medical Research Council's Common Cold Research Centre in the UK that a particular rhinovirus will give specific protection against the homologous strain and such data were obtained only by active challenge experiments in human volunteers. It is felt quite strongly in some countries, however, that the challenge must be made with small doses of wild virus not subjected to tissue culture passage. Only in this way will the natural disease be simulated and challenge experiments using laboratory passaged material requiring a large virus dose may give different clinical symptoms and lead to spurious results.

When once a correlation between protection or antibody response in animals and protection in man has been established much greater reliability can be placed on animal tests but the more recent virus vaccines and certainly the future virus vaccines will require clinical trials for the assessment of efficacy.

THE BALANCE OF RISKS

No vaccination procedure, nor indeed the injection of an antibiotic or saline, is free from all risk. Thus the acceptability of vaccination against any disease is an assessment of the balance of the risk against benefits expected from it.

In order to assess the benefits from vaccination each disease must be considered separately for its severity and the chance that a non-immune subject may contract the disease. On the other hand, the vaccine must be judged from its efficacy and severity of undesirable reactions to the vaccine. These factors differ from place to place, time to time, and vary in different social and economic groups. Reactions to a vaccine giving good long-lasting protection against a serious disease would certainly be tolerated by the community, but where the disease is mild the vaccine must be virtually free from danger.

Some risks in vaccinating are inherent in the nature of the vaccine and the variability of the human responses. Some risks may be either inadvertently or negligently introduced during the course of manufacture although safety tests are designed to eliminate these. Failure to recognize contraindication is also a risk but even after all precautions have been taken there will remain the unpredictable episode in the individual.

Though safety must be a cardinal factor in the development of vaccines it is essential that our tests are based on fact and not on theoretical considerations which may hamper progress in the field of preventive medicine. It is equally important however that the necessity for a vaccine is also assessed on facts and not speculation. It is the responsibility of scientists to present such balanced judgements.

STAGES OF DEVELOPMENT AND TESTING OF A VIRUS
VACCINE

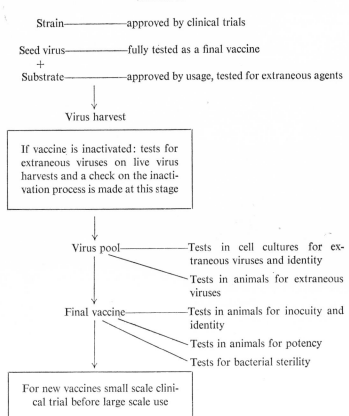

REFERENCES

BEALE A.J. & MASON P.J. (1962) The Measurement of the D. antigen in poliovirus preparations. *J. Hyg., Camb.* **60**, 113.

EDDY BERNICE, BORMAN G.S., GRUBBS G.E. & YOUNG R.D. (1962) Identification of the oncogenic substance in rhesus monkey kidney cell cultures as simian virus 40. *Virology* **17**, 65

ENDERS J.F., KATZ S.L. & HOLLAWAY ANN (1962) Development of attenuated measles virus vaccines. *Am. J. Dis. Child.* **103**, 335.

GARD S., WESSIEN T., FAGRAEUS A., SOEDMYR A. & OLIN G. (1956) The use of guinea-pigs in tests for immunogenic capacity of poliomyelitis virus preparations. *Arch. ges. Virusforsch.* **6**, 401.

GIRARDI A.J., SWEET B.H., SIOTNICK V.B. & HILLEMAN M.R. (1962) Development of tumours in hamsters inoculated in the neonatal period with vacuolating virus, SV 40. *Proc. Soc. exp. Biol. Med.* **109**, 649.

HILLEMAN M.R. & GOLDNER H. (1962) Perspectives for testing safety of live measles vaccine. *Am. J. Dis. Child.* **103**, 484.

HULL R.N., MINNER J.R. & MASCOLI C.C. (1958) New viral agents recovered from tissue cultures of monkey kidney cells. III. Recovery of additional agents both from cultures of monkey tissues and directly from tissues and excreta. *Am. J. Hyg.* **68**, 31.

HULL R.N. (1968) *Virology Monog. 2. The Simian Viruses.*

KOPROWSKI H., PONTEN J.A., JENSEN F., RAVDIN R.G., MOORHEAD P. & SAKSELA E. (1962) Transformation of cultures of human tissue infected with simian virus SV 40. *J. cell. comp. Physiol.* **59**, 281.

MEDICAL RESEARCH COUNCIL (1958) Freeze Dried BCG Vaccines: Results of laboratory tests and of trials among school children in Middlesex. *Br. med. J.* **i**, 79.

SABIN A.B., HENNESSEN W.A. & WINSSER J. (1954) Studies on variants of poliomyelitis virus: experimental segregation and properties of avirulent variants of three immunologic types. *J. exp. Med.* **99**, 551.

SHEIN H.M. & ENDERS J.F. (1962) Transformation induced by simian virus 40 in human renal cell cultures. I. Morphology and growth characteristics. *Proc. natn. Acad. Sci., U.S.A.* **48**, 1164.

STANBRIDGE E.J. & PERKINS F.T. (1969) Nature **221**, 80.

SWEET B.H. and HILLEMAN M.R. (1960) The vacuolating virus SV 40. *Proc. Soc. exp. Biol. Med.* **105**, 420.

CHAPTER 12

Biochemical Tests in Toxicology

A.E. STREET

INTRODUCTION

Studies of toxicity to animals have become a basic requirement in almost all countries, prior to the introduction of a new drug, food additive or pesticide, and data on clinical biochemistry has become an integral part of new tests. Clinical biochemistry is therefore called upon to provide an early warning of signs of toxicity, to identify target organs, if possible, and to provide evidence of reversibility of changes. In this way emphasis is placed on tests of organ function, particularly of the liver and kidney. The measurements made are similar to those carried out in any hospital clinical chemistry laboratory as a diagnostic service to the clinician. Indeed most of the techniques are the same as those used in human medicine, modified as and where necessary to suit the particular circumstances in terms of numbers of samples and the peculiarities of any species of animal that may be under test. The toxicologist will not be using the tests for diagnostic purposes, but in most cases will be looking for group effects related to the varying doses being used. The toxicologist has the great advantage of having control subjects, housed and handled under identical conditions, with which to compare results. Nevertheless he requires a greater methodological precision than is necessary in clinical medicine, since small group differences, even when they are within the accepted normal ranges, may be significant.

A number of factors may influence the outcome of biochemical observations, and control of these factors is important in the assessment of the significance of any changes that are encountered. In particular regularity and accuracy of dosing, the close control of conditions in the animal house, and the control of intercurrent

313

disease all bear on the significance of biochemical results, and need constant care. Any given series of experiments may vary in duration from a few days or weeks up to perhaps as much as 5 to 7 years. In these circumstances it is difficult or impossible for the biochemist to introduce new methods of analysis during one series of tests. Normal ranges depend so much on the method of choice: the laboratory may thus find itself with more than one method of analysis of the same parameter, running side by side in the laboratory for long periods of time. Moreover, since the animals under toxicological experiment may be receiving as much as 100 times the prospective human dose rate of any given compound, the risk of interference with the assay by the drug or chemical that is being given to the animal or by one of its metabolites must always be borne in mind and whenever thought or found necessary the method of analysis must be chosen to eliminate such risks. This may well be apparent during the initial planning of the experiment and the protocol therefore suitably amended. The risk is obviously considerably less for blood analysis than it is for urine analysis.

In addition to concurrent control groups initial values are obtained from all animals that are to be used for long term experiments. These must, of course, be within normal limits. These baseline data should preferably be obtained on two or more separate occasions during the acclimatization period, when the animals are being held under observation before the actual commencement of the experiment. Where this is not possible background information on normal values can be used to enable any deviation to be followed up, resulting in the replacement of the animal for experimental purposes should it be found unsuitable.

Normal Ranges

The normal range given by an analytical technique will be a composite of analytical precision for the chemical constituent under analysis, the effects, if any, given by the type of diet, the care with which the samples were obtained, and indeed the route by which the blood samples were obtained, environmental temperatures, the degree of acclimatization to handling and perhaps most importantly the age and species upon which the experiment is being performed. Published normal values are therefore only of limited importance to the toxicologist since he *must* establish them for his own laboratory in order to be able to detect slight deviations reliably.

The values given in the tables at the end of this chapter are therefore for guidance purposes only where it is proposed to use an analytical procedure without previous experience or where the species of animal to be used is one with which the laboratory has not previously been working. It is for this reason that standard deviations and 95% confidence limits will not be quoted, since they can only be pertinent to the laboratory producing them.

Precision and Choice of Laboratory Analytical Procedures

It may not greatly affect a clinical diagnosis if blood glucose is reported as being 350 mg/100 ml when its true value may be either 300 or 400 mg/100 ml. By contrast very much smaller group differences, even variations within the accepted normal range, may be indicative to the toxicologist of an early change. Great emphasis must therefore be placed on the quality control programme of the biochemistry department. In the author's laboratory every sixth sample to be analysed, whether by the Auto Analyser or by some manual procedure, is a control sample. These controls consist of lyophilized freeze-dried, commercially available serum, the chemical composition of which is known to the chief technician only, or of aqueous pure standard prepared in the laboratory as a check on instrumental drift. The control samples may be varied by purchasing different batches with differing compositions and from different manufacturers, or by altering dilution and either calculating the expected result or by using the diagram published by Thiers & Cole (1965). With the commercially available control sera however, the mean and acceptable limits of values quoted by the manufacturer may well be at variance with one's own results, particularly in enzymology. The biochemist must analyse these samples by the techniques in use in his own laboratory, in order to establish for himself a mean and an acceptable range of deviation from that mean.

Apart from availability and suitability of the types of instrumentation installed in the laboratory, other factors have to be borne in mind. First and foremost perhaps is the volume of sample required, since it is seldom that the toxicologist can afford to use even 1 ml of serum for a single analytical procedure. Indeed this volume may well represent the total available for a complete biochemical profile from the smaller species. This in some circumstances is not such a disadvantage as might at first appear when one considers that the normal alkaline phosphatase for a young rat is of the order of tenfold that of the human normal range. It may be possible to work on diluted samples, about 1:5 to 1:10.

SPECIMEN COLLECTION

Urine and faecal specimens can be collected from experimental animals without too much difficulty, even for quantitative work, by the use of suitably designed metabolism cages. An adequate acclimatization period to the metabolism cage is essential as is a constant environmental temperature (Worden & Waterhouse, 1956). Without this acclimatization it would not be uncommon for a dog to be placed in a metabolism cage nightly for up to five nights running without passing any urine whilst in the cage but, after acclimatization. normal habits are resumed. This problem is now being minimized at the Huntingdon Research Centre laboratories by the simple conversion of the ordinary runs into metabolism units. Each run can be converted into one or two metabolism cages, in the case of animals that are housed in pairs, by the simple insertion of the necessary grids and collecting devices for urine and faeces. This not only saves the space otherwise required for separate metabolism cages, but also allows the animals to remain in their own environment, thus avoiding the stress associated with removal to a completely strange room. The collection of blood specimens from laboratory animals such as the dog, the rabbit, and the pig and the smaller sub-human primates, presents very little difficulty. However, from small laboratory animals, and from extremely strong animals such as the baboon, blood often has to be collected under anaesthesia and the choice of anaesthetic may affect the results of subsequent biochemical estimations as has been shown by Kellett & Street, who examined some baseline biochemical parameters under varying conditions of anaesthesia and found that the changes reflected the stress associated with the induction of anaesthesia. The transaminases are particularly susceptible to stress effects as was shown by Pearl, Ballazs, & Buyske

(1966). They restrained rats for a period of 6 hours and followed the SGOT and SGPT which were remarkably elevated, the SGOT not having returned to basal level within a period of 6 days. Young rats should be handled to the same degree before an experiment commences as will be the case during the course of the work. It is important that the same people dose, feed, and weigh these animals as take the blood samples from them, and where intubation is to be the mode of administration, the animals should be conditioned to this procedure prior to their use in short-term studies. Additionally any control groups should have the same procedures carried out on them using saline, or the carrier, if one has to be used for the dosed compounds (Sanchez, Miya & Bousquet, 1966).

Urinalysis

In view of the diagnostic importance of urinalysis it should not be regarded as one which any junior trainee technician can perform. This attitude has perhaps been handed down over the ages and has been intensified by the introduction and widespread acceptance of the tablet or dip type tests. These are extremely valuable as a first screen but must always be regarded with an open mind as to the possibilities of false positive or negative results brought about by the dosed compound or a metabolite.

One of the easiest procedures for checking interference with urine analysis, when a dosing schedule is for less than 7 days a week, is to collect confirmatory urine samples after a weekend when no dose has been given. All positive results given by tablet or dip tests should be checked by the use of a standard chemical procedure, the chemistry of which is different to that originally used in the tablet or dip test.

Care and attention to detail is of the utmost importance for the possible detection of renal or hepatic disfunction by urine analysis. Careful scrubbing of the collection cages and grids without detergent and the use of disposable waxed carton collection pots are essential precautions. Indication from the animal house that a rat was found with blood oozing from a torn claw or that an animal is in oestrus saves much time and effort collecting further samples to check on the presence of blood or unusual cells.

Rat and dog urines are naturally acid, whereas those of sub-human primates and pigs naturally alkaline. Rat urine almost invariably contains protein, the type and amount of which varies with the sex and age of the animal. This was well documented for the Wistar rat by Perry (1965). Examination of the centrifuged deposit is almost impossible with rabbit urine owing to the presence of amorphous debris which makes cellular contents difficult to observe. Pigs appear to pass the majority of their urine immediately after feeding and tend to trample faecal material through the grids. It is thus important to remove urine from their cages as soon as it is passed, each succeeding sample being stored and bulked under suitable conditions before taken to the laboratory.

On every urine sample the following tests should be performed:

The colour should be noted and the volume measured.
pH recorded on a pH meter (not by pH papers).

Specific gravity may be measured by one of three main means depending on the volume available: (1) hydrometer for volumes of 25 ml or more, (2) by weighing in a pycnometer, (3) refractometer. This technique is invaluable when only a single drop of urine is available such as by direct expression onto the prism of the refractometer from the bladder; a precalibrated instrument for this purpose is manufactured by Otago Ltd, and can be obtained from Chemlab Instruments Ltd, Chigwell, Essex. Specific gravities below 1,010 or above 1,075 by the latter technique should be checked by pycnometric weighings if the greatest accuracy is necessary and sufficient sample can be obtained.

Screening tests for reducing substances, true glucose, ketones, bile in its various forms, and for free haemoglobin may be carried out using the reagents supplied for these purposes by the Ames Company Ltd. They are sufficiently well known not to require further description, but the need for care and cross checks as already described should be remembered. In addition it is worth stating that on many occasions quite normal dogs excrete sufficient bile pigment to give a two plus positive reaction.

Protein in urine can be screened for by the 'Albustix' technique but quantitative measurement must be carried out by precipitation with sulphosalicylic acid and the resultant turbidity compared with permanent protein standards. An extremely valuable diagnostic aid is to type the protein present by electrophoresis. The majority of urine samples will need concentration before this can be carried out. Dialysis, by inserting a small amount of carbowax in a very small membrane sac, the whole of which can be placed into a conical centrifuge tube containing the urine sample, will give rapid and satisfactory concentration of the urine.

Examination of the spun deposit must be carried out by extremely experienced technologists. Only relatively light centrifugation is essential (10 min at 1,000 r.p.m. is ample); staining of the deposit, after decantation of the supernatant, with methylene blue greatly helps differentiation of cell types as does the use of phase contrast microscopy. Types of cast present must be noted as must any unusual crystal forms.

The most useful and simple procedure for detecting renal damage is to withhold water for an overnight period of about 16 hours, then to measure the specific gravity of the urine passed during that period as an index of renal concentration. In the dog the value should be 1,040 or above. Values between 1,035 and 1,040 are grounds for suspicion of poor renal function. Consistent values of less than 1,035 are indicative of renal damage. As with most simple tests it is imperative that any low specific gravity samples should be re-run on at least three separate occasions to confirm the original observation. The procedure for rats is basically similar, with the exception that owing to the protein content of rat urine, specific gravity is found according to the formula:

$$\text{True SG} = \text{SG found} - (\text{mg protein}/100 \text{ ml} \times 0 \cdot 003)$$

Even when this is done it is not possible to give limiting ranges similar to those given for the dog.

Urinary glutamate-oxalate-transaminase (UGOT) analyses have been used in an attempt to assess renal damage. The method used was adapted from that advocated for blood analysis, details of which are contained in the Sigma bulletin 505. Blanks are essential when using urine. UGOT and a quantitative Addis cell count as described by Balazs (1963) should undoubtedly help to differentiate marginally abnormal results.

The inclusion of either or both of these as standard procedures cannot be justified in terms of laboratory time and therefore expense when the simple water deprivation and specific gravity will be adequate in the great majority of cases.

Urinary creatinine may also be of some value, if used as a measure of the completeness of a 24 hour collection period. This, of course, is because of its constancy in health. The technique for serum analysis on the Auto Analyser works with minor modifications extremely well, and can usefully be used in checking the completeness of collection of urine over 24 hour periods when following excretion of such electrolytes as sodium and potassium by flame photometry. The insensitivity of urinary creatinine levels to changes in renal function make this test of little use to detect kidney damage.

The detection of hyperfunctional liver enlargement as opposed to toxic liver enlargement has been assessed by measurement of the excretion of urinary ascorbic acid (Gaunt, 1965). There is a very considerable day to day variation in the ascorbic acid excretion, some of which is probably related to the degree of handling and the acclimatization of the animals concerned. It is therefore important that no firm conclusions are drawn from the technique unless a considerable series of strictly comparative assays are performed. This, of course, somewhat limits the usefulness of the test as a check when some treated animals are found to have enlarged livers and yet normal biochemistry. Since this is only detected at termination of the experiment in the post-mortem room, to start the experiment again would be prohibitively expensive. If, however, follow up work is planned for any compound and hyperfunctional liver enlargement is suspected, the test is well worth serious consideration.

Faecal Samples

Perhaps the most important toxicological procedure performed on faecal samples, apart from metabolic studies, is the examination for occult blood to detect intestinal bleeding. This has caused considerable difficulty owing to the fact that samples from dogs and rats are invariably positive for blood by all the standard techniques that we have applied to faecal homogenates. The sensitivity of the *ortho*-toluidene method of Smith (1958) may be reduced by titrating normal faeces from each species of animal against reagent concentrations until they just give a negative reaction after 2 min exposure. The faecal homogenates must be boiled and with some species filtered prior to this testing. All reactions taking longer than 2 min to develop are reported as negative.

Faecal stercobilinogen is occasionally useful in cases of suspected liver damage in animals. The standard technique of Maclagen (1946) has been used, albeit infrequently, without difficulty. The best standard is Terwens alkaline phenolphthalein and matching the colour by eye is more satisfactory than attempts to use colorimetry.

BLOOD ANALYSIS

Urea

For many years now it has been the procedure in our laboratory to estimate urea concentration from the plasma sample supplied for the analysis of total reducing substances on a dual-channel Auto Analyser system. The test used for urea is that of Moore (1963). By this means we have avoided some of the errors that may easily remain undetected owing to blockages in pulse suppressors when whole blood is used for analysis; this advantage more than offsets the larger samples required in order to separate plasma from the cells.

Blood urea concentration is one of the best indicators of renal function in man. In the dog it is perhaps less valuable, particularly in detecting minimal changes, unless care is taken. It has been shown for example that the blood urea of the beagle dog is significantly raised for a number of hours after feeding, the maximum being a 100% rise over approximately a 6 hour period, only approaching return to baseline after 16 hours (Street, 1968). These findings do not agree with other published opinions (Coles, 1967; Canterow & Trumper, 1962; Hoe & O'Shea, 1965), who consider that in the dog, as in man, the level of the blood urea in the normal subject reflects the general state of protein nutrition, rather than the direct influence of the subject's last meal.

Climatic changes may also affect the blood urea concentration in the dog. During a short hot spell when shade temperatures of 90°F were encountered, blood samples taken from some 30 dogs on the second day of the heat-wave gave values 39% higher than was found some 2½ days later when the temperature had returned to lower levels.

As in man, the blood urea levels in animals are not elevated until renal damage is well advanced, owing to the very high reserve capacity of the kidneys.

Blood Glucose

For many years since the Auto Analyser became standard equipment in toxicological biochemistry laboratories, the ferricyanide reduction method for estimating total reducing substances as in Technicon Method Sheet N2b adapted from Hoffman (1937) has gained almost universal usage. There can, however, be no really valid reason for using a non-specific method of analysis where highly specific methods exist. The glucose oxidase reaction was adapted for use with the Auto Analyser in our laboratories by Street & Richards. Cramp (1967) has published a similar method, including the precipitation of the fluoride by ammonium sulphate.

The most satisfactory source of enzyme for both manual and automated technique has been 'Fermcozyme' supplied by Hughes & Hughes Limited.

Cleanliness of the manifold is imperative or partial blockages of narrow inlets to the glass cactus pieces may occur. Rotational replacement of these for thorough manual cleaning ensures smooth trouble free operation of the manifold.

As mentioned briefly in the discussion of blood urea, all analyses are performed on plasma samples. The results obtained may be some 20 or more mg per cent above those for whole blood. This figure will vary somewhat with the circulating level of glucose as was shown by McDonald (1964).

Plasma analysis is now generally favoured for glucose determinations. Because of the differences between plasma levels and those for whole blood it is essential to note which technique has been used.

Serum Enzymes

Alkaline phosphatase has been in use as a diagnostic aid for the detection of liver damage for many years and numerous methods are advocated for analysis. However, that adapted from the method of Kind & King (1954) for the Auto Analyser, particularly as a dual channel system simultaneously recording blank and test values, works extremely well and has proved to be invaluable, particularly in the dog whose range of normal values are akin to those found in men. In the rat, however, values of 100 King-Armstrong units or more in the young, rapidly growing animal reduce to a range of 30–50 King-Armstrong units as the animal matures. This gives rise to a high degree of scatter and the difficult task to the biochemist of attempting to detect marginal increases in the enzyme. This renders the test rather less sensitive in acute experiments. In baboons the picture is more complicated. Values of 200–350 King-Armstrong units in the young, rapidly growing animal have been recorded in our laboratories, again with a steep fall-off towards maturity. Alkaline phosphatase is not a liver specific enzyme and many other sources can contribute to the circulating levels. For the rat and the baboon particularly, a good case could be made out for substituting for alkaline phosphatase a more specific liver enzyme such as 5′-nucleotidase, in view of the levels of serum alkaline phosphatase found in young animals.

SERUM GLUTAMATE PYRUVATE TRANSAMINASE (SGPT)

Measurement of the circulating level of SGPT is one of the most sensitive indicators of liver function, nevertheless it poses a number of problems to the analytical laboratory. Undoubtedly, the best analytical procedure is the classical method of Wroblewski & LaDue (1955) involving use of an ultra-violet spectrophotometer. However, the colorimetric method of Reitman & Frankel (1957) has gained very wide acceptance due to its simplicity and applicability to the type of instrument that most laboratories possess. The adaptation of this method by the Sigma Chemical Company Limited, as fully described in their leaflet No. 505, can be recommended.

The measurement of the SGPT suffers several disadvantages, one being the inherently high blank values leading to a reduction of sensitivity at lower levels of activity, and a second being the number of occasions on which isolated animals including untreated control group animals, will show raised transaminase activity. These animals often return to normal values within 2 or 3 days. It is important therefore in cases such as this that repeated samples from the animals be examined.

Many attempts have been made to automate the colorimetric transaminase procedures. In our hands none of these have so far proved satisfactory in that direct adaptation of the manual methods requires tremendously long running periods before the baseline becomes stable. This is because the coloured complex is absorbed into the plastic tubing of the Auto Analyser manifold and this leads to variation of the baseline and recorder settings, a high noise level; additionally the tubes will require saturating afresh each time a series of analyses is to be run. This is due to the fact that during the washout of the manifold prior to shut down of the instrument, some of this colour complex will be eluted.

The introduction of flow cell spectrofluorimeters has influenced this situation favourably and can be expected to obviate the difficulties encountered when values fall in the suspicious zone, where the colorimetric procedures are least sensitive and as yet most reliance may have to be placed on them.

Many laboratories have adapted instruments already in their possession for this purpose. Locarte produce a small, yet remarkably stable, fluorimeter, the flow cell of which only contains 0·05 ml, thus giving good wash and no detectable interface interferences.

The full standard curve by the Sigma technique should be checked regularly and rather frequently in our experience, for the greatest confidence in results.

Quality control of the transaminase determinations must, as briefly mentioned, be performed by each individual laboratory to establish its own acceptable range of values since those quoted by the manufacturers of commercial freeze-dried control sera are often unacceptably wide for toxicological purposes.

SERUM GLUTAMATE OXALOACETATE TRANSAMINASE (SGOT)

The comments under the heading SGPT apply almost equally well throughout the analyses for SGOT and the methodology used by us is, again, that of the Sigma Company in their bulletin 505. This technique is, however, much more subject to interference by marginal levels of haemolysis than is that of the SGPT and unfortunately in the toxicological evaluations carried out on small animals it is not always possible for the laboratory to reject samples as unsuitable for analytical purposes. It is therefore our practice to analyse such sera using a visual appraisal of the degree of haemolysis and of which samples are haemolysed. It is then possible to indicate where a measured increase of the enzyme activity may be due to the haemolysis, and fresh samples obtained. Equally, the knowledge that if the result is not abnormal with haemolysis present, it could not possibly be abnormal on a non-haemolysed sample from the same animal will be of value in aiding any decision to be made as to the necessity of further blood sampling.

The rise of circulating SGOT is sometimes more spectacular and stays elevated for longer periods than does the SGPT, for instance, in response to a single dose of carbon tetrachloride in the rat (Ruckebusche, 1966). However it should be stated that the type of rise of serum enzymes and their duration may well vary from species to species and from compound to compound.

ISOCITRIC DEHYDROGENASE (ICID)
ICID is a valuable indicator of active heptacellular damage. The colorimetric method for determination of this enzyme (Bell & Baron, 1960) is applied to animal blood samples without modification. We prefer to use this technique for supporting evidence, rather than dye clearance tests. A young dog will have normal levels of 20–30 Bell & Baron units, gradually dropping until adulthood when values of around 10 units/100 ml blood will be found.

Serum Bilirubin

The measurement of the circulating levels of bilirubin is not as valuable in the animal field as it is in the human. This is mainly because the dog and the rat have a very low renal threshold for bilirubin; it is not uncommon to find clinically healthy and apparently biochemically normal dogs that secrete enough bilirubin to give a two plus reaction to Fouchet's reagent (Harvey, 1967). He gives a normal range from 0–0·6 mg/100 ml and finds greater than 1 mg/100 ml extremely rare. All this is borne out in our own experience with the exception that our normal range is about half that quoted. Thus we are concerned with very low levels initially and only marginal changes on which to base our conclusions.

For many years we successfully used the direct spectrophotometric technique devised by White (1958). Although great care had to be taken over the preparation of the diluent and in operating the spectrophotometer since relatively small changes of optical density could be highly significant. The development of an efficient scale expansion circuit for the recorders of the Auto Analyser in our workshop has enabled us to automate our total bilirubin measurements, using the technique for increasing the colour developed after diazotisation described by Van den Bosch (1965). Therefore we are now able to quantitate reliably changes of bilirubin concentration as small as 0·2 mg/100 ml. This technique has quite often been of value when a degree of anaemia has been shown to be present by the haematological studies, the liver function shown to be entirely normal by the serum enzyme measurements, but bilirubin slightly raised as a result of the haemolytic condition.

At these extremely low levels there is little point in attempting to measure direct and indirect bilirubin.

Total Protein and Electrophoresis

These two analytical procedures are grouped together because of the usefulness of the albumin:globulin ratio in tests of liver function. The measurement of total protein on its own is of little value. The measurement of the albumin fraction by an automated technique is relatively simple, but it does miss a great deal of information on changes of the minor components when used as a standard procedure; therefore we measure the total protein and perform electrophoresis on all sera.

Total protein is most easily and economically performed on the Auto Analyser utilizing the Technicon basic methodology N. 14b derived from the method of Weichselbaum (1946). By increasing the reaction time using longer coils immersed in a constant temperature water bath, a greater degree of sensitivity can be achieved enabling us, as mentioned before, to analyse for serum total protein on the same dilution of serum that has been used for the alkaline phosphatase determinations. The handling characteristics of cellulose acetate when large numbers of assays are required, and when the records must be retained render this an impracticable technique except for the investigation of samples that have shown an unusual pattern by standard paper electrophoretic techniques.

The Millipore phoroslide electrophoretic system offers great advantages in terms of speedy availability of the analytical results and in the storage and handling of the electrophoretograms. This system is currently being run side by side with the existing paper electrophoresis system in an evaluation programme by our laboratory. The support medium is basically a celluloid strip coated with a cellulose acetate powder. With the small electrode and buffer chambers designed for use with this support medium, no equilibration period is necessary and good separation of the major components can be demonstrated after as little as 16 min current application at 100 volts for the dog. Pig and man require about 20 min; for the rat, in order to obtain good separation of the α_1 globulin from the albumin fraction, use a Barbitone-Acetate buffer system, pT 8·6, ionic strength 0·075. Buffer solutions should be prepared 24 hours before required in order to obtain optimum resolution. The prepared buffers should be discarded weekly with most electrophoretic systems but daily when using phoroslides.

Quantitation of the electrophoretograms from the phoroslide system can be achieved with the Chromoscan, but for the best results a special gear ratio should be cut. We are therefore using the Phoroscope, a completely electronic instrument with essentially no mechanical working parts. This instrument presents the pattern of the separated proteins on an oscilloscope. Additionally it gives a direct read out of the percentage composition of each protein fraction, thus halving the necessary mathematics for computing the analytical results. By this technique it is estimated that two people should be able to perform 72 electrophoretic separations per day if required.

The album:globulin ratio by these two techniques is almost identical, but there are differences in the calculated results for α_2, β and γ globulin, for instance, the dog by phoroslide shows a higher α_2 and a lower β globulin in comparison to paper methods.

Dye Excretion Tests

BROMOSULPHTHALEIN CLEARANCE (BSP)

In experimental animals as in man the bromosulphthalein clearance test is used most frequently. The excretion of BSP is extremely rapid both in the dog and the rat, but especially so in the rabbit. In this species it is not always possible to get a satisfactory result, even by increasing the amount of dye administered. Dosages of BSP recommended by different authors vary from 5 mg/kg to as much as 50 mg/kg. This in itself is indicative of the difficulties experienced by laboratories in trying to adapt the technique to animal species. A 100% blood level is virtually unobtainable. One way to circumvent this is to calculate a theoretical 100% level from the bodyweight of the animal, and known percentage body composition in terms of blood volume. Notwithstanding this, the sheer mechanics of organizing the injection of the dye and the sampling of the blood are extremely critical, and the difficulty of achieving accurately timed periods for large groups of animals renders this test impracticable as a screening procedure. A difference as small as 20 sec in the time at which blood is withdrawn can mean the difference between a normal and an abnormal result. This is seen quite clearly by the inspection of the curves of BSP clearance published by Ruckebusch (1966).

INDOCYANINE GREEN CLEARANCE (ICG)
Indocyanine green clearance as a test for hepatic function has also been investigated, particularly by Vogin (1965, 1967), but this technique entails blood sampling on a minimum of two or more often three occasions at between 2 and 10 minute intervals after the ICG administration. The exact time of these blood samples must be known and half-life clearance can then be calculated.

These techniques, to be properly performed, therefore require venepuncture on three or four separate occasions which is, of course, an impossible workload in most animal houses that use large groups of animals.

These techniques are extremely valuable for evaluation of experiments that do not present a clear picture by standard enzyme techniques, or where a further function test is thought to be necessary. However, we find it preferable to extend our observations by the inclusion of the isocitric dehydrogenase estimation, rather than by using one of the clearance techniques.

Some of the criticisms that have been mentioned in the preceding paragraphs have been met in the human patient, at least, by the application of dichromatic ear densitometry (Levy, 1967). Use of this technique enables blood levels of ICG to be followed without taking a blood sample and serially at more than one concentration of ICG.

The dosages of BSP used in our laboratory when the test has to be used are 20 mg/kg for the dog, 25 mg/kg for the rat and 40 mg/kg for the rabbit. Blood is sampled at a standard 15 min after injection of the dye. The 100% level is calculated from theory.

PHENOL RED TEST OF KIDNEY FUNCTION
Under the heading of dye tests some mention should be made of the phenol red test for kidney function. Catheterization of animals that are on long-term toxicity tests is unwise because of the risk

of infection or mechanical damage. Experience with the phenol red excretion test is therefore limited in our laboratory to small rodents, where the bladder can be approximately emptied by digital pressure. Phenol red of neutral pH is injected into the caudal vein; 0·2 ml of a solution which contains 0·01 mg of dye is injected per 100 g bodyweight of the animal, after the bladder has been emptied. Thirty minutes later the bladder is emptied again, the whole of the urine sample made up to 10 ml with dilute alkali and the extinction read and compared with a calibration curve made from previously known volumes of phenol red. Approximately 47% of the injected dose is excreted in the first 30 min in the normal animal.

Tests Used in Human Medicine, Little Applied in Toxicology

THE LIVER, TURBIDITY, AND FLOCCULATION TESTS

These tests depend on alterations in the type of protein present in the serum or plasma and are most frequently related to changes in one or more of the globulin fractions.

The Thymol Turbidity test of Maclagen (1944) has been used quite extensively in the past. However, it proved insensitive in use for both the dog and the rat. It is probably superfluous when electrophoresis is performed on all sera, but it should be remembered that the results of this type of test do not always parallel alterations in the albumin:globulin ratio.

Many other reagents have been used in human medicine such as zinc sulphate, cephalin, cholesterol, and colloidal gold. It is often advocated that a combination of two of these will give easier diagnostic interpretation, but they have been little used in toxicology.

HIPPURIC ACID SYNTHESIS

This test is designed to assay the efficiency of the liver in converting benzoic acid to hippuric acid, excreted in the urine where the amount passed in a fixed period can be measured. Difficulties in obtaining urine specimens from animals at fixed periods have prevented the use of this test.

CARBOHYDRATE METABOLISM

Galactose or fructose tolerance tests have not gained a place in toxicology because of the necessity of taking serial blood samples at fixed intervals from large numbers of animals.

THE KIDNEYS

Urea clearance, inulin, sodium thiosulphate, or *p*-aminohippurate clearance have all been found useful in human medicine. All these tests require that urine specimens be obtained at fixed intervals. For this reason they have been little used in toxicology.

BLOOD LIPIDS

Investigation of the circulating lipids is reasonably straightforward. The normal values encountered are generally much lower than those found in man. Cholesterol determinations on the Auto Analyser suffer from two considerable drawbacks. Firstly, the material to be pumped is extremely acid, with consequent risks to instruments and staff when a tubing junction blows. Secondly, although repeat analysis of a serum sample by a manual procedure over a period of many days shows no deterioration, the results by Auto Analyser on the same sample at the same time intervals show a steady loss of measurable cholesterol. Under the same conditions pure standards are stable. The manual procedure of Pearson (1965) is therefore our standard technique.

Lipid phosphorus determinations were at one stage rather troublesome, both during digestion and colour development. Since changing to the method of Zilversmit (1950) no further difficulties have been encountered.

Triglyceride by the semi-automated method of Loffland (1964) is relatively simple to apply provided one uses the amendments as reported by the same author (Loffland, 1965).

Occasionally it is valuable to know the ratio of the α and β lipo-proteins. The prestaining technique of Swahn (1952), followed by electrophoresis on paper support medium has been used without modification by us. The Poroslide manual gives a method for separating lipo-protein which we have tried, but all developed colour on the bands lost during clarification in the solvent recommended, an ethyl acetate-acetic acid mixture. We shall continue to work on this problem.

Pancreatic Function

The determination of serum amylase for the study of pancreatic function has been used intermittently over the past years. The rat has an extremely high and variable level of this enzyme. It is therefore of somewhat doubtful value. The technique described by Stuart & Dunlop (1962) can be used without modification if required.

Thyroid Function

Protein bound iodine is the usual technique for the study of thyroid function, but great care must be taken to ensure that there is no contamination from atmosphere, particularly in an open-plan laboratory, or where continuous-flow wet chemistry instrumentation and iodinated reagents are in use. Our experience has been confined to Ackland's method (1957) which works very well, provided enough care is taken in cleaning the glassware, and against atmospheric contamination.

On the other hand it is worth noting that a totally enclosed system for oxygen consumption, or indeed a full BMR or small animals, such as rats and mice, is made and marketed by Carlo-Erba of Milan. The principle of operation is that the system, being closed circuit, generates oxygen electrolytically. If too much gas is produced the positive pressure blows the electrolyte from contact with the electrode. Oxygen is therefore generated to replace that consumed by the animal. Exhaled carbon dioxide is removed by chemical scrubbing. The current consumed by the electrolysis may be converted to cubic centimetres of oxygen or to calories. CO_2 may be determined by chemical analysis of the scrubbers (Capraro, 1953).

ELECTROLYTES

Although, as has been shown by Richards (1967), there is an overall trend for metabolic acidosis to occur in nephritic dogs, the possible causes of upsets in the acid base balance are considerably more widespread both in human medicine and in toxicological experimentation. It is therefore wise to include as a basic minimum estimations sodium, potassium, chloride, and carbon dioxide and only estimate calcium, magnesium, and phosphorus where detailed investigations are called for.

The Astrup (1960) technique is obviously attractive to the biochemical toxicologist, but so far as is known no nomograms for the animal species with which we work have been published. It is on these theoretical grounds that we still use the classical techniques of flame photometry for sodium and potassium, the Van Slyke manometric technique for carbon dioxide, the Technicon Auto Analyser method for chloride from their sheet N5B, serum calcium by the colorimetric technique of Spare (1964), inorganic phosphate by the Technicon method sheet N4B and finally because of the well-known difficulties with reproductibility of batches of Titan yellow, the Mann and Yoe dye technique published by Bahnon (1962) for serum magnesium.

METHAEMOGLOBIN

The quantitative determination of methaemoglobin by the method of Evelyn & Malloy (1938) is perfectly satisfactory in the dog, but in the rat, turbidity almost invariably develops after addition of the neutralized cyanide reagent. This is due in all probability to the difference in the α_1-globulin protein fractions between these two species. This can be overcome by using the Tritan X 100 in boric buffer solution and by not neutralizing the sodium cyanide as described by Hainline (1965). In addition, in toxicology it is always wise to be alive to the possibility that both methaemoglobin and sulphaemoglobin may be present at one and the same time in any given blood sample. Whenever this is suspected we use the technique of Hodge (1967) which continuously records the light absorption before and after the addition of sodium cyanide by recording spectrophotometry through the wavelengths 400–650 mμ.

CHOLINESTERASE

There are numerous techniques for performing cholinesterase determinations. Some changes in technique are rendered necessary by the newer carbamate insecticides, and because of the use of this determination as a test of liver function, the levels being depressed in liver damage.

The determination of cholinesterase by the delta pH method of Michel (1949) is probably best suited for handling relatively large numbers of samples at a time. However, using the buffer strength described for a human plasma or cells only low levels of activity are indicated. By modifying the buffer and substrate concentration, Williams (1957) was able to devise a technique whereby the inhibition of cholinesterase by organo-phosphorous insecticides could be detected readily in samples derived from experimentally poisoned animals, and this is now our routine method. But, when working with the newer carbamate insecticides, one must be aware that the enzyme-inhibitor complex dissociates rapidly on dilution and especially during the prolonged incubation times used in the majority of techniques. These permit complete dissociation with little evidence of inhibition. For these compounds therefore we use a titrimetric method with the apparatus supplied by Radiometer Ltd, adding the samples to the buffer and substrate and measuring the initial velocity for just a few minutes. It is possible to follow the dissociation by increasing the incubation time, but working over the initial linear point of the titration curve gives us something of the order of 104% recovery of added enzyme for either plasma or erythrocyte measurement. This technique was described by Casterline & Williams (1967) for the rat erythrocyte. They were unsuccessful in applying it to plasma since they found far too much variation. We have, however, adapted this and have employed it routinely for plasma, erythrocyte and brain samples from both rats and dogs.

SUMMARY

It will now be apparent that because of the importance of the liver for metabolizing and detoxicating administered compounds, very heavy emphasis has been placed on liver and kidney function tests. (This is because the kidneys, in addition to playing a part in metabolic processes are the site of readsorption of the break-down products.) These tests may now be assembled into an order of sensitivity and applicability to the problem at hand.

The most sensitive and diagnostic tests for liver function are glutamate oxalate transaminase, alkaline phosphate, and glutamate pyruvate transaminase. Next in order of sensitivity and priority are bilirubin and the electrophoresis of proteins, because of the additional information they can provide in cases of drug induced reaction other than liver damage. Isocitric dehydrogenase is preferred to dye excretion tests, unless the latter can be performed to give full elimination curves, when difficulties arising from timing can be eliminated.

The most useful renal function tests are: the concentrating power of the kidney under water deprivation and water loading conditions; blood urea; and standard urine analysis with particular emphasis on the examination of well-prepared specimens of deposits under the microscope. Supporting tests that may be particularly valuable in borderline cases are the urinary glutamate oxalate transaminase and quantitative cell count tests.

CONCLUSION

The aim of the discussion of various tests has been to provide practical advice to those who are not fully experienced in the application of clinical biochemical tests to toxicological experiments, and, for those more experienced, to describe the advantages and disadvantages that have been found with particular tests with which they may not be familiar. Several general points emerge from the particular discussions and merit specific mention.

Several important differences exist between the applications of biochemical tests to clinical medicine, and application to toxicological experiment. The most obvious of these differences is the species on which the test is to be performed. It is clearly essential to validate any particular test by large numbers of observations on normal animals of the species to be used in an experiment, both to demonstrate that the test, if necessary appropriately modified, is in fact detecting the biochemical effect it is supposed to, and also to provide figures for normal ranges for that species in the particular circumstances of the laboratories performing the experiment and carrying out the tests.

It may also be of importance to detect very small differences in organ function between experimental and control groups—differences which might well be insignificant in the application of the test to human medicine. The design of toxicological experiments should be such as to provide a statistically sufficient basis for the detection of small differences, and it is important that the test methods chosen should be sufficiently precise and well controlled for reliance to be placed on small differences in their outcome.

Toxicological experiments impose logistic problems on laboratories undertaking them, and particularly on the biochemical laboratory. Often very large numbers of individual observations must be made, and it is important that these large numbers of observations be made at the same time, and on frequently repeated occasions. Automated methods are therefore essential and especially those methods that use only very small amounts of biological material. Even when the methods are available, a highly efficient laboratory organization is required to ensure the smooth integration of specimen collection, performance of tests, and reporting of results within the conduct of the total experiment.

A fundamental difference between the clinical and experimental application of biochemical tests arises in the interpretation of results. In clinical medicine, biochemical tests are undertaken to help to confirm or exclude a particular diagnosis, and they are not usually employed as a method for screening for abnormality. The result of a biochemical test is therefore evaluated against the diagnostic expectations which prompted its performance. In toxicological experiments, however, biochemical tests are performed primarily as a screening mechanism in order to detect organ damage earlier or more certainly than would be the case with other methods, and positive results from such tests must often be evaluated in the absence of other indications of organ dysfunction.

While positive results in properly chosen and conducted biochemical tests will usually indicate damage to specific organs, other possible factors must be remembered. The demonstration of a dose/response relationship of the results of a test is essential confirmatory evidence that the deviation from control values is due to the compound administered. The further elucidation of a positive finding will often demand additionally more specific tests than those performed initially. Finally, the experimental toxicologist always has the possibility, usually happily denied to the clinician, of examining the organs of his subjects *post-mortem*. Histology with both light and electron microscopes, histochemistry, and biochemical studies on fresh tissue will, when used appropriately, enable unusual biochemical test results to be interpreted with assurance. It is obviously important, at the conclusion of toxicological experiments to review the evidence provided by biochemical studies during the course of them, and to determine what studies must be made at the time the animals are killed.

REFERENCES

ACLAND J.D., *Biochem J.* (1957) **66**, 177.

ASTRUP P., SIGGAARD-ANDERSON O., JØRGENSON K. & ENGEL K. (1960) *Lancet* **i**, 1935.

BAHNON C. (1962) *Clinica chim. Acta* **7**, 811.
BALAZS T., HATCH A., ZAWIDZKA Z. & GRICE H.C. (1963) *Toxic. appl. Pharmac.* **5**, 661.
BELL J.L. & BARON D.N. (1960) *Clinica chim. Acta* **5**, 740.
CANTERON A. & TRUMPER M. (1962) *Clinical Biochemistry*. 6th Edition. London, Saunders.
CAPRARO V. (1953) *Nature* **172**, 815.
CASTERLINE J.L. & WILLIAMS C.H. (1967) *J. Lab. clin. Med.* **69** (2), 325.
CHASSON A.I., GRADY H.J. & STANLEY M.A. (1961) *Am. J. clin. Path.* **340**, 83.
COLES E.H. (1967) *Veterinary Clinical Pathology*. London, Saunders.
GAUNT I.F., FEUER G., FAIRWEATHER F.A. & GILBERT D. (1965) *Fd Cosmet. Toxicol.* **3**, 433.
HAINLINE A. (1965) *Stand. Meth. clin. Chem.* **5**, 143.
HARVEY D.G. (1967) *J. Small Anim. Pract.* **8**, 473.
HODGE H.C., DOWNS W.L., PANNER B.S., SMITH D.W., MAYNARD E.A., CLAYTON J.W. & RHODES R.C. (1967) *Fd Cosmet. Toxicol.* **5**, 513.
HOE C.M. & O'SHEA J.D. (1965) *Vet. Rec.* **77**, 210.
KELLETT D.N. & STREET A.E. (to be published).
LEEVY C.M., SMITH F., LONGUEVILLE J., PAUMGARTINER G. & HOWARD M.M. (1967) *J. Am. med. Ass.* **200**, 236.
LOFLAND H.B. (1964) *Anal. Chem.* **9**, 393.
LOFLAND H.B. (1965) *Analyt. Biochem.* **10**, 1.
MACLAGEN N.F. (1946) *Br. J. exp. Path.* **27**, 190.
MCDONALD G.W., FISHER G.F. & BURNHAM C.E. (1964) *Publ. Hlth Rep.* **79**, No. 6.
MICHEL H.O. (1949) *J. Lab. clin. Med.* **34**, 1564.
MODELL W. (1967) *Science* **156**, 346.
MOORE J.J. & SAX S.M. (1965) *Clinica chim. Acta* **11**, 475.
PEARL W., BALAZS T. & BUYSKE D.A. (1966) *Life Sci.* **5**, 67.
PEARSON S., STERN S. & MCGOVAC T.H. (1953) *Anal. Chem.* **25**, 813.
PERRY S.W. (1965) *J. Path. Bact.* **89**, 2.
RICHARDS M.A. & HOE C.M. (1967) *Vet. Rec.* **80**, 640.
RUCKEBUSCH Y. (1966) *Rev. Med. Vet.* **117**, 8–9, 667.
SANCHEZ C., MIYA T.S. & BOUSQUET W.F. (1966) *Proc. Soc. exp. Biol. Med.* **123**, (2) 615.
SIGMA METHOD SHEET No. 505.
SMITH R.L. (1958) *Br. med. J.* **1**, 1336.
SPARE P.D. (1964) *Clin. Chem.* **10**, 726.
STREET A.E., CHESTERMAN H., SMITH G.K.A. & QUINTON R.M. (1968) *J. Pharm. Pharmac.* **20**, 325.
STREET A.E., RICHARDS B. (Unpublished) similar to CRAMP D.G. (1967) *J. clin. Path.* **20**, 910.
STUART C.P. & DUNLOP D. (1962) *Clin. Chem.* 6th edition. Livingstone.
SWAHN B. (1952) *Scan. J. path. clin. Invest.* **4**, 98.
TECHNICON METHOD SHEET METHODS
  HOFFMAN W.S. (1937) Technicon Method Sheet N2B. *J. biol. Chem.* **120**, 51.

FISK G.H. & SUBBARROW Y. (1925) Technicon Method Sheet N4B. *J. biol. Chem.* **66**, 375.

ZALL D.M., FISHER D. & GARNER M.O. (1956) Technicon Method Sheet N5B. *Anal. Chem.* **28**, 1665.

KIND P.R.N. & KING E.J. (1954) Technicon Method Sheet N6A. *J. clin. Path.* **1**, 324.

WEICHSELBAUM T.E. (1946) Technicon Method Sheet N14B. *Am. J. clin. Path.* **7**, 40.

THIERS R.F. & COLE R.R. (1965) *Clin. Chem.* **2**, 1036.

VAN DEN BOSSCHE H. (1965) *Clinica chim. Acta* **11**, 379.

VAN SLYKE D.D. & NEIL J. (1924) *J. biol. Chem.* **61**, 523.

VARLEY H. (1967) *Practical Cinical Biochemistry*, 4th Edition, Heinemann.

VOGIN E.E., SCOTT W. & MATTIS P.A. (1965) *Proc. Soc. exp. Biol. Med.* **119**, 2.

VOGIN E.E., SKEGGS H.R. BOKELMAN D.L. & MATTIS P.A. (1967) *Toxicol. Appl. Pharmac.* **10**, 577.

WHITE D., HAIDA G.A. & REINHOLD J.G. (1958) *Clin. Chem.* **4**, 189.

WILLIAMS M.W., FRAWLEY J.P., FUYAT H.W. & BLAKE J.R. (1957) *J. Ass. off. agric. chem.* **40**, 4.

WOOTTON I.D.P. (1964) *Micro Analysis in Medical Biochemistry*, 4th Edition, p. 106. London, J. & A. Churchill.

WORDEN A.N. & WATERHOUSE C.E. (1956) *ATA Jl* **7** (3), 64.

WROBLEWSKI F. & LADUE J.S. (1955) *Ann. int. Med.* **43**, 345.

ZILVERSMIT D.B. & DAVIES A.K. (1950) *J. Lab. clin. Med.* **35**, 155.

CHAPTER 13

Haematological Studies During Toxicity Tests

S.R.M. BUSHBY

EFFECTS ON
HAEMOPOIETIC SYSTEM

Toxic effects of drugs on the cellular elements of the blood can be divided into those that affect the circulating cells and those that interfere with the development of these cells. Of the circulating cells it is the erythrocytes that are usually affected whereas interference with development may affect any of the classes of cells of the haemopoietic system.

Blood is the principal transport system of the body and drugs may cause changes in the non-cellular constituents. Except for those that affect coagulation, these changes are usually regarded as secondary and do not fall within the field of haematology. Examples of these secondary changes are alterations in the concentrations of enzymes, urea, and electrolytes and are dealt with elsewhere in this book.

Effects on Erythrocytes

HAEMOLYTIC ANAEMIAS

Toxic effects on the circulating red cells may lead to haemolysis which can occur either intravascularly or extravascularly. Intravascular haemolysis is a relatively rare event in man, except in persons whose red cells are deficient in glucose-6-phosphate dehydrogenase; apart from the latter condition, intravascular haemolysis may result from direct toxic effects on erythrocytes. More commonly the haemolytic process occurs extravascularly due to the red cells being altered by the drug so that they are destroyed by the

338

normal physiological process for removing effete cells, i.e. phago-
cytosis by the cells of the reticulo-endothelial system; the net result
of this type of toxicity is to shorten the normal life-span of the
cells.

With either form of haemolysis, there is usually a compensating
hyperplasia of the erythropoietic tissue and many young red cells,
the reticulocytes, appear in the peripheral blood; if the process is
severe, nucleated red cells may also be present in the circulating
blood. Besides these changes there are usually increases in unconjugated bilirubin in the plasma and of coproporphyrin I in the
faeces. The bilirubin is derived from the haemoglobin of the destroyed cells and the coproporphyrin is a by-product of the compensating increased erythropoiesis; the excretion of coproporphyrin
III may also be increased due to interference with its conversion
to haemoglobin. Hyperplasia of the erythropoietic tissue is also
associated with a raised serum lactic dehydrogenase (Hoffbrand
et al., 1966).

Some intravascular haemolysis occurs normally and the haemoglobin is taken up by serum haptoglobins to be eliminated as bilirubin. When there is increased haemolysis and the haptoglobins
become saturated, some of the free haemoglobin passes through
the kidneys and the remainder dissociates within the circulation
to liberate haem which combines with albumin to form methaemalbumin. The molecule of methaemalbumin is too large to pass
through the kidneys and its presence in the plasma is detectable
by Schumm's test. A fall in the normal concentration of haptoglobins is a sensitive indicator of increased haemolysis but the
concentration can fall through other causes, e.g. in cirrhosis of the
liver (Owen *et al.*, 1959); under these conditions haemoglobinuria
can occur without there being increased haemolysis.

If the increased erythropoiesis which occurs in these haemolytic
conditions cannot compensate for the increased destruction,
anaemia develops.

Toxic effects on the circulating cells may be associated with
changes in the haemoglobin, leading to formation of Heinz bodies
within the cells and to oxidation of the intracorpuscular haemoglobin to methaemoglobin. The presence of methaemoglobin in
blood, as distinct from methaemalbumin which occurs extracorpus-
cularly, is indicative of intracorpuscular changes. Drugs may also
affect red cells during maturation in the bone marrow and lead to

changes in basophilic material of the reticulocyte so that the young cells appear as stippled red cells in a Romanowsky-stained film.

An indirect cause of haemolysis may be changes in the antigenicity of the cells through the action of the drug so that they stimulate the production of autoantibodies; cells sensitized with these antibodies are then destroyed by the reticulo-endothelial system. Sensitization can be detected by the antiglobulin test. This sensitization of cells usually changes their shape so that they are thicker than normal (spherocytosis) and this change lowers their *in vitro* resistance to lysis by hypotonic saline. In man, another indirect cause of haemolysis by drugs is their effect on cells with reduced glucose-6-phosphate dehydrogenase activity; this deficiency is an inherited (X-linked) condition and the normal enzyme is apparently replaced by one of a different structure. This enzyme is responsible for the conversion of glucose-6-phosphate to phosphogluconate and the liberated protons maintain glutathione and nicotinamide adenine dinucleotide phospate in the reduced forms which are apparently essential for integrity of the cells. The role of reduced glutathione may be the reduction of methaemoglobin; it also plays a part in the maintenance of the structure of both the red cell stroma and the globin part of the haemoglobin molecule through influencing the sulphydryl groups of cysteine (Lehmann & Huntsman, 1966). However, the exact connection between the reduced activity of the enzyme, the drug, and the haemolysis is not yet clear as the cells of persons with this type of sensitivity have other biochemical abnormalities (Brewer *et al.*, 1962). Under normal circumstances, the conditions within the defective cells are sufficient to keep glutathione in the reduced state but in the presence of drugs or their metabolites that can act as proton acceptors, the system breaks down. When this happens, oxidative end-products of haemoglobin appears as Heinz bodies within the cells and methaemoglobin accumulates. The deficiency of glucose-6-phosphate dehydrogenase is most marked in older cells; the changes therefore occur in these older cells and lead to a shortening of the average life-span of the cells. The role of the drug in this haemolytic process seems to be merely that of an oxidant.

HYPOPLASTIC AND APLASTIC ANAEMIAS

Haemolytic anaemias are associated with a compensating hyperplasia of the bone marrow and are thus of the regenerative type; when the anaemia is due to interference with the development of the cells, it is of the non-regenerative type. In this latter type of anaemia, there are few if any young red cells present in the circulating blood, the excretion of coproporphyrin I is within or below normal limits, and the erythropoietic tissue is either hypoplastic, consisting mainly of only primitive cells indicating interference with maturation, or aplastic with few or no precursor cells present.

MACROCYTIC ANAEMIAS

In some instances, interference with maturation occurs at the erythroblastic level, so that the cells do not divide to form normoblasts but mature into abnormally large red cells, the macrocytes or megalocytes. This effect is due to blocked synthesis of deoxyribonucleic acid through deficiency of or interference with the metabolism of vitamin B_{12} (cyanocobalamin) or of folic acid. As both these co-enzymes are derived from food or bacterial metabolism within the gut, a drug can interfere with their production, absorption, transportation, or utilization. When this interference occurs the bone marrow contains many erythroblasts showing abnormally large nuclei and polychromatic cytoplasm due to early haemoglobinization; these abnormal cells are termed megaloblasts. Although an increase in the mean diameter of the cells of the peripheral blood is characteristic of this type of anaemia, a more dominant feature is marked anisocytosis, i.e. abnormal variation in cell size. If there is concomitant iron deficiency, the cells tend to be smaller. The effects of interference with B_{12} or folic acid metabolism are not only on the maturation of red cells. Neutrophil leucocytes and their precursors are abnormally large and the former show hypersegmentation; megakaryocytes are also affected, and giant platelets are formed.

Effects on B_{12} metabolism are not confined to the haemopoietic tissue; B_{12} is also essential for normal growth of young animals, the production of the epithelial cells of the gastrointestinal tract, and the maintenance of myelin in the central nervous system. It is also involved in fat and carbohydrate synthesis, the conversion of homo-cysteine to methionine, the persistence of sulphydryl groups, and protein synthesis. Drugs that interfere with metabolism involving B_{12} may therefore have widespread effects.

The aetiology of macrocytic anaemias is further complicated by the enlarged cells having an abnormally short life-span, so that the anaemia has a haemolytic component; in consequence, iron-binding capacity of the plasma is decreased; as the total iron content is increased the bilirubin content of the plasma is raised. Haemosiderin is present in the reticulo-endothelial cells and there is a raised serum lactic dehydrogenase. The thicknesses of large cells are, relative to their diameters, less than normal and in consequence the cells are more resistant to the lytic action of hypotonic saline.

Besides deficiency of B_{12} and folic acid, pyridoxine and related substances are known to be concerned with red cell production; riboflavin and nicotinic acid are probably involved. Thiamine, thymidine, and choline are also intimately concerned with the role of folic acid in erythropoiesis. In thyroid deficiency, there may be anaemia but this is probably an indirect metabolic effect and the cells are not always macrocytic. Toxic effects on the liver may affect red cell production as this organ plays an important part in the production of essential proteins and is the largest store of iron.

HYPOCHROMIC ANAEMIAS

Toxicity may affect haemoglobinization of the red cells; in these circumstances the red cells are low in haemoglobin concentration and stain poorly, i.e. show hypochromia. Although drug interference may occur at any one of the complex stages that lead to haemoglobinization, the commonest failure is due to deficiency of iron. Examples not directly involving iron metabolism are interference within the normoblast involving the synthesis or utilization of protoporphyrin (the non-iron-containing moiety of haem) and deficiencies of first-class proteins or trace metals, e.g. copper and cobalt.

Lead affects haemoglobinization apparently through interference intracorpuscularly with the metabolism of delta-aminolaevulic acid and leads to excessive excretion of this acid in the urine (Haeger-Aronsen, 1960). Copper appears to assist in the incorporation of inorganic iron into haemoglobin but the daily need is extremely low (Cummings & Earl, 1960). Cobalt is also essential for haemoglobin production and its absorption or utilization could be affected; the daily need is even less than that of copper, being 5–8 µg for man.

Iron deficiency can arise through insufficient iron in the diet, interference with absorption from the alimentary tract, failure in transportation to the site of erythropoiesis or ineffective utilization. In adult animals, dietary iron deficiency is not a usual cause of hypochromia except when there is an excessively large demand, as after haemorrhage; this is because iron from effete cells is conserved and re-used. Dietary iron is therefore only necessary to replace incidental losses, which in adult man amount to 0·5–1·0 mg daily (McCance & Widdowson, 1943); during growth, however, the demand for this iron is considerably greater. Dietary iron is absorbed mainly in the ferrous state by the mucosal cells; although its absorption can be influenced by substances that affect the electronic state of the iron or form insoluble complexes, it is uncommon for drugs to cause hypochromic anaemia through interference with absorption.

The conservation of iron is maintained through the action of transferrin, a special iron-binding glyco-β-globulin, present in plasma. Iron, in the ferric form, passes from the mucosal cells into the plasma where it immediately combines with transferrin, and in this form it is carried either to the tissue depots or to the sites of erythropoiesis. The depots are mainly in the liver and spleen and consist of the reticulo-endothelial cells, which also destroy effete red cells and store iron complexed with a protein (apoferritin) as ferritin.

The concentration of transferrin in the plasma represents the iron-binding capacity of the plasma and in man it is normally utilized to the extent of about 33%. This degree of saturation varies physiologically, both diurnally and with sex; for the iron to be readily available for erythropoiesis, there is a minimum degree of the transferrins, which in man is about 30%. When the saturation rises to a critical level, iron is deposited in the tissue depots, especially in those of the liver; when saturation is exceptionally high, as occurs with excessive haemolysis, the ferritin may aggregate to form coarse granules of haemosiderin. In the absence of transferrin, iron is heavily deposited in all tissues except the bone marrow.

Drug-induced hypochromic anaemia can arise not only through interference with the transport of iron but also through interference with its utilization. At the sites of erythropoiesis the ferritin is taken up by reticulum cells and passed to the normoblasts.

Effective haemoglobinization, therefore, depends on properly functioning iron-storing reticulum cells; the refractory or myelophthisic anaemias are apparently due to failure at this stage in the transport of iron.

In simple chronic iron deficiency anaemias, the iron-binding capacity of plasma is usually increased, in spite of a low total iron content. It is also reduced in haemolytic anaemias, in macrocytic anaemia due to B_{12} or folic acid deficiency, and in aplastic anaemias; in these conditions, there is an increase in the total plasma iron and similar changes may also occur in hepatic cirrhosis. When there is a bone marrow block or when there is an increase in iron absorption, as in haemochromatosis, there is marked decrease in the unsaturated iron-binding capacity and the total plasma iron is increased. Determinations of the iron-binding capacity and the total content of the plasma therefore help to identify the site of toxic action of drugs causing anaemia, and further useful information can be obtained by measuring the rate at which ^{59}Fe is removed from the plasma and incorporated into the red cells after the intravenous injection of autogenous plasma which has been incubated with the radioactive iron; with depression of erythropoiesis, there is an abnormal delay in disappearance of radioactive iron from the plasma. The ferrioxamine test is another useful means of detecting iron deficiency, as it enables a deficiency to be discerned before anaemia develops.

Effects on Leucocytes

Depression of leucopoiesis is the commonest toxic action of drugs on leucocytes, but a rise in the number of circulating neutrophils may occur; it has been noted with a variety of drugs, e.g. salicylates, quinine, phenyl hydrazine, antipyrine, phenacetin, salvarsan, and benzol derivatives. Apart from mitotic poisons which interfere with leucopoiesis, idiosyncrasy in man seems to be a greater danger than toxicity attributable to the action of a drug. Leucopenia may be secondary to toxic changes in other organs, e.g. in uraemia (Jensson, 1958).

Neutrophilia, without toxic effects on leucopoiesis, is usually associated with changes in the appearances of the circulating cells due to the out-pouring of young cells. The nuclei of these cells are less segmented than those of older cells and show little or no condensation of the chromatin; they are larger than normal mature neutrophils and may be unsegmented (the 'juvenile' cells of Schilling). When there is toxic depression of leucopoiesis, the circulating neutrophils show abnormal maturation; instead of the nuclei developing from the juvenile to the normal multi-lobed mature form, with condensed chromatin and lobes connected together by fine threads of chromatin, the nuclei show little or no segmentation although the chromatin is condensed. The nuclei of these abnormal cells often remain as a band and if lobes do form they remain connected by relatively broad bands of chromatin; these cells are the 'stab' cells of Schilling. In addition to these nuclear changes, they are smaller than 'juvenile' cells and often contain many basophilic granules, i.e. show toxic granulation. B_{12} and folic acid deficiencies may also affect the morphology of neutrophils (p. 341).

Except for the lymphopenia that occurs with drugs that interfere with cell division and usually cause pancytopenia, lymphocytes are not often affected. However, lymphopenia does occur with increase of adrenocortico-steroid excretion and it may occur in uraemia.

Reduction in the number of circulating eosinophils can also occur as a secondary effect to adrenocortical stimulation. Eosinophilia may occur under conditions associated with histamine release.

Haemorrhagic Disorders

Basically these disorders arise through failure to prevent loss of blood from the blood vessels. The arrest of haemorrhage is complex; the degree of complexity depends on whether the leakage is from capillaries following minor injury, as occurs in purpura, from superficial cuts, or from relatively large vessels. Leakage from capillaries is due to defective endothelium or platelets failing to form plugs through being reduced in number or changed in adhesiveness. Arrest of bleeding from ruptured or cut capillaries depends primarily on the ability of platelets to form plugs and possibly to release the vaso-constricting substance, serotonin, but ultimately on coagulation of the blood.

PLATELETS

The number of platelets must be considerably reduced before there is clinical evidence of defects in their functions. Being derived from the megakaryocytes, their numbers in the circulation are reduced by drugs that suppress the multiplication of marrow cells, and thrombocytopenia can often be the first evidence of toxic effects on haemopoiesis. Thrombocytopenia can, however, occur without a decrease in the number of megakaryocytes in the marrow, and the cause is usually attributed to inhibition of platelet formation by a splenic factor. Although it is theoretically possible for drugs to produce thrombocytopenia by such a mechanism, a more likely cause of thrombocytopenia, without reduction in megakaryocytes, is through the drug behaving as a haptene. In these circumstances, the drug may form a drug-platelet complex which is antigenic, and the resulting autoantibodies combine with the sensitized platelets causing clumping and lysis (Schen & Rabinovitz, 1958). Complement is necessary for these changes to be demonstrated *in vitro* (Ackroyd, 1962).

Platelets are also essential for the contraction of blood clots, which is a vital step in the effective arrest of haemorrhage.

COAGULATION

Although coagulation of blood depends on the rapid conversion of prothrombin to thrombin, which enzymatically converts fibrinogen to fibrin, thrombin formation is a highly complex process which involves, as MacFarlane so aptly states, 'a cascade of proenzyme transformations' (MacFarlane, 1964). Opinions vary as to the precise role of the various factors involved and it is not pertinent to the present discussion to consider them in detail. However, including the initial step, which involves contact between normal platelets and a surface other than the normal vascular endothelium, it is theoretically possible for drugs to affect each of the factors and so modify coagulation; eight factors are involved in clotting and modification of any would lead to defective clotting.

Coagulation defects from drug toxicity can be secondary to effects on other systems. At least five of the factors are derived from the liver and their concentrations in plasma can be reduced with liver disease; these factors are fibrinogen, prothrombin, proconvertin (Factor VII), plasma thromboplastin component (factor IX), and Stuart-Power factor (factor X). Vitamin K is the precursor of prothrombin and conditions which affect its absorption may lead to prothrombin deficiency. Calcium is essential for clotting and its concentration in the ionic form can be indirectly affected by drugs.

Sedimentation of Red Cells

An increase in the rate at which red cells settle in plasma is often used as a non-specific test for evidence of organic disease as distinct from functional disease. An increase in sedimentation rate during toxicity testing of drugs may be regarded as evidence of an organic change.

The rate at which the cells settle depends on their concentration and on the extent that they form rouleaux, i.e. aggregate in an orderly fashion with their concave, flattened sides adjacent. Excessive rouleaux formation is generally due to increased concentrations of fibrinogen and cholesterol and may also occur with increased concentrations of globulins; decreased formation occurs in association with falls in the concentration of albumin, nucleoprotein, or lecithin. In toxicity studies of drugs, an increase in rouleaux formation, without an obvious cause, should be regarded as an indication for more extensive investigation.

Blood Volume

The quantity of blood in the circulation and in the splenic reservoir does not vary greatly under normal physiological conditions. In pregnancy there is a relatively greater increase in plasma than in cells and this produces an apparent anaemia. Changes can, however, occur with a variety of pathological conditions; the volume may be increased in nephrosis, diabetes, cirrhosis of the liver, hyperthyroidism, and protein deficiency, and it may decrease with glomerular nephritis. Because the fluid and cellular constituents are not altered proportionally, these changes can cause apparent polycythaemia or anaemia, and for these reasons estimations of haemoglobin concentration in anaemic conditions may not reveal the real deficiency of total haemoglobin.

HAEMATOLOGICAL INVESTIGATIONS

The foregoing account summarizes the principal haematological changes that may occur in man as side-effects from drug therapy and the majority of these changes should be predictable from animal experiments. The circumstances under which these changes are sought in animals, however, differs greatly from those in man; in toxicity tests in animals, the drugs are administered in relatively large doses for prolonged periods in order that any changes may become pronounced and therefore detectable by a few relatively simple tests, whereas in man, during the clinical trial stages of a drug, the choice of tests should aim at detecting early changes, which usually requires extensive and more complicated methods.

In practice, the essential haematological investigations to be performed during sub-acute and chronic tests are those that enable anaemia and alterations in leucocytes and platelets to be detected. If changes are detected, further observations aimed at elucidating the direct cause should be undertaken. Measurement of the sedimentation rate of the red cells is valuable in helping to exclude organic changes, but investigations of effects on clotting mechanisms are probably unnecessary except when there are clinical signs of haemorrhagic disease.

The haematological studies may therefore be divided into two categories; those that are essential for detecting damage, and those that may throw light on the probable site of action when damage is revealed. Some investigations of the second category, however, will rarely be used in toxicity tests for they have been primarily developed for diagnostic use in man, aimed at detecting deficiencies before the development of clinical signs or symptoms or for identifying the biochemical site of injury; in Table 13.1, in which these categories are summarized, the investigations are divided into three groups. The exact status of some of the various investigations is obviously a matter of opinion; for example, some tests used in the investigation of haemorrhagic disorders are performed routinely by certain investigators and would therefore be included by them in group I. Chart 13.1 shows a sequential development in the application of these tests.

There are no standard techniques for these investigations but this is no handicap provided that the chosen methods give reproducible results and that untreated animals are always included as controls in the studies. Technique must be applicable to the size of the animal and this may necessitate using micro-methods, but in practice they do not differ essentially from those described in standard haematological text books to which the reader is referred

aematological values.[a]

Leuco-cytes	Neutro-phils	Eosino-phils	Basophils	Lympho-cytes	Mono-cytes	Platelets	No. of animal
11·6 5·0–27·2	7·5 3·0–18·7	0·52 0·12–2·25	0·01 —	2·8 0·8–9·0	0·53 0·20–1·42	323 106–986	40
12·8 5·3–30·8	8·7 3·3–23·1	0·57 0·03–1·16	0·01 —	2·4 0·5–10·9	0·57 0·18–1·83	357 153–833	51
6·9 2·7–18·0	1·7 0·6–4·5	0·08 0·01–2·98	0·01 —	4·4 1·4–13·7	0·46 0·12–1·71	522 277–988	130
7·2 3·1–17·0	1·7 0·7–4·4	0·15 0·01–1·47	0·01 —	4·6 1·8–11·7	0·50 0·2–1·3	501 210–1197	61
4·7 1·7–13·0	1·6 0·5–5·6	0·15 0·10–1·3	0·01 —	2·4 0·8–7·5	0·30 0·08–1·2	633 391–1024	73
12·7 4·2–38·1	6·9 1·5–32·7	0·46 0·04–5·97	0·01 —	4·0 1·2–13·0	0·62 0·17–2·26	440 203–951	111
14·8 6·6–33·0	8·7 3·4–22·2	0·40 0·01–10·2	0·01 —	4·4 1·8–11·2	0·70 0·20–2·1	412 191–890	60
8·3 3·5–20·0	3·4 0·7–16·5	0·16 0·01–5·72	0·01 —	3·8 1·6–9·1	0·49 0·11–2·21	264 63–1122	25
9·0 4·5–18·1	3·2 0·8–12·2	0·46 0·07–3·16	0·02 0·01–2·08	4·3 1·8–10·4	0·41 0·01–1·84	323 165–635	10
16·5 7·9–34·7	9·5 3·2–28·4	1·0 0·10–10·5	0·01 —	4·5 1·9–10·2	0·56 0·11–0·30	371 157–876	114
8·0 4·0–12·0	2·0 0·7–4·0	0·15 0·0–0·5	0·05 0·0–0·10	5·5 3·0–8·5	0·30 0·0–1·3	278 246–339	
10·0 7·0–19·0	4·2 2·0–7·0	0·4 0·2–1·3	0·07 0·0–0·30	4·9 3·0–9·0	0·43 0·3–2·0	783 525–900	

alculated from results obtained in the author's laboratory. The mean values are the
alues for mice and guinea pigs were taken from data published by Spector (1956).

for technical details.* Table 13.2 shows the mean values and their p95 limits observed in the author's laboratory for the parameters commonly used in detecting damage to the haemopoietic system; these values are similar to those by Wintrobe (1961), Spector (1956), and Schermer (1967), who have each consolidated the results of several investigators. The table shows that there are wide variations among the individual animals; this is especially so with the total leucocytes of the rat and the mean value given in the table is somewhat lower than that usually reported but it is well within the range. The results reported by Schermer are included in a monograph entitled 'Blood Morphology of Laboratory Animals' and this work is particularly valuable because in it the peculiarities of the various animals are discussed.

The remainder of this chapter is confined to a general discussion of various haematological tests that are useful in toxicity studies.

Collection of Blood

With few exceptions, unclotted samples of blood are required for haematological investigations and sequestrin is a suitable and convenient anticoagulant; used at the correct concentration, it does not affect the size of the red cells or cause clumping of leucocytes or platelets. The di-potassium salt of ethylenediamine tetra-acetic acid (EDTA) is a convenient form and it should be used at a concentration of 4 mg/2 ml of blood. This quantity can readily be obtained by drying 0·1 ml of a 4% aqueous solution in a suitable tube at 80°C.

The blood can be taken from a convenient vein and added directly to the tube containing EDTA and, although this anticoagulant has little effect on the morphology of leucocytes, films of the fresh blood are preferably made directly from the syringe if detection of subtle changes in morphology are considered necessary; EDTA can affect the appearances of the nuclei of lymphocytes and monocytes. Unless a rapid flow of blood can be obtained from a vein, the blood should be taken by heart puncture; in the case of small animals, the methods should be adapted to the volume of blood obtainable from individual animals rather than to use pooled samples of blood from each dose group. Convenient veins are the jugular, ulnar, or saphenous of the dog and the

---

* See References for recommended books.

femoral vein in the inguinal region of the monkey. The venous plexus of the ocular orbit, using the simple procedure described by Halpern and Pecaud (1951) and by Riley (1960), is convenient for obtaining blood from rats and mice.

Detection of Anaemia

Anaemia implies a fall in the haemoglobin content of blood. Although theoretically this can occur without a fall in the number of red cells, it is rare in practice for changes in the haemoglobin, red cells, and packed cell volume to occur independently. Therefore, for the exclusion of anaemia, it is usually unnecessary to determine more than one of these values, and that of the haemoglobin is the simplest and most accurate. However, when changes occur, information will be required regarding the haemoglobin content and size of the red cells, and unless these values have been ascertained, the whole toxicity test may have to be repeated.

Changes in packed cell volume (PCV) are due to alterations in the number of the cells and/or their size. Although unlikely, in the initial stages an increase in size could balance a reduction in number so that a fall in the red cell count would not be shown by a lowered PCV. However, if the duration of the experiment is sufficiently long, the effects on red cell formation will become apparent from the haematocrit readings. In practice, therefore, decreases in the number of red cells are detectable either by red cell counts or PCV determinations.

The number of red cells can be determined by direct counting in a haemocytometer after making a suitable dilution, e.g. 1:200 in a Thoma pipette or preferably in an automatic Trenner pipette. However, because only relatively few cells are counted, the variation due to random distribution, personal bias in counting, and uneven flow when filling the chamber, can be as much as 0·8 million with a red cell count of 5 million per mm³. This large variation is based on statistical analysis ($+2\sigma$) and applies to the counting of the cells in 80 small squares with 1:200 dilution (Magath *et al.*, 1936; Biggs & Macmillan, 1948; Hynes, 1947–8). The use of an electronic counter increases precision, but as it still entails careful mixing and diluting of the blood, significant errors can arise from faulty technique. The determination of the PCV is simple and less prone to technical error than enumeration of

the cells; in practice, therefore, it is preferable to rely on haematocrit readings and haemoglobin determinations for excluding
anaemia.

As changes in the PCV do not necessarily parallel changes in
the red cell count, through alterations in cell size, and as these
latter changes may indicate the stage of erythropoiesis on which
the drug is acting, cell size should be examined. Critical inspection
of the stained film is usually adequate for detecting macrocytosis
and thus avoiding a relatively small fall in the PCV being mis-
interpreted. If there is a doubtful change in cell size this can be
confirmed only by direct measurements with either a microscope
micrometer scale or preferably by means of a projection microscope; a rapid method for direct measurement of red cells is that
described by Hynes & Martin (1936). Calculation of the mean
corpuscular volume by dividing the packed cell volume by the
total number of red cells is of little value with questionable macrocytosis because of the inaccuracies of the red cell count.

The method used for estimating haemoglobin content is not important provided that it gives reproducible results. However, a
standard procedure is preferable and the cyanmethaemoglobin
method is recommended; estimations by this method include the
concentration of normal oxy- and reduced haemoglobin and
methaemoglobin. The concentration can be measured by direct
vision or spectrophotometrically.

The main advantage of the cyanmethaemoglobin method lies in
the high stability of this haemoglobin derivative so that it can be
used as the reference standard. The standard can be obtained
either from commercial sources or prepared in the laboratory. The
only disadvantage of the method is the use of sodium cyanide but
at the strength that it is used in the diluent, there is no risk of
inadvertent poisoning (Wootton, 1964a).

In iron deficiency anaemias, red cells are not fully saturated
with haemoglobin and calculation of the concentration of haemoglobin per unit volume is therefore valuable. The concentration is
usually expressed as the mean corpuscular haemoglobin concentration (MCHC) and is calculated by dividing the haemoglobin in
grams per 100 ml by the volume of packed cells from 100 ml of
blood. Cells that are not saturated with haemoglobin are hypochromic and in stained films their centres are paler than normal; in

severe hypochromic anaemias the cells may appear mainly as pale rings.

Less informative than the MCHC is the mean corpuscular haemoglobin (MCH). This value is expressed in $\mu\mu g$ and it is calculated by dividing the haemoglobin content of a unit volume of blood by the number of red cells present in that volume. Because cells cannot be super-saturated with haemoglobin, a rise in MCH is indicative of macrocytosis; the converse is, however, not true, for a low MCH can occur in macrocytic hypochromic anaemias.

An increase in the number of circulating reticulocytes and the appearance of nucleated red cells in the peripheral blood occurs under a variety of conditions of bone marrow stress, especially in haemolytic anaemias. Abnormal forms of red cells, e.g. variation in size (anisocytosis) and irregular shapes (poikilocytosis) may also occur and their presence should be noted when examining stained films. The nucleated red cells, which should be identified as normablasts, erythroblasts, or megaloblasts, are usually expressed as a percentage of the number of leucocytes and are conveniently noted during the differential leucocyte count.

RETICULOCYTES

The number of circulating reticulocytes is a sensitive indicator of erythropoietic activity. These cells are a little larger than the normal red cell and usually appear as purple stained cells (polychromasia) in Romanowsky stained films. In some toxic conditions, e.g. lead poisoning, the basophilic material which gives the cell its purple hue may be condensed into granules to give stippling or punctuate basophilia.

A more sensitive method of demonstrating these cells is by staining supravitally with brilliant cresyl blue, when the basophilic material appears as a reticulum. The simplest procedure is to prepare charged coverslips with the dye by spreading an 0·3% alcoholic solution of the dye over one surface and when dry to polish to remove any excess dye by lightly rubbing on a piece of smooth paper. A very small drop of blood, which can be taken from a sequestrin sample, is placed on the charged surface of the coverslip and a second similarly charged coverslip is then placed diagonally across the first. After about one minute the coverslips are gently pulled apart to make even smears of the blood. The films are counterstained with any Romanowsky stain, and the number of reticulocytes counted as a percentage of the total number of red cells. The charged coverslips will keep indefinitely. An alternative method consists of mixing on a slide one drop of a freshly prepared saturated solution of the dye in saline with one drop of blood. The mixing is done with a glass rod, and the mixture is then spread as a film by the usual method. Any Romanowsky stain is suitable as a counterstain.

HEINZ BODIES

These inclusions can readily be seen in wet preparations of red cells either by direct examination under phase-contrast microscopy, when the bodies appear as highly refractile particles about $1-2\mu$ in diameter, or after staining by mixing equal volumes of blood with 0·5% methyl-violet in normal saline when the bodies are pale purple. They also stain feebly, with brilliant cresyl blue and so appear as pale blue bodies in well-stained reticulocyte preparations.

OSMOTIC FRAGILITY TEST

Red cells swell in sypotonic saline. The thinner the cell, relative to its diameter, the greater is its resistance to lysis. In practice, changes in osmotic fragility are measured by suspending the cells in decreasing concentrations of sodium chloride ranging from 0·7 to 0·1%. The percentage of haemolysis that occurs in each concentration is recorded and plotted graphically against the results with control normal red cells. Alternatively, the results can be recorded as the concentration of sodium chloride in which 50% of the cells lyse, but because only a small proportion of the cells may show increased fragility, the results are more informative when shown graphically. Cells that contain oxy-haemoglobin are less fragile than those containing reduced haemoglobin; therefore in fragility tests the cells should be fully oxygenated. Also, as changes in pH can affect lysis, it is better to use whole blood rather than washed red cells, to take advantage of the buffering action of the plasma protein; alternatively, a buffer solution, osmotically equivalent to the sodium chloride can be used, e.g. NaCl 180 g, Na_2HPO_4 27·31 g, $NaH_2PO_42H_2O$ 4·86 g/2,000 ml corresponds to 10% sodium chloride.

Cells of different animal species vary in diameter-thickness ratios, and comparison with cells of untreated animals is therefore essential.

LIFE-SPAN OF RED CELLS

The most satisfactory method of measuring alterations in the life-span of red cells is by labelling some of the cells with ^{51}Cr. Blood is taken from the subject into sodium citrate and after removing most of the plasma, radioactive sodium chromate is added. The cells are left at room temperature for 30 min, washed thoroughly in saline, and reinjected intravenously into the same subject. At intervals, samples of blood are withdrawn and the rate of disappearance of the radioactivity measured (Weinstein & LeRoy, 1953; Mollison & Veal, 1955).

SEDIMENTATION RATE

Although the sedimentation rate can be measured in the Wintrobe haematocrit tube after standing vertically for 1 hour, changes in the rate are exaggerated if blood is diluted with sodium citrate solution as used in the Westergren method; in this method, one part of 3·8% trisodium citrate solution is added to nine parts of blood. In human studies, the Wintrobe method has the advantage that allowances can be made for the effects of anaemia by reference to correlation charts (Wintrobe & Landsberg, 1935; Hynes & Whitby, 1938); although similar charts are not available specifically for animals, those for man probably apply equally well.

AUTOANTIBODIES

These antibodies are the result of an allergic autoimmune response and they are usually present in the circulation united with the red cell. They are therefore detectable only by the direct antiglobulin test; in this test the globulin-coated cells agglutinate when they are suspended in antiglobulin serum. It is essential that the antiserum be derived from an animal immunized with globulin homologous with the species of the animal in which the toxicity test is made, i.e. when the drug is administered to dogs, the serum used in the test must be anti-dog globulin.

The antiglobulin test is extremely sensitive and its performance requires particular attention to detail at every stage, the most important details being the removal of all free globulin from the cells and the cleanliness of glassware.

In practice, this test will rarely be required in toxicity testing for the development of autoantibodies depends on the idiosyncrasy of an individual animal.

BILIRUBINAEMIA

Because bilirubin is the breakdown product of haemoglobin, excessive intravascular or extravascular haemolysis leads to a rise in the unconjugated form in the plasma and this can readily be detected and measured by the indirect van den Berg reaction. A micro-method suitable for animal investigations has been described by Wootton (1964b).

An increase in the intensity of the colour of the plasma is an indication of bilirubinaemia. Although this can be measured as the Icterus Index by comparing the colour with that of 1 : 10,000 aqueous solution of potassium dichromate, it is preferable in practice merely to note the colour of the plasma in the haematocrit tube and if the intensity is increased, to perform a van den Berg reaction which will indicate whether the jaundice is hepatic or haemolytic in origin.

PORPHYRINS

During the synthesis of porphyrin III for the formation of haemoglobin, coproporphyrin I is produced (apparently as a by-product) and excreted in the bile, urine, and faeces.

Although the detection of porphyrins in urine is a simple procedure, the identification and quantitative estimation of the isomers I and III depend on fluorometric analysis after chromatographic separation (Schwartz *et al.*, 1947). The method is involved and is rarely justified in toxicity tests solely to acquire evidence of excessive erythropoiesis or interference with conversion of porphyrin III to haemoglobin.

HAEMOGLOBINAEMIA

The amount of free haemoglobin in plasma can be measured by the micro-benzidine method of Crosby & Furth (1956), but special care is necessary during the taking of the sample of blood in order to avoid any spontaneous lysis.

ABNORMAL HAEMOGLOBIN

Methaemoglobin, which is normally present in concentrations of less than 1%, can be detected in concentrations of 5% or more by direct vision spectroscopy but only if the cells are lysed and examined in concentrations sufficiently high to allow only the orange-red part of the spectrum to be transmitted. Under these conditions, an absorption band of this part of the spectrum at 6,3000 Å indicates the presence of methaemoglobin and this band should disappear if a suitable reducing agent, e.g. sodium hydrosulphite, is added. Persistence of the band indicates that it is due to the presence of sulphaemoglobin. A quantitative method is that of Evelyn & Malloy (1938). This method requires the use of a spectrophotometer; it depends on measuring absorption at 635 mμ before and after the addition of sodium cyanide and it will detect a concentration as low as 1%.

Methaemalbumin, which indicates intravascular haemolysis, can be detected by Schumm's method in which 9 volumes of serum is overlaid with ether, 1 volume of a saturated solution of ammonium sulphide is added, and after thorough mixing the serum is examined spectroscopically for an absorption band at 558 mμ.

GLUCOSE-6-PHOSPHATE DEHYDROGENASE

Although the haemolytic anaemia that develops in patients whose red cells are deficient in glucose-6-phosphate dehydrogenase (G-6-PD) and who are treated with oxidizing drugs such as primaquine, is undoubtedly related to low enzymatic activity, there is little that at present can be done to forecast which drugs will produce this effect in man. Brewer's methaemoglobin reduction test, in which methaemoglobin remaining in red cells is measured after three hours' incubation with sodium nitrite and methylene blue, detects G-6-PD deficiency in man but the results of this test in animals show no correlation with G-6-PD activity; sheep cells are particularly low in G-6-PD activity but show high activity in this dye test (Salvidio *et al.*, 1963) and they are not particularly sensitive to primaquine. There is, therefore, no justification for choosing a particular animal for forecasting effects of drugs in persons deficient in G-6-PD. Also, primaquine induces methaemoglobinaemia more readily in dogs than in other animals but this difference is probably related to the low catalase activity of dog red cells (Allison, 1957).

Probably any drug which acts as an oxidant should be regarded as a potential inducer of haemolytic anaemia in persons deficient in G-6-PD. Primaquine and one of its metabolites have been shown

13—M.I.T.

by Brodie & Undenfriend (1950) to produce methaemoglobin when incubated with red cells and this observation can perhaps form a basis of a test; the results will need careful control as methaemoglobin forms in normal blood when it is incubated *in vitro* even without an oxidant.

An alternative basis for a screening test could be the increased oxidation of glucose through the pentose pathway which occurs in normal red cells when in the presence of most of the drugs known to produce haemolytic anaemia in G-6-PD deficient persons (De Loecker & Prankerd, 1961; Szeinberg & Marks, 1961). When red cells are incubated in the presence of these drugs, Heinz bodies form but this effect is less specific than the increased oxidation of glucose.

Effects on Leucocytes

Although gross changes in the number of leucocytes can be detected by inspection of stained films, variations can be followed only by direct counting. As with the red cells, this can be done by counting in haemocytometers or by electronic methods. With either method the sources of error are the same as with the red cell counts, but physiological variations are greater; time after feeding is a principal cause of variation, so it is important that the taking of samples of blood should be strictly comparable in the treated and untreated animals.

Changes in the proportions of the different types of normal leucocytes and the presence of primitive leucocytes can only be detected in films, preferably stained by a Romanowsky stain. These cells are counted as a percentage of the total number of leucocytes, but as the figures are much more informative when converted to absolute figures from the total leucocyte count, this procedure should always be followed; it avoids the need for the conception of relative changes in one of the leucocytic components, e.g. relative lymphocytosis.

Apart from those that occur during infections, changes in the number of lobes of neutrophils can give indications of abnormal maturation due to toxic effects and interference with utilization of B_{12} or folic acid; these effects are shown, respectively, by abnormal segmentation and hyper-segmentation. They can be noted during the making of differential counts or more quantitatively by performing either an Arneth-Cooke count or a Schilling count; the former is based solely on the number of lobes separated by a fine strain of chromatin and the latter places more emphasis on the size of the cell and the nuclear structure.

PLATELETS

Changes in platelets can be qualitative or quantitative. Gross quantitative changes are readily detected in stained films and as physiological changes occur rapidly this examination is often adequate. However, absolute numbers are generally preferred and these can be determined with blood containing EDTA which prevents clumping. The number can be determined by counting in a haemocytometer after lysing the red cells as in Kristenson's method (Lempert, 1935). Platelets can also be counted electronically, but technical difficulties are often encountered because of their small size.

Platelets contain factors involved in the formation of thrombin and in order to reveal changes in these factors, resort may have to be made to the complicated thromboplastin generation test (Biggs & Douglas, 1953). Liberation of these factors and thrombus formation depends on the adhesion of platelets to surfaces other than the normal endothelium of blood vessels, and changes in adhesiveness can be measured by counting the number of platelets in platelet-rich plasma before and after exposure to a water-wettable surface, e.g. glass (Payling-Wright, 1941) or, in the presence of adenosine diphosphate, to a non-wettable surface, e.g. polystyrene (Eastham, 1964), or more simply by observing the clumps of platelets present in stained smears prepared from fresh blood without an anticoagulant. With the latter method, if groups of three or more platelets occur frequently, it can be assumed that the adhesive function is reasonably normal.

The animals undergoing test should be inspected for evidence of easy bruising or petechiae, which may indicate platelet deficiency or capillary abnormality. If there is doubt, confirmatory evidence should be obtained by applying a tourniquet to a shaven limb or by using the suction method of Elliott (1938), suitably modified for the particular animal; by either of these methods typical petechiae form when platelet deficiency or capillary abnormality exists.

Haemorrhagic Disorders

In routine chronic toxicity testing it is not feasible to test for alterations of each of the factors involved in haemorrhagic disorders. In practice, it is probably sufficient to rely on clinical observations and, when changes are suspected, to determine the prothrombin time and the partial thromboplastin time; changes in the number of platelets will usually be detected in the routine counts.

A normal prothrombin time will indicate that there is no defect in factors I (fibrinogen), II, V, VII, X, XI, and XII. This is a simple test requiring only oxalated or citrated plasma from the test animal and a solution of calcium chloride and dehydrated brain as a source of tissue thromboplastin (Quick, 1957); rabbit brain is generally used, but brain from any species is satisfactory.

The partial thromboplastin time test differs from the prothrombin time test in using 'partial' thromboplastin which requires, in addition to the factors needed for a normal prothrombin time estimation, factors VIII and IX. The original partial thromboplastin was either cephalin, Russell viper venom, or platelets (Langdell et al., 1953), but there is now available a commercial product, Thrombofax (Nye et al., 1962). Some investigators prefer to treat the test plasma with kaolin before adding the partial thromboplastin and the calcium. This treatment activates factors XI and XII, and it is claimed to improve the uniformity of the test especially when identifying deficiencies of the haemopoietic factors XIII and IX (Nye et al., 1962; Matchett et al., 1965). In toxicity investigations the partial thromboplastin test could most profitably be done with or without kaolin activation. The partial thromboplastin time test also differs from the prothrombin time test in being unaffected by the deficiencies of factors VII.

Normal times recorded by these two tests will exclude defects in factors I, II, V, VII, VIII, IX, X, XI, and XII; the tests therefore cover all likely clotting errors except changes in the platelets. The deficient factor causing abnormalities in these tests can be identified by demonstrating the inability of the affected plasma to correct known deficient plasma.

Blood normally contains coagulation inhibitors, antithrombins; the proper functioning of the clotting mechanism depends on a delicate balance between these factors and those involved in the formation of fibrin. Excess of antithrombins occurs in some pathological conditions, and they can usually be identified by the ability of a minute amount of the abnormal blood or plasma when added to normal blood or plasma to prolong a coagulation time, prothrombin time, or partial thromboplastin time. The proportion of abnormal blood added to the normal blood should be approximately 1 : 10.

If there is evidence of bruising and delay in clotting, coagulation time should also be determined. Although prolongation in this test is usually due to deficiencies of factors VIII and IX, it can also be due to reduced prothrombin (factor II) or fibrinogen (factor I), and to probably any of the other factors, except factor VII, provided the reduction is gross. Several methods have been described for measuring coagulation time; they all involve determining the time that freshly withdrawn blood takes to clot. Two methods, simple in practice, are those of Lee & White (1913) and Dale & Laidlaw (1911–12); the former method employs a tube of 8 mm and the latter a capillary tube containing a small movable lead shot. As with all methods used for this purpose, reliable results are obtained only by careful attention to detail.

The ability of a blood clot to retract should also be noted. This can be done qualitatively by merely observing the amount of serum that exudes from the contracted clot in the Lee & White coagulation tube, 1 hour after coagulation has occurred, or quantitatively by measuring the amount of serum exuded. The simplest procedure for this quantitative estimation is to allow the blood to clot around a glass rod so that the coagulum may be removed after 1 hour at 37°C from the time of clotting, and the volume of serum then measured (MacFarlane, 1939).

Proper retraction depends on an adequate number of platelets, but the amount of serum exuded depends also on the fibrinogen content and on the size of the red cell mass.

EXAMINATION OF BONE MARROW

In man, examination of bone marrow during life is often of diagnostic value but this is seldom justified in animals during toxicity testing because marrow can readily be obtained at autopsy. If examination of biopsy material is undertaken sections will be more informative than smears although both should be employed because they reveal the architecture and cellularity of the tissue although abnormal cells will be more easily recognized in smears.

Biopsy is feasible only with the larger animals, e.g. dogs and monkeys. Tissue can be removed by trephining or by needle. Although better sections are obtained from the trephined marrow and impression smears can be readily made from this tissue by pressing the marrow onto slides, needle biopsy is simpler and usually adequate. With the animals under general anaesthesia, marrow can be collected from the iliac crest or from the tibia by using the needles developed for marrow aspiration of human infants. Smears should be made immediately after collection by placing a few drops of the aspirate on a slide and then with a capillary pipette carefully withdrawing fluid blood so as to leave behind as many solid particles of marrow tissue as possible. From these particles, smears can be spread over a small area by means of a second slide; after fixation with methanol and washing in ether to remove fat, the smears are stained with a Romanowsky stain. Histological examinations can be made on particles of marrow from the aspirate, collected after addition of heparin. Collection is aided by centrifuging at 1,500 rev/min and then collecting the buffy layer. The tissue may be fixed and processed by any suitable procedure, e.g. that described by Clayden (1962).

Interpretation of changes in the marrow requires recognition of the different types of cells and knowledge of their normal proportions within the marrow.

IRON METABOLISM

Except perhaps for the differential ferrioxamine test, investigations of iron metabolism are of little value in toxicity tests except for elucidating the mechanism by which a drug interferes with haemoglobinization. The ferrioxamine test measures the iron stores as ferritin-haemosiderin and also the iron newly released from haemoglobin (Fielding, 1965); the test is of prognostic value, for according to Fielding *et al.* (1965) depletion of iron stores can occur without detectable anaemia.

The ferrioxamine test consists of injecting intravenously desferrioxamine methanesulphonate together with ferrioxamine labelled with 2 μC ^{59}Fe, and then collecting a single 6 hour specimen of urine. Two values are measured: (1) the excreted ferrioxamine, derived from body iron by chelation with the desferrioxamine (F_t), which can be estimated chemically; and (2) the proportion of injected ferrioxamine (F_{ex}) which can be estimated radiologically. From these data, chelation *in vivo* is calculated from F_t/F_{ex}, which in iron deficiency approaches zero. Much of the isotope is excreted within 3 days and the test may therefore be repeated as desired.

SERUM IRON

The serum iron can be estimated spectrophotometrically after its liberation from transferrin, using o-phenanthroline in the presence of sodium hydrosulphite (Davies *et al.*, 1952) or tripyridyl in the presence of ascorbic acid (Wootton, 1964c). Normal serum iron in man is in the range of 60–220 µg/100 ml, and this wide variation is not entirely dependent on the time of day or taking of food; information on levels in animals is scanty.

SERUM IRON-BINDING CAPACITY

The iron-binding capacity of serum can be estimated by the methods of Davies *et al.* (1952) or Ramsey (1957) in which excess iron, sufficient to saturate the transferrin, is added to the serum, the unbound iron being then removed and the bound iron estimated as for total iron.

Williams & Conrad (1966) have described a one-tube method for measuring serum iron concentration and unsaturated iron-binding capacity. In this method, iron is released from transferrin in acid solution and chelated to a chromogen which binds iron only between pH values of 2 and 5. After measuring the intensity of the colour, the mixture is made alkaline, which permits the iron to recombine with transferrin, and excess iron is added. The surplus unbound iron is estimated by complexing it with a chromogen which reacts in alkaline conditions.

UTILIZATION OF RADIOACTIVE IRON

Rubin *et al.* (1960) described a simple procedure using radioactive iron which is claimed to permit early detection of erythropoietic damage. The method entails measuring the rate of disappearance of ^{59}Fe from plasma and the rate of appearance of radioactivity in the circulating red cells. A decrease in the rate at which the radioactivity disappears from the plasma, associated with delay in its appearance in the red cells, will indicate erythropoietic depression.

SIDEROCYTES

Siderocytes are red cells containing small granules that give a prussian blue reaction. Their absence from the marrow is probably a more reliable indication of iron deficiency than a change in total serum iron (Beutler *et al.*, 1958).

The cells are readily demonstrated by immersing methanol-fixed films in a freshly prepared mixture of equal parts 0.2 N HC1 and 2% potassium ferrocyanide for 5 min and then counterstaining with 0.1% eosin.

HAPTOGLOBINS

A decrease in the concentration of serum haptoglobins is a sensitive test for increased intravascular haemolysis. The concentrations can be measured electrophoretically on filter paper, cellulose acetate, or agar gel, advantage being taken of the differences in mobility of free and haptoglobin-combined haemoglobin. Known quantities of haemoglobin are added to the serum in order to determine the amount necessary to saturate the haptoglobins (Herman, 1961; Brus & Lewis, 1959; Rowe, 1961; Owen *et al.*, 1960).

FOLIC ACID AND B_{12} DEFICIENCIES

Although the mechanism is unknown, rises in serum lactate dehydrogenase have been observed in a variety of anaemias but especially in those caused by folic acid or B_{12} deficiency (Hoftbrand *et al.*, 1966); estimations of this enzyme could therefore be useful in toxicity testing but as an increase is a reflection of an increased turnover of cells, it is unlikely that they would add to information obtainable by more routine investigations.

The FIGLU test is generally regarded as a specific test for detecting deficiency or interference with the utilization of folic acid. In this test, the subject is given an oral dose of histidine; if there is a deficiency of folic acid or a defect in its metabolism, formiminoglutamic acid (an intermediate in the conversion of histidine to glumatic acid) accumulates and is excreted in the urine. Methods for measuring the excretion have been described by Kohn (1964) and by Chanarin & Bennett (1962).

The concentration of folic acid in serum can be measured microbiologically using *Lactobacillus casei* (Waters & Mollin, 1961) and that of B_{12} by using *Euglena gracillis* (Anderson, 1964).

BLOOD VOLUME

The volume of circulating blood is usually determined by measuring either the volume of the red cells or that of the plasma and calculating the total volume from the proportion of these two constituents, measured in a haematocrit. Alternatively the volumes of both the cells and the plasma are determined.

The volume of the red cells can be determined isotopically. The radioactive iron method involves administering ^{59}Fe to the donor to allow incorporation of the iron in the red cells and the subsequent transfusion of the labelled blood in the subject (Gibson *et al.*, 1946; Hahn *et al.*, 1942). In the radioactive phosphorous method, red cells are labelled *in vitro* with ^{32}P and then returned to the circulation. Radioactive chromium, as used for measuring the life-span of red cells, can also be used. With these methods the dilution effect is measured after allowing a sufficient interval of time for adequate mixing within the host.

The plasma volume can be measured by injecting a non-toxic dye, e.g. T-1824 (Evans blue), which becomes firmly bound to the plasma albumin so preventing rapid elimination from the blood stream, and then determining the concentration in the plasma at various intervals. A time-concentration curve is constructed and extrapolation enables the concentration of the dye at the time of injection to be calculated (Campbell *et al.*, 1958). The plasma volume can also be determined isotopically by labelling serum albumin with ^{131}I (Gregerson & Rawson, 1959).

All these methods depend on measuring the dilution of marker that occurs in one of the two main constituents of the blood. The calculated total volume depends on uniform mixing with that constituent and also on the ratio of the two constituents being constant throughout the circulation. The former requirement can only be met by allowing a sufficient interval of time to elapse after injection of the marker and by measuring its concentration on several occasions; the investigator has no control over the second requirement other than to avoid making these observations during severe circulatory collapse.

CONCLUSIONS

Although in prolonged toxicity testing a few simple observations will usually exclude damage to the cells or coagulation of blood, extensive and involved investigation may be necessary to identify the site of action.

RECOMMENDED TEXT BOOKS

BRITTON C.J.C. (1969) *Disorders of the Blood*, eds. WHITBY & BRITTON. 10th Edition. London, J. & A. Churchill Ltd.

DACIE J.V. (1968) *Practical Haematology*. 4th Edition. London, J. & A. Churchill Ltd.

DAVIDSON I. & WELLS B.B. (1969) *Clinical Diagnosis by Laboratory Methods*, ed. TODD-SANFORD, 14th Edition, Philadelphia, W.B. Saunders Company.

SCHERMER S. (1967). *The Blood Morphology of Laboratory Animals*, 4th Edition. Philadelphia, F.A. Davis Company.

WINTROBE M.M. (1969) *Clinical Haematology*, 6th Edition. London, Henry Kimpton.

REFERENCES

ACKROYD J.F. (1962) The immunological basis of purpura due to drug hypersensitivity. *Proc. roy. Soc. Med.* **55**, 30.

ALLISON A.C., REES W. AP., & BURN G.P. (1957) Genetically controlled differences in catalase activity of dog erythrocytes. *Nature, Lond.* **180**, 649.

ANDERSON B.B. (1964) Investigations into the *Euglena* method for the assay of the vitamen B_{12} in serum. *J. clin. Path.* **17**, 14.

BEUTLER E., ROBSON M.J. & BUTTENWEISSER E. (1958) Comparison of the plasma, iron, iron-binding capacity, sternal marrow iron and other methods in the clinical evaluation of iron stores. *Ann. intern. Med.* **48**, 60.

BIGGS R. & DOUGLAS A.S. (1953) The thromboplastin generation test. *J. clin. Path.* **6**, 23.

BIGGS R. & MACMILLAN R.L. (1948) The error in the red cell count. *J. clin. Path.* **1**, 288.

BREWER J.G., TARLOV A.R., KELLERMEYER W. & ALVING A.S. (1962) The haemolytic effect of primaquine XV role of methaemoglobin. *J. Lab. clin. Med.* **59**, 905.

BRODIE B.B. & UNDENFRIEND S. (1950) Metabolites of Pamaquine in urine. *Proc. Soc. exp. Biol. Med.* **74**, 845.

BRUS I., & LEWIS S.M. (1959) The haptoglobin content of serum in haemolytic anaemia. *Brit. J. Haemat.* **5**, 348.

CAMPBELL T.J., FROHMAN B. & REEVE E.B. (1958) A simple, rapid and accurate method of extracting T-1824 from plasma, adapted to the routine measurement of blood volume. *J. Lab. clin. Med.* **52**, 768.

CHANARIN I. & BENNETT M.C. (1962) A spectrophotometric method for estimating formimino-glutamic and uroconic acid. *Brit. med. J.* **1**, 27.

CLAYDEN E.C. (1962) *Practical Section Cutting and Staining*, 4th edition, p. 130. London, J. & A. Churchill Ltd.

CROSBY W.H. & FURTH F.W. (1956) A modification of the benzidine method for the measurement of haemoglobin in plasma and urine. *Blood* **11**, 380.

CUMMINGS J.N. & EARL C.J. (1960) Caeroplasmin as demonstrated by starch gel electrophoresis. *J. clin. Path.* **13**, 69.

DALE H.H. & LAIDLOW P.P. (1911–12) A simple coagulometer. *J. Path. Bact.* **16**, 351.

DAVIES G., LEVIN B. & OBERHOLZER V.G. (1952) The micro estimation of serum iron and iron-binding capacity in normals and in disease. *J. clin. Path.* **5**, 312.

DE LOECKER W.C.J. & PRANKERD T.A.J. (1961) Factors influencing the hexose monophosphate shunt in red cells. *Clinica chim. Acta* **6**, 641.

EASTHAM R.D. (1964) Rapid adhesive platelet count in whole blood. *J. clin. Path.* **17**, 45.

ELLIOTT R.H.E. (1938) The suction test for capillary resistance in thrombocytopenia purpura. *J. Am. med. Ass.* **110**, 1177.

EVELYN K.A. & MALLOY H.T. (1938) Microdetermination of oxyhemoglobin, methemoglobin, and sulfhemoglobin in a single sample of blood. *J. biol. Chem.* **126**, 655.

FIELDING J. (1965) Differential ferrioxamine test for measuring chetatable body iron. *J. clin. Path.* **18**, 88.

FIELDING J., O'SHAUGHNESSY M.C. & BRUNSTRÖM G.M. (1965) Iron deficiency anaemia. *Lancet* **ii**, 9.

GIBSON J.G., WEISS S., EVANS R.D., PEACOCK W.C., IRVINE J.W. Jr., GOOD W.M. & KIP A.F. (1946) The measurement of the circulating red cell volume by means of two radioactive isotopes of iron. *J. clin. Invest.* **25**, 616.

GREGERSEN M.I. & RAWSON R.A. (1959) Blood volume. *Physiol. Rev.* **39**, 307.

HAEGER-ARONSEN B. (1960) Studies on urinary excretion of δ-aminolaevulic acid and other haem precursors in lead workers and lead-intoxicated rabbits. *Scand. J. clin. Lab. Invest.* **12**, 47.

HAHN P.F., ROSS J.F., BALE W.F., BALFOUR W.M. & WIPPLE G.H. (1944) Red cell and plasma volumes (circulating and total) as determined by radio iron and by dye. *Am. J. Physiol.* **141**, 363.

HALPERN B.N. & PACAUD A. (1951) *Technique de prélèvement d'échantillons de sang chez les petits animaux de laboratoire par ponction du plexus ophthalmique*. *C. r. Séanc. Soc. Biol.* **145**, 1465.

HERMAN E.C. (1961) Serum haptoglobins; their semi-quantitative estimation by a paper electrophoretic technique. *J. Lab. clin. Med.* **57**, 825.

HOFFBRAND A.V., KREMENCHUZKY S., BUTTERWORTH P.J. & MOLLIN D.L. (1966) Serum lactic dehydrogenase activity and folate deficiency in myelosclerosis and other haematological diseases. *Br. med. J.* **1**, 577.

HYNES M. (1947–48) Distribution of leucocytes on the counting chamber. *J. clin. Path.* **1**, 25.

HYNES M. & MARTIN L.C. (1936) A rapid method of measuring erythrocyte diameters. *J. Path.* **43**, 99.

HYNES M. & WHITBY L.E.H. (1938) Correction of the sedimentation rate for anaemia. *Lancet* **ii**, 249.

JENSSON O. (1958) Observation on the leucocyte blood picture in acute uraemia. *Br. J. Haemat.* **4**, 422.

KOHN J. (1964) Quantitative estimations of formiminoglutamic acid in urine. *J. clin. Path.* **17**, 466.

LANGDELL R.D., WAGNER R.H., BRINKHOUS K.M. & HILL C. (1953) Effect of antihemophilic factor on one-stage clotting tests. *J. Lab. clin. Med.* **41**, 637.

LEE R.I. & WHITE P.D. (1913) A clinical study of the coagulation time of blood. *Am. J. med. Sci.* **145**, 495.

LEHMANN H. & HUNTSMAN R.G. (1966) *Man's haemoglobins*, p. 183. Amsterdam, North Holland Publishing Company.

LEMPERT H. (1935) A modified technique for the enumeration of blood platelets. *Lancet* **i**, 151.

MACFARLANE R.G. (1939) A simple method for measuring clot-retraction. *Lancet* **i**, 1199.

MACFARLANE R.G. (1964) Haematology—an enzyme cascade in the blood clotting mechanism and its function as a biochemical amplifier. *Nature, Lond.* **202**, 498.

McCANCE R.A. & WIDDOWSON E.M. (1963) Iron excretion and metabolism in man. *Nature, Lond.* **152**, 326.

MAGATH T.B., BERKSON J. & HURN M. (1936) The error of determination of the erythrocyte count. *Am. J. clin. Path.* **6**, 568.

MATCHETT M.O. & INGRAM G.I.C. (1965) Partial thromboplastin time test with kaolin. *J. clin. Path.* **18**, 465.

MOLLISON P.L. & VEAL N. (1955) The use of the isotype ^{51}Cr as a label for red cells. *Br. J. Haemat.* **1**, 62.

NYE S.W., GRAHAM J.B. & BRINKHOUS K.M. (1962) The partial thromboplastin time as a screening test for the detection of latent bleeders. *Amer. J. Med. Sci.* **243**, 279.

OWEN J.A., BETTER F.C. & HOBAN J. (1960) A simple method for the determination of serum haptoglobins. *J. clin. Path.* **13**, 163.

OWEN J.A. MACKAY I.R. & GOT C. (1959) Serum haptoglobins in hepatobiliary disease. *Brit. med. J.* **1**, 1454.

QUICK A.J. (1957) *Haemorrhagic Diseases.* Philadelphia, Lea & Febiger.

RAMSEY W.N.M. (1957) Determination of the total iron-binding capacity of serum. *Clinica chim. Acta* **2**, 221.

RILEY V. (1960) Adaptation of orbital bleeding technique to rapid serial blood studies. *Proc. Soc. expt. Biol. Med.* **104**, No. 4, 751.

ROWE D.S. (1961) A rapid method for the estimation of serum haptoglobin. *J. clin. Path.* **14**, 205.

RUBIN D., WEISBERGER A.S. & CLARK D.R. (1960) Early detection of drug induced erythropoietic depression. *J. Lab. clin. Med.* **56**, 453.

SALVIDIO E., PANNACCIULLI I. & TIZIANELLO A. (1963) Glucose-6-phosphate and 6-phosphogluconic dehydrogenase activities in red blood cells of several animal species. *Nature, Lond.* **200**, 372.

SCHEN R.J. & RABINOVITZ M. (1958) Thrombocytopenic purpura due to quinidine. *Brit. med. J.* **2**, 1502.

SCHERMER S. (1967) *The Blood Morphology of Laboratory Animals,* 4th edition, Philadelphia, F.A. Davis Company.

SCHWARTZ S., HAWKINSON V., COHEN S. & WATSON C.J. (1947) A micro-method for the quantitative determination of the urinary coproporphyrin isomers (I and III). *J. biol. Chem.* **168**, 133.

SPECTOR W.S. (1956) *Handbook of Biological Data,* p. 275. Philadelphia & London, W.B. Saunders Company.

SZEINBERG A. & MARKS P.A. (1961) Substances stimulating glucose catabolism by the oxidative reactions of the pentose phosphate pathway in human erythrocytes. *J. clin. Invest.* **40**, 914.

WATERS A.H. & MOLLIN D.L. (1961) Studies on the folic acid activity of human serum. *J. clin. Path.* **14**, 335.

WEINSTEIN I.M. & LEROY G.V. (1953) Radio-active sodium chromate for the study of survival of red blood cells. *J. Lab. clin. Med.* **42**, 368.

WILLIAMS H.L. & CONRAD M.E. (1966) A one-tube method for measuring serum iron concentration and unsaturated iron-binding capacity. *J. Lab. clin. Med.* **67**, 171.

WINTROBE M.M. (1961) *Clinical Haematology,* p. 1128. London, Henry Kimpton.

WINTROBE M.M. & LANDSBERG J.W. (1935) A standardized technique for the blood sedimentation test. *Amer. J. med. Sci.* **189**, 102.

WOOTON I.D.P. (1964) *Micro-analysis in Medical Biochemistry,* (a) p. 120, (b) p. 80, (c) p. 124. London, J. & A. Churchill Ltd.

WRIGHT H.P. (1941) The adhesiveness of blood platelets in normal subjects with varying concentrations of anti-coagulants. *J. Path.* **53**, 255.

Appendixes

A. Normal ranges found with various biochemical tests at Huntingdon Research Centre

PLASMA UREA

(mg%)

	Mean	Range
Dogs	30	15–44
	Significantly lower in young animals	
Baboons	30	17–42
Rats	43	26–60
Pigs	26	15–55

PLASMA GLUCOSE BY GLUCOSE OXIDASE

(mg%)

	Mean	Range
Dogs	95	82–106
Baboons	100	63–134
Rats	121	86–149
Pigs	95	80–118

PLASMA GLUCOSE BY FERRICYANIDE REDUCTION

(mg%)

	Mean	Range
Dogs	99	86–100
Baboons	103	60–166
Rats	146	101–184
Pigs	91	60–135

SERUM ALKALINE PHOSPHATASE

(King Armstrong units)

	Mean	Range
Dogs	17	14–28
	Significantly lower in adult animals	
Baboons	173	75–300
	Sharp fall in values as animal matures	

	Mean	Range
Rats	61	40–95
	Significantly lower in adult animals	
Pigs	16	7–30

SERUM GLUTAMATE PYRUVATE TRANSAMINASE

(Sigma Frankel units)

	Mean	Range
Dogs	25	12–38
	Significant increase in adult animals	
Baboons	33	23–45
Rats	30	21–52
	Small increase in adult animals	
Pigs	35	20–65

SERUM CHOLESTEROL

(mg%)

	Mean	Range
Dogs	161	106–212
Baboons	140	90–194
Rats	128	90–150
Pigs	145	103–198

PLASMA CHOLINE ESTERASE

Adapted Michel Technique

(pH/hour)

	Mean	Range
Dogs	0·80	0·4–1·3
Rats ♂	0·66	0·4–0·9
Rats ♀	1·53	1·0–2·3
	Sex difference not present in young rats	

RED CELL CHOLINE ESTERASE

Adapted Michel Technique

(pH/hour)

	Mean	Range
Dogs	0·80	0·4–1·3
Rats	0·51	0·35–0·60

Slight sex difference only

PLASMA CHOLINE ESTERASE

TITRIMETRIC

(μmols/ml/min)

Dogs	1·56	0·93–2·84
Rats ♂	0·66	0·45–1·00
Rats ♀	1·44	1·00–2·50

Sex difference not present in young animals

RED CELL CHOLINE ESTERASE

TITRIMETRIC

(μmols/ml/min)

Dogs	1·96	1·30–2·50
Rats	1·50	1·00–2·50

Small sex difference only

SERUM GLUTAMATE OXALO-ACETATE TRANSAMINASE

(Sigma Frankel units)

	Mean	Range
Dogs	33	19–41
Baboons	47	20–70
Rats	132	96–200

Significant increase in adult animals

Pigs	44	21–60

SERUM ISOCITRIC DEHYDROGENASE

(Bell & Baron units)

Dogs	16	10–25

Significant reduction in adult animals

Baboons	15	9–25
Pigs	13	6–29

SERUM BILIRUBIN

(mg%)

Dogs	0·15	0·1–0·3
Baboons	0·20	0·1–0·3
Rats	0·15	0·1–0·3

SERUM PROTEINS

(g%)

		Total protein	Alb	L_1	L_2	B	Y
Dogs	Mean	5·5	3·0	0·4	0·6	1·1	0·4
	Range	4·8–7·0	2·7–3·6	0·2–0·5	0·4–0·8	0·9–1·5	0·3–0·7
Baboons	Mean	7·0	3·7	0·3	0·8	1·2	1·1
	Range	6·0–8·6	2·9–4·8	0·1–0·4	0·5–1·1	0·8–1·4	0·6–1·5
Rats	Mean	6·2	2·6	1·2	0·6	1·3	0·9
	Range	5·4–6·9	2·6–3·2	0·7–1·7	0·4–1·0	0·9–1·8	0·5–1·4
Pigs	Mean	6·0	2·1	0·4	1·2	1·2	0·9
	Range	5·0–6·4	1·6–2·6	0·2–0·6	0·9–1·8	0·9–1·5	0·5–1·3

Most protein values change significantly with age

SERUM SODIUM
(mEq/l)

	Mean	Range
Dogs	134	129–149
Baboons	145	130–155
Rats	134	126–142
Pigs	140	130–158

SERUM CHLORIDE
(mEq/l)

	Mean	Range
Dogs	110	104–117
Baboons	107	96–114
Rats	104	94–110
Pigs	101	90–113

SERUM POTASSIUM
(mEq/l)

Dogs	4·3	3·7–5·0
Baboons	4·7	3·5–5·8
Rats	4·7	3·8–5·4
Pigs	5·6	4·2–7·0

PLASMA CARBON DIOXIDE
(mEq/l)

Dogs	25·0	20–32
Baboons	22·0	17–27
Pigs	28·0	20–35

SERUM CALCIUM
(mEq/l)

	Mean	Range
Dogs	5·1	3·8–6·4
Rats	4·0	3·1–5·2
Pigs	4·2	3·3–5·2

B. Report forms used at Huntingdon Research Centre

BLOOD CHEMISTRY (Rats)

Group:
Compound:
Level (   ):

Group/ rat no.	Week no.	Urea (mg %)	Total red subs. (mg %)	SAP (KA units)	SGPT (SF units)	SGOT (SF units)	Bilirubin (mg %)	Cholest. (mg %)	Electrolytes (mEq/1)			Serum proteins (g%)								
									Na	K	Cl	Total	Alb	α_1	α_2	β	γ			

Schedule No.:

HRC 181

BIOCHEMISTRY DEPARTMENT
(Dogs, pigs, and primates)

REPORT NO.
Date of report

EXPERIMENT
SPECIES
DATE OF SAMPLE

No./sex	Dose (mg/kg/day)	Urea (mg%)	Total red. sub. (mg%)	Serum proteins (g%)						A/G ratio -:1	SAP (KA units)	SGPT (SF units)	Bili-rubin (mg%)
				Total	Alb	α_1	α_2	β	γ				

HRC 73

BIOCHEMISTRY DEPARTMENT

REPORT NO.
Date of Report

EXPERIMENT
SPECIES
DATE OF SAMPLE

No./ sex	Dose (mg/kg/ day)	SGOT (SF units)	Chol- esterol (mg%)	ICD (S units)	Creatinine (m%)	Cholinesterase Δ pH				
						Plasma	RBC			

HRC 74

BIOC: 52: 65:

URINALYSIS (all species)

Group:
Compound:
Level (   ):

Group/ rat no.	Week no.		Volume ml/rat	pH	SG	Protein mg %	Tot. red. sub.	Glucose	Ketones	Bile pigs.	Bile salts	Urobilin	Blood pigs.	Microscopy						
														E	P	M	R	O	C	A

Schedule No:

Index